MEASURING WHAT MATTERS

Allocation, Planning, and Quality Assessment for the

Ryan White CARE Act

Committee on the Ryan White CARE Act:
Data for Resource Allocation, Planning, and Evaluation

Board on Health Promotion and Disease Prevention

INSTITUTE OF MEDICINE
OF THE NATIONAL ACADEMIES

THE NATIONAL ACADEMIES PRESS
Washington, D.C.
www.nap.edu

THE NATIONAL ACADEMIES PRESS 500 Fifth Street, N.W. Washington, DC 20001

NOTICE: The project that is the subject of this report was approved by the Governing Board of the National Research Council, whose members are drawn from the councils of the National Academy of Sciences, the National Academy of Engineering, and the Institute of Medicine. The members of the committee responsible for the report were chosen for their special competences and with regard for appropriate balance.

This study was supported by Contract No. 200-2000-00629 Task Order #9 between the National Academy of Sciences and the Health Resources and Services Administration (HRSA) and the Centers for Disease Control and Prevention (CDC). Any opinions, findings, conclusions, or recommendations expressed in this publication are those of the author(s) and do not necessarily reflect the view of the organizations or agencies that provided support for this project.

Library of Congress Cataloging-in-Publication Data

Measuring what matters : allocation, planning, and quality assessment for the Ryan White Care Act / Committee on the Ryan White CARE Act: Data for Resource Allocation, Planning and Evaluation, Board on Health Promotion and Disease Prevention.
p. ; cm.
Includes bibliographical references.
ISBN 0-309-09115-2 (pbk.)
1. United States. Ryan White Comprehensive AIDS Resources Emergency Act of 1990. 2. AIDS (Disease)—Patients—Services for—United States—Finance.
[DNLM: 1. United States. Ryan White Comprehensive AIDS Resources Emergency Act of 1990. 2. Acquired Immunodeficiency Syndrome—United States. 3. HIV Infections—United States. 4. Financing, Government—United States. 5. Public Health—United States. 6. Quality of Health Care—standards—United States. WC 503 M484 2004] I. Institute of Medicine (U.S.). Committee on the Ryan White CARE Act: Data for Resource Allocation, Planning and Evaluation.
RA643.83.M43 2004
2004005892—dc22

2004005892

Additional copies of this report are available from the National Academies Press, 500 Fifth Street, N.W., Lockbox 285, Washington, DC 20055; (800) 624-6242 or (202) 334-3313 (in the Washington metropolitan area); Internet, http://www.nap.edu.

For more information about the Institute of Medicine, visit the IOM home page at: **www.iom.edu**.

Printed in the United States of America.

The serpent has been a symbol of long life, healing, and knowledge among almost all cultures and religions since the beginning of recorded history. The serpent adopted as a logotype by the Institute of Medicine is a relief carving from ancient Greece, now held by the Staatliche Museen in Berlin.

"Knowing is not enough; we must apply.
Willing is not enough; we must do."
—Goethe

INSTITUTE OF MEDICINE
OF THE NATIONAL ACADEMIES

Adviser to the Nation to Improve Health

THE NATIONAL ACADEMIES

Advisers to the Nation on Science, Engineering, and Medicine

The **National Academy of Sciences** is a private, nonprofit, self-perpetuating society of distinguished scholars engaged in scientific and engineering research, dedicated to the furtherance of science and technology and to their use for the general welfare. Upon the authority of the charter granted to it by the Congress in 1863, the Academy has a mandate that requires it to advise the federal government on scientific and technical matters. Dr. Bruce M. Alberts is president of the National Academy of Sciences.

The **National Academy of Engineering** was established in 1964, under the charter of the National Academy of Sciences, as a parallel organization of outstanding engineers. It is autonomous in its administration and in the selection of its members, sharing with the National Academy of Sciences the responsibility for advising the federal government. The National Academy of Engineering also sponsors engineering programs aimed at meeting national needs, encourages education and research, and recognizes the superior achievements of engineers. Dr. Wm. A. Wulf is president of the National Academy of Engineering.

The **Institute of Medicine** was established in 1970 by the National Academy of Sciences to secure the services of eminent members of appropriate professions in the examination of policy matters pertaining to the health of the public. The Institute acts under the responsibility given to the National Academy of Sciences by its congressional charter to be an adviser to the federal government and, upon its own initiative, to identify issues of medical care, research, and education. Dr. Harvey V. Fineberg is president of the Institute of Medicine.

The **National Research Council** was organized by the National Academy of Sciences in 1916 to associate the broad community of science and technology with the Academy's purposes of furthering knowledge and advising the federal government. Functioning in accordance with general policies determined by the Academy, the Council has become the principal operating agency of both the National Academy of Sciences and the National Academy of Engineering in providing services to the government, the public, and the scientific and engineering communities. The Council is administered jointly by both Academies and the Institute of Medicine. Dr. Bruce M. Alberts and Dr. Wm. A. Wulf are chair and vice chair, respectively, of the National Research Council.

www.national-academies.org

COMMITTEE ON THE RYAN WHITE CARE ACT: DATA FOR RESOURCE ALLOCATION, PLANNING, AND EVALUATION

PAUL D. CLEARY, Ph.D. (*Chair*), Professor, Department of Health Care Policy, Harvard Medical School

RONALD BAYER, Ph.D., Professor, Joseph L. Mailman School of Public Health, Columbia University

ERIC G. BING, M.D., Ph.D., M.P.H., Director, Drew Center for AIDS Research, Education and Services, Charles R. Drew University of Medicine and Science

SAMUEL A. BOZZETTE, M.D., Ph.D., Director, Health Services Research Section, Veteran Affairs Health Care System, San Diego; Professor of Medicine, University of California San Diego; Senior Natural Scientist, The RAND Corporation

DAVID D. CELENTANO, Sc.D., Professor and Director, Infectious Diseases Program, Department of Epidemiology, Johns Hopkins Bloomberg School of Public Health

VICTOR G. DE GRUTTOLA, S.M., Sc.D., Professor, Department of Biostatistics, Harvard School of Public Health

CARLOS DEL RIO, M.D., Professor of Medicine and Chief of Medical Service, Grady Memorial Hospital, Emory University School of Medicine

AIDA GIACHELLO, Ph.D., Associate Professor, Jane Addams College of Social Work, University of Illinois at Chicago

WILLIAM HOLZEMER, R.N., Ph.D., F.A.A.N., Professor and Associate Dean, International Programs, Department of Community Health Systems, University of California San Francisco School of Nursing

SANDRAL HULLETT, M.D., M.P.H., Acting CEO, Jefferson Health System

WENDY K. MARINER, J.D., L.L.M., M.P.H., Professor, Health Law, Boston University Schools of Public Health, Law and Medicine

BETH MEYERSON, M.Div., Ph.D., President, Policy Resource Group, LLC

A. DAVID PALTIEL, Ph.D., Associate Professor, Division of Health Policy and Administration, School of Public Health, Yale University

HAROLD POLLACK, Ph.D., Associate Professor, Social Service Administration, University of Chicago

GEORGE W. RUTHERFORD, III, M.D., Salvatore Lucia Professor of Preventive Medicine and Epidemiology, Department of Epidemiology and Biostatistics, University of California San Francisco School of Medicine

EILEEN SALINSKY, M.B.A., Senior Research Associate, National Health Policy Forum

DAVID R. SMITH, M.D., Chancellor, Texas Tech University System and President, Texas Tech University Health Sciences Center

Liaison from the Board on Health Promotion and Disease Prevention

ROBERT B. WALLACE, M.D., Irene Ensminger Stecher Professor of Epidemiology and Internal Medicine, Department of Epidemiology, College of Public Health, University of Iowa, College of Medicine

Study Staff

ALICIA R. GABLE, M.P.H., *Study Director*
REBECCA KLIMAN HUDSON, M.P.H., *Research Associate*
ANNIE O'CONNELL, *Senior Project Assistant*
DONNA ALMARIO, M.P.H., *Research Associate*
AMY GROSSMAN, *Senior Project Assistant*
ROSE MARIE MARTINEZ, Sc.D., *Director, Board on Health Promotion and Disease Prevention*

Consultants

AMY FINE, *Health Policy Program Consultant, Washington, DC*
JOHN G.H. PALEN, Ph.D., M.P.H., *Associate Research Professor, Department of Health Policy, George Washington University, School of Public Health*
MICHAEL STOTO, Ph.D., *Senior Statistical Scientist, The RAND Corporation, Washington, DC*

Reviewers

This report has been reviewed in draft form by individuals chosen for their diverse perspectives and technical expertise, in accordance with procedures approved by the National Research Council's (NRC's) Report Review Committee. The purpose of this independent review is to provide candid and critical comments that will assist the institution in making its published report as sound as possible and to ensure that the report meets institutional standards for objectivity, evidence, and responsiveness to the study charge. The review comments and draft manuscript remain confidential to protect the integrity of the deliberative process. We wish to thank the following individuals for their review of this report:

Mariella Cummings, Results Incorporated
Haile Debas, University of California San Francisco School of Medicine
David Fleming, Bill and Melinda Gates Foundation
Lawrence Gostin, Georgetown University
Jennifer Kates, Kaiser Family Foundation
Stephen Lagakos, Harvard School of Public Health
Thomas Louis, Johns Hopkins Bloomberg School of Public Health
Bruce Schackman, Weill Medical College of Cornell University
Renslow Sherer, University of Chicago Hospitals
Martin Wasserman, GlaxoSmithKline
Gregory Zaric, University of Western Ontario

Although the reviewers listed above have provided many constructive comments and suggestions, they were not asked to endorse the conclusions or recommendations nor did they see the final draft of the report before its release. The review of this report was overseen by **Maureen Henderson**, University of Washington, and **Henry Riecken**, University of Pennsylvania. Appointed by the NRC and Institute of Medicine, they were responsible for making certain that an independent examination of this report was carried out in accordance with institutional procedures and that all review comments were carefully considered. Responsibility for the final content of this report rests entirely with the authoring committee and the institution.

Acknowledgments

This report represents the collaborative efforts of many organizations and individuals, without whom this study would not have been possible. The Committee extends its most sincere gratitude to all those mentioned below.

The Committee thanks the sponsors of this study, the Health Resources and Services Administration (HRSA) and the Centers for Disease Control and Prevention (CDC). We extend special gratitude to our project officers, Steven Young of HRSA, and Patricia Sweeney and Monina Klevens, from CDC. They were extremely helpful and patient in handling the Committee's numerous requests for information. Several other people at HRSA and CDC helped the Committee in various ways, such as participating in site visits and conference calls and responding to data requests. The Committee would particularly like to thank the following people from HRSA: Jill Ashman, Douglas Morgan, Deborah Parham, Kathy Marconi, Magda Barini, Hilda Douglas, Richard Conviser, Faye Malitz, Idalia Sanchez, and John Milberg. People who were central to CDC's efforts to assist the Committee include Matthew McKenna, Patricia Fleming, Rob Janssen, Bob Frey, Lisa Lee, Hazel Dean, John Karon, Kate Glynn, and Irene Hall. We thank the other HRSA and CDC staff who helped with data requests and provided other support.

The Committee conducted several information-gathering activities throughout the course of the study. We thank the following individuals for their helpful and insightful testimony during public sessions of the Committee's first three meetings:

A. Cornelius Baker, Whitman-Walker Clinic, Washington, DC
Guthrie Birkhead, New York State Department of Health AIDS Institute
G. Stephen Bowen, Broward General Medical Center, Fort Lauderdale, FL
Michael Bursaw, County of San Diego Health and Human Services Agency
A. Gene Copello, CAEAR Coalition and Florida AIDS Action, Tampa, FL
Sharen Duke, AIDS Service Center of Lower Manhattan, New York, NY
Geno Dunnington, Whitman-Walker Clinic, Washington, DC
Charles Henry, County of Los Angeles Department of Health Services
Robert Janssen, Centers for Disease Control and Prevention
Jack Jourden, Washington State Department of Health
James G. Kahn, Institute for Health Policy Studies, University of California San Francisco
Janice Kopelman, Pennsylvania Department of Public Health
Matthew McClain, McClain and Associates, Inc., Silver Spring, MD
Matthew McKenna, Centers for Disease Control and Prevention
Michael Montgomery, California Department of Health Services
Judy Owen, North Carolina Department of Health and Human Services
John Palen, George Washington University
Liza Solomon, Maryland Department of Health and Mental Hygiene
Laura Thomas, San Francisco Department of Public Health
Craig Thompson, Mississippi State Department of Health
Fikirte Wagaw, Chicago Department of Public Health
Steven Young, Health Resources and Services Administration

The Committee thanks attendees of the discussion session at the HRSA All-Titles Meeting on August 15, 2002. Representatives from the following Title I Eligible Metropolitan Areas (EMAs) attended: Atlanta, GA; Detroit, MI; Dutchess County, NY; Maricopa County, AZ; Miami-Dade, FL; Minneapolis, MN; Philadelphia, PA; Riverside/San Bernardino, CA; and San Juan, PR.

A similar discussion session was held with Title II representatives during the annual meeting of the National Alliance of State and Territorial AIDS Directors on May 20, 2002. We would like to thank the AIDS Directors from Puerto Rico, Colorado, Nebraska, Georgia, Kentucky,

South Carolina, Maryland, Kansas, California, and New Hampshire who participated in this discussion.

The Committee would like to thank the numerous (almost 70) HIV/AIDS surveillance coordinators and health department staff from over 40 CARE Act grantee areas who participated in a conference call with the committee on July 24, 2003, and shared their "hands-on" experiences of conducting surveillance at the state and local levels. Others from National Alliance of State and Territorial AIDS Directors (NASTAD) and CDC also participated in this call.

The Committee commissioned two papers during the course of the study. The first paper by Mike Stoto provided a very helpful assessment of the history of public health surveillance. The second paper, by John Palen, provided a very useful overview of the legislative history of the Ryan White CARE Act and provided significant detail and information for Chapter 2.

The Committee wishes to thank the liaison panel members: Terje Anderson, A. Cornelius Baker, Christopher Bates, Ignatius Bau, Guthrie Birkhead, G. Stephen Bowen, Mary Ann Chiasson, Richard Conviser, Gene Copello, Sharen Duke, Helen Fox Fields, Debra Fraser-Howze, Robert Fullilove, Kenneth T. Jones, Jennifer Kates, Seth Kilbourn, Monina Klevens, Christopher Labonte, Miguelina Ileana León, Marsha Martin, Jean McGuire, Jesse Milan, Thomas L. Milne, Murray Penner, Kees Reitmeijer, Matt Salo, Jane Silver, Paul Simon, Wayne Smith, Tim Westmoreland, Joy Johnson Wilson, David Wunsch, and Steven Young. The Committee is grateful for their guidance.

The following people also provided the Committee with guidance and further understanding of complex study issues: Jennifer Kates, Tim Westmoreland, Thomas Louis, Tom Jabine, Connie Citro, Sandy Berry, and John Fanning. We also would like to thank Steven Asch and Doug Owens who provided a technical review of select chapters of the report.

Throughout the course of the study, several people from NASTAD were exceptionally helpful in providing information to the Committee. In particular, the Committee would like to thank Julie Scofield, Arnie Doyle, Murray Penner, Chris Aldridge, and Connie Jorstad. The Committee thanks NASTAD for collecting information on states' HIV surveillance funding and the the 41 state AIDS directors and staff who responded to NASTAD's request for information.

Donna Glebatis (New York State Department of Health), Polly Thomas (New York City Department of Health and Mental Hygiene), Sandra Schwarz (San Francisco Department of Public Health), and their staff members provided helpful information on HIV surveillance in their areas.

The Committee thanks representatives from the Alabama Department of Public Health and several Ryan White Title III clinics who, during site visits, provided valuable insight about the experience of HIV/AIDS surveillance and providing care in Alabama: Health Services Center (Anniston); Franklin Primary Care Center (Mobile); Montgomery AIDS Outreach; Copeland Care Clinic (Selma, Tuskegee); Maude Whatley Health Services (Eutaw, Livingston); Alabama State Health Department; Jefferson County Health Department; St. George's Clinic (Jefferson County).

The Committee would like to thank the numerous staff members of the Institute of Medicine (IOM), the National Research Council, and the National Academies Press who contributed to the development, review, production, and dissemination of this report. The committee is most grateful to Alicia Gable, who did an outstanding job of directing this very complex study. She was assisted by Rebecca Kliman Hudson, Annie O'Connell, Donna Almario, and Amy Grossman, all of whom provided exceptional research and administrative support. Natane Singleton also provided excellent project support as an intern. Amy Fine served as a consultant to the project and assisted the Committee and IOM staff with facilitation of discussions and report writing. We also thank Sandra Hackman for editing the report. Rose Marie Martinez and Susanne Stoiber provided valuable guidance and oversight for this study.

Contents

APPENDIXES

Executive Summary

In 1981, clusters of cases of unusual pneumonia and cancer in otherwise healthy gay men led to the identification and first reports in the United States of what we now know as Acquired Immune Deficiency Syndrome (AIDS) (CDC, 1981). Epidemiologic studies showed that the virus was transmitted by sexual contact with an infected person, exposure to infected blood and blood products, sharing of contaminated syringes and needles, and from infected mothers to infants during pregnancy, at the time of delivery or via breastfeeding (IOM/NAS, 1988). Three years later, the cause of AIDS, a newly recognized retrovirus now known as Human Immunodeficiency Virus or HIV, was identified (Barre-Sinoussi et al., 1983; Gallo et al., 1984).

HIV infection causes progressive damage to the immune system by destroying white blood cells called CD4+ T-lymphocytes. Initial infection with HIV causes a flu-like illness in some individuals. Others have no symptoms at all until 10 or more years later when they experience symptoms of infections or other diseases that take hold due to their lowered immunocompetence. These conditions can range all the way from dementia, to cancer, to chronic diarrhea (Pantaleo et al., 1993; Fauci et al., 1996).

Testing the blood for antibodies against HIV infection indicates whether the individual is infected with the virus, but does not allow one to determine the stage of the infection. This is done by measuring viral replication, or the amount of virus in the blood (HIV RNA), and the state of the immune system (CD4+ cell count). AIDS is a term used to define those persons with HIV infection that have a CD4+ count < 200 cells/μL or a specific opportunistic infection and represents the advanced stage of HIV disease (CDC, 1992; Pantaleo et al., 1993; Fauci et al., 1996).

Recent advances in treatment of HIV disease have resulted in slowing the progression of the disease, and often temporary restoration of immune functioning, in infected individuals. Early detection of HIV infection, before the infected person develops AIDS, can allow the individual to enter care and thus receive treatment and preventive services that could limit the spread of infection and prevent the morbidity and mortality of AIDS.

The Ryan White Comprehensive AIDS Resources Emergency (CARE) Act, enacted in 1990 and reauthorized and amended in 1996 and 2000, provides funding to cities, states, and other public and private entities to provide care and support services to individuals with HIV and AIDS who have low incomes and little or no insurance (Ryan White CARE Act. 42 U.S.C. § 300ff [2003]). The CARE Act was named after Ryan White, a teenager from Indiana whose struggle with HIV/AIDS and AIDS-related discrimination helped raise awareness of the disease. The CARE Act is a discretionary program that relies on annual appropriations from Congress. Since its original authorization, CARE Act funding has increased from $220 million in fiscal year (FY) 1991 to $2.0 billion in FY2003 (HRSA, 2003). The Health Resources and Services Administration's HIV/AIDS Bureau (HRSA/HAB) has lead responsibility for implementation of the CARE Act.

The CARE Act is composed of four major program titles and several other components. Title I provides grants to Eligible Metropolitan Areas (EMAs—currently 51) that have been disproportionately affected by the HIV/AIDS epidemic (HRSA, 2002a). Title II provides grants to U.S. states and territories to improve the quality, availability, and delivery of health care and support services for individuals with HIV disease, and provides access to medications through the AIDS Drug Assistance Program (ADAP) (HRSA, 2002b). Title III provides direct grants to nonprofit entities for primary care and early intervention services, and capacity building and planning grants (HRSA, 2002c). Title IV provides grants for family-centered care for infants, children, youth, and women living with HIV disease and their families (HRSA, 2002d). Other components of the CARE Act include the AIDS Education Training Centers, the Dental Reimbursement Program, and the Special Projects of National Significance.

The CARE Act operates against a backdrop of significant inequalities in access to health care in the United States. More than 43 million Americans are uninsured (Mills and Bandhari, 2003), and millions more hold insurance policies that do not cover basic medications or treatments (IOM,

2001a). Congress enacted the CARE Act in 1990 at least in part to address this challenge regarding people with HIV infection.

Uninsured and underinsured HIV-infected individuals rely on a variety of safety-net programs, including CARE Act–funded providers, community and migrant health centers, private free clinics, and public hospitals (Kaiser Family Foundation, 2000). Some individuals with private or other sources of insurance also rely on programs funded under the CARE Act because other sources of coverage are poorly coordinated and gaps often remain (Kaiser Family Foundation, 2000). Congress established the CARE Act, also referred to as RWCA, as the "payer of last resort"; the RWCA funds care for low-income, uninsured, or underinsured individuals who have no other resources to pay for care (Ryan White CARE Act. 42 U.S.C. § 300ff-11 [2003]). Funding for the CARE Act, however, has been insufficient to redress all of the inequalities and gaps in coverage for people with HIV.

CHARGE TO THE COMMITTEE

In response to a congressional mandate in the Ryan White CARE Act Amendments of 2000, HRSA and the Centers for Disease Control and Prevention (CDC) commissioned the Institute of Medicine (IOM) to conduct this study. The Committee's charge has three components (Box ES-1):

- To assess whether reported HIV cases are adequate, reliable, and sufficiently accurate for inclusion in formula grants under Titles I and II of RWCA and to make recommendations for the improvement of HIV reporting systems (discussed in Chapter 4).
- To identify data and tools for assessing a community's severity of need and how that information can be used in allocation decisions (discussed in Chapter 5).
- To identify available health outcome and other data that can be used to measure the quality of and access to RWCA-funded services (discussed in Chapter 6).

Each of the three components of the Committee's charge is discussed below.

USE OF HIV DATA IN THE TITLE I AND II ALLOCATION FORMULAS

Formulas are used to allocate 70 percent of RWCA funds through Title I and II ($1.3 billion in FY2002) (HRSA, 2003). These formula alloca-

BOX ES-1
Charge to the Committee

In the Ryan White CARE Amendments of 2000, Congress directed the IOM to examine the following issues (Ryan White CARE Act. 42 U.S.C. § 300ff-11 [2003]):

Use of HIV Data in the Title I and II Allocation Formulas

- "whether the surveillance system of each of the States regarding [HIV] provides for the reporting of cases of infection with the virus in a manner that is sufficient to provide adequate and reliable information on the number of such cases and the demographic characteristics of such cases, both for the State in general and for specific geographic areas in the State."
- "whether such information is sufficiently accurate for purposes of formula grants under parts A and B of title XXVI of the Public Health Service Act" [i.e., Title I and II of the RWCA].
- "With respect to any State whose surveillance system does not provide adequate and reliable information on cases of infection with the virus, [provide] recommendations regarding the manner in which the State can improve the system."

Information for Estimating Severity of Need for Resources

- "Existing and needed epidemiological data and other analytic tools for resource planning and allocation decisions, specifically for estimating severity of need of a community and the relationship to the allocations process."

Quality-of-Care Measures

- "The availability and utility of health outcome measures and data for HIV primary care and support services and the extent to which those measures and data could be used to measure the quality of such funded services"; and
- "other factors determined to be relevant to assessing an individual's or community's ability to gain and sustain access to quality HIV services."

NOTE: The Ryan White CARE Act Amendments of 2000 also directed the IOM to study the public financing and delivery of HIV care. HRSA commissioned a separate IOM study to address those issues.

tions are based on estimated living AIDS cases (ELCs),[1] using data from the AIDS case reporting system[2] (HRSA, 2001). Many have raised concerns that such allocations are not equitable because the epidemic is not adequately reflected by AIDS cases alone, and that areas with emerging HIV epidemics are underfunded because all cases of HIV disease are not included (U.S. Congress, 2000a,b). A related concern with basing allocations on AIDS cases is that jurisdictions are not compensated for providing early access to care and treatment (U.S. Congress, 2000b). There is a widely held perception that incorporating HIV data in the formulas would increase the equity of RWCA allocations by targeting funds according to need (U.S. Congress, 2000a,b).

Prompted by these concerns, Congress specified in the 2000 reauthorization of the CARE Act that reported cases of HIV disease should be incorporated into RWCA Title I and II formulas as early as FY2005—provided that the Secretary of Health and Human Services determines that such data are available from all eligible areas, and that they are "sufficiently accurate and reliable" (Ryan White CARE Act. 42 U.S.C. § 300ff-13 [2003]). Cases of HIV disease are to be incorporated in the formulas no later than the beginning of FY2007 (Ryan White CARE Act. 42 U.S.C. § 300ff-13 [2003]). The legislation authorized the IOM to assist the Secretary in assessing the readiness of states to produce adequate and reliable HIV case-reporting data, determine the accuracy of using HIV cases within the existing allocation formulas, and establish recommendations regarding how states could improve their HIV case-reporting systems (Ryan White CARE Act. 42 U.S.C. § 300ff-11 [2003]).

At the outset, the Committee recognized the difficulty of defining such terms as "sufficiently accurate," "adequate," and "reliable" to char-

---

[1]ELCs are calculated by applying annual survival weights to the most recent 10 years of reported AIDS cases and summing the totals. CDC updates the survival weights every two years. CDC provides both the survival weights and the most recent 10 years of reported AIDS cases to HRSA, which performs the award calculations (HRSA, 2001).

[2]Legal authority to require reporting of diseases resides primarily at the state level (Thacker, 2000). All U.S. states and territories have laws requiring health care providers and laboratories to report cases of AIDS using a standardized name-based reporting system. As a result of changes in the natural history of the disease due primarily to improvements in therapy, data from the AIDS case-reporting system have become less informative about current trends in the HIV epidemic. Many states also have passed laws, some as early as the mid-1980s, requiring the reporting of cases of HIV (non-AIDS) disease in an effort to obtain more recent information about trends in HIV epidemic and to assist in program planning, evaluation, and targeting of prevention resources. Unlike AIDS case reporting, which relies on a standardized name-based reporting system, HIV reporting practices vary substantially by state (see Chapters 3 and 4).

acterize the quality of HIV surveillance data. No absolute standards of accuracy, adequacy, or reliability exist for assessing HIV reporting data; these standards vary according to the purposes and tasks for which the data are used. Evaluating HIV reporting systems for use in resource allocation formulas requires a different set of performance criteria than evaluating these data for public health purposes (e.g., epidemic surveillance, contact tracing, and partner notification). While CDC (1999) has established performance criteria[3] for evaluating the latter function, it was not the purpose of this Committee to assess these standards. Rather, the Committee defined criteria for "sufficiency," "adequacy," and "reliability" in terms of over- and underfunding errors to RWCA grantees.

Congress specified that allocation formulas should incorporate information about HIV cases based on the belief that such information would better characterize the HIV/AIDS epidemic and areas' needs for resources than AIDS cases alone (U.S. Congress, 2000b,d). Thus, the Committee focused on whether incorporating HIV reporting into the RWCA formulas would provide a better representation of HIV disease-related resource needs across jurisdictions and more fairly channel scarce RWCA resources.

The Committee concluded that four conditions need to be met for this to occur:

- Every state would need to be capable of providing data on HIV cases for the formulas.
- The quality of HIV data across states and EMAs would have to be comparable. This means that if there are biases in HIV reporting, those biases should be of similar direction and magnitude across areas.
- Incorporating HIV case-reporting data into the formula would need to produce different and more accurate assessments of the "relative disease burden" among states and jurisdictions and their resource needs than AIDS data alone.

---

[3]CDC issued surveillance guidelines in December 1999 (CDC, 1999) outlining the performance criteria for states' HIV/AIDS surveillance systems. Several of the performance measurements had specific quantitative measurements. The criteria outlined in the document stated that the system had to be timely (66 percent of HIV/AIDS cases reported to the health department within 6 months of diagnoses), provide accurate case counts (≤5 percent mis-matched reports and ≤5 percent duplicate cases in the database), have complete ascertainment of mode of exposure to HIV (≥85 percent of reported cases, or representative sample, must have reported transmission mode after complete epidemiologic follow-up), and have complete case reporting (≥85 percent of diagnosed cases reported to the health department). In addition, states must show that they can match to other databases of public health importance, follow up on cases of public health importance, collect valid and reliable data for key data elements, and use data for public health planning (CDC, 2003).

• Including HIV data in the RWCA allocation formulas would result in significant variation in the relative size of awards to states and EMAs and more equitable allocations. If, in contrast, HIV data dampen variations in awards among jurisdictions, then the formulas may not result in more equitable allocations.

Capability of States to Provide Data for the Formula

To evaluate the capability of states to provide data for the formulas the Committee asked three questions: (1) Does each state have an HIV reporting system? (*coverage*); (2) Has the HIV reporting system of each state had sufficient time for full implementation? (*maturity*); (3) Are the data from every state with a system of HIV reporting reliable enough to be used in the formulas? (*full use of reported data*).

The Committee found that (as of October 2003) all U.S. states, territories, and cities, except Georgia and Philadelphia,[4] had implemented HIV reporting systems, but that states are not equally capable of providing high-quality data. Some have only recently implemented such systems and need time to fully implement or refine them. Furthermore, CDC does not accept data from states that use codes rather than names to report their cases, owing to a lack of methods for unduplicating those coded cases.

Comparability of HIV Reporting Data

Even if all states were capable of providing data on HIV cases, data should be of comparable quality across jurisdictions before they are used in the RWCA formulas, or the differential errors should be such that incorporating the data increases—rather than decreases—the equity of the resulting RWCA allocations. Differential rates of completeness and timeliness of HIV reporting, and the migration of people living with HIV across jurisdictions, have the potential to create significant biases in allocations. Methodological inconsistencies in the finding or reporting of HIV cases across jurisdictions, such as variations in policies on laboratory reporting and the aggressiveness of case finding, can also lead to differential biases in underlying HIV data. Due to lack of data, the Committee could not fully investigate the potential influence of possible patterns of underreporting, reporting delays, migration of people with HIV disease, or variation in laboratory reporting policies and the aggressiveness of

[4]Since the release of this report, Georgia implemented name-based reporting and Philadelphia adopted code-based reporting. All areas of the United States now have HIV reporting.

case finding on resulting formula allocations. CDC is currently conducting an evaluation that would provide information about several of these issues in selected regions, but additional studies are needed to examine the comparability of data from the HIV case-reporting system across jurisdictions for the purpose of allocating resources.

Relative Disease Burden and Ranking of Need Across Jurisdictions

Including data on HIV cases in allocation formulas would not increase the overall amount of RWCA allocations, but it could potentially shift the amounts provided to different jurisdictions. One premise underlying this possibility is that the HIV epidemic is in different stages of maturity in different areas of the country. Here maturity refers to the length of time that the epidemic of HIV infection has been established in at-risk populations. Because the risk of AIDS is low in the first years after infection and then rises over time, one would expect the ratio of reported HIV to AIDS cases to be higher in more recently infected populations than in populations where the epidemic had been established for a longer period of time, and most infected individuals acquired the HIV virus many years ago. Thus, assuming very different stages of maturity of the epidemic would lead one to expect significant variation in this ratio across jurisdictions. States that believe that their HIV epidemic was established relatively recently suspect that the current measure (based on AIDS cases alone) places them at a disadvantage in RWCA formula allocations. If, however, the epidemic is at similar levels of maturity across jurisdictions, and therefore the ratio of reported AIDS cases to reported HIV cases is relatively constant, including data on HIV cases in the formula will, in fact, have little influence on the relative measure of disease burden, and hence little influence on the resulting awards.

Although it seems reasonable to assume that the epidemic is in various stages of maturity in different jurisdictions, it is difficult to confirm this belief. Some data do suggest the possibility of regional variation—specifically that the epidemic may be growing more quickly in the southern region of the United States than elsewhere. Between 1994 and 2001, the number of reported AIDS cases appeared to increase faster in southeastern states than in other parts of the country (Kates and Ruiz, 2002). Inspection of the cumulative distribution of AIDS cases suggests that the AIDS incidence curves have fairly similar—though not identical—shape across states over time (Chapter 4, Figures 4-1 and 4-2); similarity in shape implies roughly similar epidemic dynamics. These figures also illustrate shifts over time in these curves, implying that the stage of epidemic maturity differs somewhat from state to state (and from EMA to EMA). The conclusion is that while we might expect a higher ratio of HIV to AIDS cases in some jurisdictions than others, this effect is not likely to be particularly large. The assumptions regarding regional variability in epidemic maturity need further assessment.

Sensitivity of Formula Allocations to Changes in the Underlying Input Data

For HIV reporting data to more fairly channel resources, allocation formulas need to be sensitive to changes in the underlying data. The Committee could not examine the impact of including HIV data in the formula because data on HIV cases were not available from all states, including several key states with a high disease burden. Since data from those states could have a large influence on results, any analyses based on partial data could be very misleading. Instead, using a combination of data from states for which reported HIV cases are available and estimated HIV cases in others, the Committee examined what the current allocation is using the ELCs (the measure now used for RWCA resource allocation) and combined estimates of HIV prevalence and AIDS prevalence (see Appendix C).[5]

In its analyses, the Committee examined allocations per case (using Title I and II funds) across states and EMAs as a point of departure. The Committee acknowledges that there are many reasons why an equitable system would depart from this standard, including unequal costs of care, unequal need, differences in the efficiency with which jurisdictions apply funds, differences in the quality and comprehensiveness of the existing resource base from one jurisdiction to another, and differences in economies of scale.

Similar to the findings from a previous General Accounting Office (GAO) study (2000), the Committee found substantial variations in the amount of Title I and II funds received per ELC across states and EMAs. This appeared to stem primarily from the Title II formulas, which give an advantage to states with EMAs. Such variations persist regardless of the measure of disease burden used.

The Committee also found that except for San Francisco, Title I formula allocations per ELC are uniform across EMAs. The large allocation to San Francisco reflects the influence of the hold-harmless provision; removal of this provision would reduce San Francisco's allocation to within the reported range for other EMAs, but would have a small impact

[5]The Committee also examined current allocations using AIDS prevalence alone. The differences in allocations using estimated AIDS prevalence and ELCs were not informative, suggesting that any methodological differences between the calculation of ELCs and the calculation of AIDS prevalence is not important for the purposes of identifying allocation variations.

on other EMAs, which would observe a 2.6 percent increase in their allocation if San Francisco's dropped. As noted by the GAO (2000), the hold-harmless provision has a small overall effect on allocations to EMAs, except for San Francisco.

The Committee identified a number of structural features of the Title I and Title II funding formulas (including hold-harmless provisions, set-asides, minimum funding thresholds, and the eligibility criteria for EMAs) that have a large influence on resulting allocations. These features may dampen the influence of and obviate the potential benefits of adding HIV data to the RWCA formulas.

The Committee also used multiple regression analysis to examine cross-state variations in Title I and Title II RWCA funding allocations. Similar to previous GAO findings (GAO, 2000), these analyses indicated that the presence of an EMA was a significant factor in determining funding allocations. States whose reported AIDS cases were concentrated within EMAs received greater combined RWCA funding per case than did other jurisdictions. Appendix C provides further details.

The Committee notes with concern that southeastern states appear to receive the smallest allocations, per estimated living AIDS case, under the current formulas. While southeastern states might benefit more than other states from a measure that includes reported HIV cases, the structure of RWCA formulas, which favors states with EMAs, is more important in explaining the relative disadvantage of southeastern states.

RWCA funds are intended for individuals who are low income and uninsured or underinsured. Insofar as the current RWCA case reporting–based formula counts patients that have other sources of insurance or funding, it overestimates the number of cases that qualify for RWCA services, just as it may underestimate the needs of a particular jurisdiction with greater proportions of patients with HIV. In addition, the current formulas do not account for variations in costs of care or fiscal capacity across Title I and II jurisdictions (GAO, 1995).

The Committee makes several recommendations for improving the quality and completeness of HIV case-reporting systems for the purposes of allocating RWCA resources. Greater use of electronic laboratory reporting, and potentially the use of data from pharmacies, could enhance the comparability of HIV reporting data across states in terms of completeness and timeliness.

Name-based reporting is cited as one way to facilitate elimination of duplicate reports (CDC, 1999). However, it is unclear if name-based reporting is intrinsically superior to code-based reporting for eliminating duplicate reports. Due to name variations, even name-based systems do not permit complete unduplication. In addition, code-based reporting systems were developed by some states after substantial political debate, and altering those systems would require significant legislative changes, time, and effort. For this reason, and because name-based reporting is not clearly superior to code-based reporting for the specific goal of accurately estimating the number of known cases for determining RWCA allocations, better methods for unduplicating reports for both code- and name-based reporting states need to be developed and implemented so allocation formulas can include data from all states. At the same time, the Committee recognizes that there are strong feelings, both pro and con, about the use of name-based reporting for other surveillance functions (Colfax and Bindman, 1998; Osmond et al., 1999; Hecht et al., 2000). The Committee did not take a position on these issues because its charge limits its scope of activity to reporting for allocation purposes.

Other techniques for estimating the prevalence of HIV infection and the differential disease burden among states and EMAs, such as modeling and survey-based approaches, should also be explored. Such approaches have the potential of providing estimates that are more accurate, more timely, and more consistent across jurisdictions than complete enumeration. The Committee further emphasizes knowing the size and distribution of the undiagnosed HIV-infected population is an important marker of our success in providing care for all patients with HIV.

The Committee makes the following recommendations to address these issues.[6] The Committee targets these and subsequent recommendations to several different entities including Congress, the Secretary of Health and Human Services (HHS), HRSA and CDC, and independent bodies. The Committee directs several recommendations (4.5, 5.2, 6.2c) to Congress that are related to the intent of the Ryan White CARE Act program. Many of the recommendations (4.2a, 4.2c, 4.4, 5.4, 6.2, and 6.3) are targeted to the Secretary of HHS, who has broad oversight responsibilities for the implementation of the CARE Act. The Committee also targeted recommendations to the Secretary of HHS when the recommendations involved coordination among multiple agencies. Several recommendations involving specific technical issues are targeted to HRSA (4.1, 5.1, 5.3, 6.1, 6.2a, 6.2b) and CDC (4.2a, 4.2b, 4.2c, 4.3, 6.2b). In a few instances, the Committee makes recommendations that assessments be undertaken, or reviewed, by an independent body (4.3, 4.4). An independent body was specified when the recommendations required a broad assessment of the science base or when the Committee thought that an independent entity could protect the federal entities from any appearance of vested or conflict of interest, since those agencies would be applying

[6]All recommendations (4-1 through 6-3) found in the Executive Summary are identified by chapter number and recommendation number within that chapter.

the resulting methods. In some situations, an independent body was specified when it was thought that such an arrangement would minimize any inappropriate pressure on an agency from groups with vested interests in the outcomes of deliberations. Such pressure could inappropriately influence scientific assessments and/or result in strained relationships between agencies and their grantees or constituents. Additional resources may be required to implement some of the Committee's recommendations.

Recommendation 4-1 For at least the next four years, HRSA should continue to use ELCs in the RWCA Titles I and II formulas. During that period, concerted effort should be devoted to improving the consistency, quality, and comparability of HIV case reporting. Specific attention should be paid to two, complementary approaches in this regard: (1) the attainment of coverage, maturity, and comparability standards and the development of de-duplication strategies that permit full use of all reported HIV cases; and (2) implementation of alternative strategies for estimating HIV cases, such as survey or model-based estimation.

Recommendation 4-2 The following steps should be taken by states as quickly as possible to improve the consistency, quality, and comparability of HIV case reporting for RWCA allocation purposes.

a. The CDC should accept reported HIV cases from all states. Until this occurs, large numbers of HIV cases will not be included in the national HIV reporting system, and there will be no reliable centralized way to use reported HIV cases to apportion CARE Act funds. CDC should work with all states to develop and evaluate methods for unduplicating HIV cases regardless of whether such cases are code- or name-based. The Secretary of HHS should provide CDC with the funding to provide the technical assistance to states necessary to support the integration of code with name-based data into the national HIV reporting database. Because of the importance of obtaining consistent data from all jurisdictions, the CDC should include HIV reporting data from code-based states and estimate the degree of overcounting due to duplication while procedures and infrastructure for definitive unduplication are developed.

b. CDC should collaborate with all states to periodically assess and compare the completeness and timeliness of their HIV reporting systems.

c. The Secretary of HHS should provide additional funds to CDC to assist states in improving the completeness and timeliness and overall comparability of their HIV reporting systems. Enhancing electronic laboratory reporting in all states is critical in achieving this goal. Pharmacy-based surveillance, with a focus on the ADAP, is another potential source of information for enhancing completeness.

Recommendation 4-3 CDC should obtain estimates of total HIV prevalence (including the undiagnosed population) and evaluate methods other than case reporting for use as an alternative or supplement in estimating HIV cases for RWCA Titles I and II formula allocations, with advice and review by an independent body. This assessment should address the accuracy and costs of different strategies and should be repeated periodically.

Recommendation 4-4 Prior to future reauthorizations of the CARE Act, the Secretary of HHS should initiate studies to improve the evidence base for understanding how well HIV case-reporting and other methods for estimating HIV cases reflect the relative burden of disease and the relative resources necessary to respond to those needs in different areas. The Secretary should engage an independent body to estimate the dollar allocations that would result for Titles I and II grantees from alternative input data and allocation formulas. Specifically:

a. "What-if" assessments should be reported every five years on the range of each EMA's and state's RWCA formula allocation, depending on whether estimated living AIDS cases or total HIV cases are used as the measure of disease burden.

b. Analyses should be conducted to estimate the dollar allocations that would result from modifying different structural elements of the formula, such as:
   - Hold-harmless provisions,
   - The eligibility requirements for becoming an EMA,
   - The percentage set-aside in the Title II base award for non-EMA states (currently 20 percent),
   - The minimum base Title II award (now $500,000 for states and $50,000 for territories),
   - The eligibility criteria for becoming a Tier 1 and Tier 2 Emerging Community.

c. Evaluate the extent of interregional variability in HIV epidemic maturity and its effect on relative resource needs.

These activities should be repeated periodically.

> **Recommendation 4-5** In keeping with the CARE Act's intent as a payer of last resort, Congress should reevaluate the RWCA formulas to determine whether they allocate resources in proportion to the estimated number of individuals with HIV/AIDS who are uninsured or underinsured in states and EMAs. Readily available data on the insurance coverage of the general population may mirror insurance coverage of people with HIV/AIDS, but additional estimation will likely be required.

These recommendations should be implemented in a timely manner to provide evidence to either (1) justify inclusion of reported HIV cases in RWCA allocations formulas by FY2007, as contemplated by Congress, or (2) conclude that reported HIV cases do not result in more equitable resource allocation so that Congress can reconsider its recommendation prior to implementation in FY2007.

ESTIMATING RESOURCE NEEDS

RWCA attempts to direct funds to areas in greatest need of financial assistance through several discretionary grants programs, including Title I supplemental awards, Title II ADAP supplemental awards, and Titles III and IV awards. These programs attempt to take into account factors other than estimates of living AIDS cases that can affect severity of need. HRSA/HAB defines "severity of need" as "the degree to which providing primary medical care to people with HIV disease in any given area is more complicated and costly than in other areas due to several factors, including the adverse health and socio-economic circumstances of the populations to be served" (HRSA, 2001).

When assessing "existing and needed epidemiological data and other analytic tools for resource planning and allocation decisions, specifically for estimating severity of need of a community and the relationship to the allocations process," the Committee focused on Title I supplemental awards, the largest of these discretionary grant awards. To date, HRSA has relied on a qualitative process in assessing the relative severity of need, or resource needs, of jurisdictions in making these awards. In its 2000 reauthorization, Congress emphasized to HRSA the need to use standard, quantitative indicators of severe need to determine supplemental awards (U.S. Congress, 2000c).

In addressing its charge, the Committee organized its work into the following tasks:

1. Developing a conceptual framework for factors affecting resource needs and criteria for evaluating measures of resource needs.

2. Evaluating the process and data now used to award Title I supplemental funds.

3. Proposing a potential new way to identify predictors of resource needs.

Conceptual Framework

Resource needs of an area are determined by a broad array of individual and social factors. The Committee grouped these factors into three categories: disease burden, the costs of providing care, and available resources. Resource needs can be viewed as a product of disease burden and cost of care minus available resources:

Resource needs = (Disease burden * Costs of providing care) – Available resources

These factors vary substantially across jurisdictions, but these variations are not fully captured in current RWCA allocation strategies.

Current Process for Awarding Funds

All Title I grantees must complete an application for the Title I supplemental award, which is scored competitively. Scoring of that application is based on demonstrated severity of need and other factors, such as compliance with Title I administrative requirements, planning council responsibilities, and quality management guidelines. The severity-of-need section of the application is worth one-third of the total possible points. Grantees are asked to provide data and descriptive text on the following aspects of the HIV/AIDS epidemic in their jurisdiction: (1) HIV/AIDS epidemiology; (2) comorbid conditions, poverty, and insurance status; and (3) populations with special needs.

The Committee reviewed Title I applications and found little consistency in the factors described by grantees. Even when grantees do describe comparable factors, there is tremendous variability in the types of indicators they use. Thus, it is virtually impossible to make objective comparative assessments of relative needs across areas. Furthermore, except for some information about insurance status and poverty rates, the application does not ask for information describing variations in the costs of providing care in different areas, or the availability of other resources. HRSA/HAB provides a scoring guide for reviewers of applications, but it also emphasizes the importance of reviewer judgment. Perhaps as a result of the difficulty in assessing variation in resource needs across regions, over and above those due to differences in the prevalence of AIDS, EMAs' Title I supplemental awards are highly correlated with their Title I base award. Given the high correlation between supplemental and base awards, the effort required for grantees to complete the application seems unjustified. Accordingly, the Committee recommends the following:

Recommendation 5-1 HRSA should modify the Title I supplemental application process. The severity-of-need component of the Title I supplemental award should be based on two components:

- Quantitatively defined need, based on a small number of measures that can be calculated by HRSA/HAB.
- Locally defined need described in a short narrative by the applicant.

Recommendation 5-2 A predominance of the weight for determining Title I awards should be given to the quantitative measure of resource needs that reflect variations in costs of care and fiscal capacity across EMAs.

Proposed New Approach

The Committee notes that either direct or indirect measures of resource needs could be developed. The Committee also describes a way to develop indirect indicators. This approach—sometimes referred to as social-area analysis—attempts to relate the characteristics of geographically defined populations to variations in disease or the use of services (Shevky and Bell, 1955; Pittman et al., 1986; Kessler, 1998).

The first step in the latter approach would be to identify direct measures or predictors of resource needs that meet acceptable standards of scientific importance, soundness, and feasibility. The second step is to develop a more explicit definition of the factors that are considered when defining resource needs. Once useful predictors of need have been identified, it will be necessary to assess the extent to which that information predicts variations in resource needs among areas. (Details of this analysis are presented in Chapter 5 and Appendix D.) Accordingly, the Committee recommends the following:

Recommendation 5-3 HRSA/HAB should evaluate the feasibility and usefulness of using social-area indicator models that are based on publicly available data that are collected in standardized ways across jurisdictions, to estimate EMA-level resource needs for the Title I supplemental award. This approach also might be useful in assessing resource needs for other RWCA discretionary grant programs.

Recommendation 5-4 The Secretary of HHS should evaluate the cost and utility of redesigning and coordinating studies conducted by HRSA/HAB and CDC to assess the specific needs and circumstances of people living with HIV. These data can be used to estimate resource needs and as part of quality assessment activities. The Secretary of HHS should also assess the cost and utility of the indirect modeling approach described in Recommendation 5-3 for assessing regional variations in resource requirements.

MEASURING QUALITY OF CARE

HRSA/HAB and RWCA grantees have undertaken a variety of quality-improvement initiatives. The 2000 reauthorization placed more emphasis on quality by requiring that all RWCA grantees establish a quality-management program. Although Titles III and IV grantees already had such programs in place, the new provision required Titles I and II grantees to implement them. The focus on quality in the most recent reauthorization reflects two national trends in quality improvement and accountability. First, the health sector has seen growing interest in measuring and improving quality (IOM, 2000, 2001b). Second, federal policy and funding decisions are increasingly being based on demonstrable performance indicators.

Progress on this broad agenda cannot be adequately measured by outcomes alone. Considering this context, the Committee interpreted this charge as a request to examine and make recommendations regarding the availability and usefulness of not only outcomes, but a broad continuum of measures for assessing and improving the quality of both primary care and support services funded through the CARE Act. Knowledge about what constitutes the best possible HIV/AIDS care is constantly changing, and the applicability of specific measures is limited by the evolving nature of the epidemic, including changes in the affected populations, the course and outcomes of infection, treatment standards, and policies and programs for financing and delivering care. Accordingly, while the Committee makes recommendations regarding measures that HRSA and grantees can use to monitor quality of care (see Recommendation 6-1), the Committee felt it could best contribute by providing a framework, criteria, and process for selecting measures that can evolve with the epidemic.

Conceptual Framework

HIV quality assessment can be thought of as having four key dimensions: the population of interest, the level assessed, the type of measures employed, and the spectrum of services to be evaluated.

Population: The HIV-infected population consists of three groups: (1) those who are not yet diagnosed (and thus are not in care), (2) those who are diagnosed but are not currently in care,[7] and (3) those who are diagnosed and are receiving care. The CARE Act traditionally has focused on individuals who are diagnosed and currently in care. The Committee believes that quality assessment in HIV disease should extend to the entire HIV-infected population. Although quality assessment typically evaluates the care provided to those already receiving services, the number of persons not in treatment in an area can be an important indicator of access to care.

Level of Assessment: Quality can be assessed at the individual patient level, at the clinic/provider level, or at the population level. When assessing the quality of a clinic or provider, analysts aggregate individual levels of quality to the program level. For example, a measure of the quality of care provided by clinics is the proportion of patients with indications for treatment who are receiving appropriate highly active antiretroviral therapy (HAART). Provider organizations, including HRSA and its grantees, now commonly employ a variety of such provider-level measures. Little attention has been paid to assessing quality for whole communities, metropolitan areas, or states.[8]

Type of Measure: The Committee adopted the widely accepted taxonomy that classifies measures into three domains: structure, process, and outcome (Donabedian, 1966). *Structure measures* assess the characteristics and resources of an organization, such as staffing, supplies, equipment, and training. *Process measures* usually focus on the actions of a provider or organization to improve care, such as promoting self-care, conducting diagnostic tests, and offering appropriate therapies. *Outcome measures* assess the changes in a patient's health status. The three elements are interrelated and theoretically causally linked; that is, structure affects the probability of good processes of care, which can in turn affect outcomes such as health status and quality of life.

Despite compelling arguments for analyzing outcomes as ultimate indicators of quality, such measures are often only weakly related to the quality of care provided by specific clinics. For this reason, process measures are often used in lieu of outcome measures at the program or clinic level, while the monitoring of outcomes is both a simpler and more compelling way of assessing the impact of all care provided in an area.

Spectrum of Services: Both primary care and support services are essential components of high-quality care. Quality measurement to date has focused almost exclusively on clinical care.

---

[7]The category of those who are "not in care" also includes those who are not in *regular care*.

[8]HRSA, however, has recently initiated some work focused on developing quality measures at the EMA level.

Review of Existing Measures

The Committee reviewed the quality measures used by key organizations and frequently cited studies (see Table 6-2 for a list), and the measures used in RWCA programs. While there is some consistency in the measures used across sources, there is also a great deal of variation in how the measures are defined and implemented. This review also shows that many sources use numerous process measures and, to a lesser extent, outcomes measures. Process measures, almost all of which were closely related to well-accepted clinical guidelines,[9] were over 10 times more frequent than outcome measures.

Comparable attention has not been devoted to measures of structure, such as the availability of clinicians with the appropriate expertise and experience, despite studies linking increased provider expertise, capacity, and number of HIV-specific services to longer patient survival and prevention of opportunistic conditions (Bennett et al., 1989; Ball and Turner, 1991; Kitahata et al., 1996; Turner et al., 1998). The Committee identified relatively few measures of support services, and no systematic efforts to assess patient experiences with care. Finally, the Committee found that all measures focused on the provider level, and that no population-level process or outcome measures of quality were in routine use, despite their importance as an indicator of the overall impact of an area's epidemic and prevention/treatment/support programs.

Based on its review of selected quality-of-care measure sets, the Committee recommends a standardized set of structure, process, and outcome quality measures for assessing and facilitating quality improvement at the clinic level and at the EMA/state levels (See Recommendation 6-1). For the well-developed process of clinical care measures, measures were selected if at least four of the nine groups included them. Other measures were identified using expert judgment. A detailed review of measures used by these sources is included in Appendix E.

The Committee also recommends several population-level measures be included in RWCA quality assessments at the EMA and state level. The Committee notes that RWCA grantees do not bear the entire responsibility for outcomes among their patients; private and public insurers and others do as well. However, population-based measures are essential in monitoring HIV care in a region and identifying areas for improvement. Rather than being interpreted as direct measures of the quality of care

---

[9]See Department of HHS guidelines (http://www.aidsinfo.nih.gov/guidelines/) and International AIDS Society-USA guidelines (Yeni et al., 2002; http://www.iasusa.org/).

provided by specific clinics, they could be interpreted as reflecting the cumulative effects of many influences on case quality and outcomes.

Overall, HRSA and RWCA-funded clinics and programs are doing an admirable job of defining, assessing, and attempting to improve the quality of care received by HIV-infected individuals. In many ways, RWCA-funded programs have a more advanced approach to measuring and improving quality of care than most general medical facilities. However, HRSA, RWCA grantees, and providers could still do much more to measure and improve quality of care by adopting a common framework and starting to standardize the assessment of quality.

A critical step in moving from the current situation of uncoordinated data collection to a more standardized approach would entail reaching a consensus on how different indicators should be defined and implemented, and then putting into place a mechanism for ensuring the quality of the ensuing data. Although there are many ways of doing this, the National Committee on Quality Assurance (NCQA) and the National Quality Forum have developed procedures and policies that could be emulated or modified. For example, NCQA has technical advisory groups that provide advice on the importance, scientific soundness, and feasibility of different measures, and maintains a standing Committee on Performance Measurement that evaluates recommendations from technical experts and staff. A comparable set of procedures should be established by HRSA. The Committee summarizes these recommendations below.

Recommendation 6-1 Quality measures: HRSA should adopt quality measures that are comprehensive with respect to populations (diagnosed in care; diagnosed but not in care; not diagnosed, not in care), level of assessment (provider and population levels), types of measures (structure, process, and outcome), and spectrum of services (clinical and supportive services). At a minimum, HRSA and grantees should strongly consider inclusion of the following standard set of measures to assess the quality of care provided by RWCA-funded providers and EMA and state-level programs. Standard definitions and detailed criteria for these measures need to be developed by HRSA in collaboration with grantees, affected communities, and other stakeholders after a rigorous examination of the importance, scientific soundness, and feasibility of potential measures.

I. CLINIC LEVEL MEASURES

A. Structure
1. Proportion of providers with appropriate expertise and experience in treating patients with HIV*
2. Availability of case management services

B. Process

Screening for:

3. Cervical cancer*
4. Hepatitis B
   a. And administration of hepatitis B vaccine if negative
5. Hepatitis C*
6. Syphilis*
7. Toxoplasmosis
8. Tuberculosis*

Performance of the following clinical monitoring tests:

9. CD4+ cell count and HIV viral load (process)*

Antiretroviral treatment:

10. Provision of indicated antiretroviral treatment*
11. Provision of adherence counseling and monitoring

Vaccinations and prophylaxis for opportunistic infections:

12. Influenza vaccination
13. Pneumoccocal pneumonia vaccination
14. Hepatitis B vaccination if patient not immune
15. If indicated, *Mycobacterium avium* complex (MAC)
16. If indicated, *Pneumocystis carinii* pneumonia (PCP)*

C. Outcomes

17. Monitoring of CD4+ and viral load values*
18. Proportion of patients with a history of an AIDS-defining opportunistic condition*
19. Proportion of patients who have >2 missed scheduled clinic appointments per year
20. Hospitalizations and emergency room visits without hospital admission*
21. Proportion of patients with unmet need for support services (e.g., assistance with obtaining housing)^

II. AREA-LEVEL MEASURES (E.G., EMA OR STATE)

Outcome measures related to access and care:

22. Proportion of HIV-infected persons in an area who are not diagnosed^
23. Proportion of diagnosed persons in area who are receiving regular care^
24. Proportion of people with HIV who died within 12 months of an HIV diagnosis*
25. Proportion of people with HIV who progressed to AIDS within 12 months of initial HIV diagnosis*

Key: * indicates high priority; ^ indicates high priority, but may require further development. Other measures are important, but of lower priority.

Recommendation 6-2 Infrastructure development: The Secretary of HHS should provide additional resources to HRSA and CDC to develop infrastructure for monitoring quality at the patient, clinic, and population levels. This infrastructure development strategy has three major components:

a. HRSA should enhance support for information technology and personnel to enable clinics to collect, aggregate, and report a focused set of clinical and patient-reported data.

b. HRSA should collaborate with CDC and other agencies to develop innovative population-based measures that can be captured using existing data sources or other community-based information gathering activities, such as surveys of unmet needs.

c. Congress should enhance flexibility in the administrative caps at the grantee level to promote infrastructure development.

Recommendation 6-3 Collaborative quality activities: The Secretary of HHS should convene a working group, not restricted to, but including the NCQA; state insurance commissioners; state Medicaid officials; and representatives from HRSA, CDC, the Centers for Medicare & Medicaid Services; providers of community, outpatient, and inpatient care; and members of the relevant research communities to consider strategies for promoting greater collaboration between public health departments and public- and private-sector providers in order to establish tools and methods to assess systems of care and quality, building on the successful collaborative models developed by the CDC for immunization (e.g., Clinic Assessment Software Application and Assessment Feedback Incentives Exchange).

SUMMARY

RWCA is a program that has provided lifesaving care to millions of persons who otherwise would not have access to adequate services, and that has helped develop an infrastructure for providing high-quality care that would not exist in its absence. Despite this success, it is critical to periodically reevaluate whether allocation strategies are an equitable and efficient way of distributing resources to jurisdictions with the greatest needs. Furthermore, it is important that activities for assessing and improving the quality of care be refined and expanded.

With the advent of HAART and the availability of a wide array of other support services and prevention efforts for HIV-infected individuals, it is essential to promote efforts to make individuals aware of their status and to facilitate their entry into care. Significant and continued improvements in long-term morbidity and mortality related to HIV will not occur unless these individuals are under appropriate care. The Committee recognizes that the last frontier to eliminate morbidity and mortality from HIV disease will be primary prevention.

The Committee proposes that overarching principles of equity be used to guide the development of a refined and more explicit framework for evaluating the distribution of RWCA resources. It proposes several specific types of analyses that could be used to guide the evaluation and improvement of allocation formulas. Similarly, it proposes a framework for assessing quality of care provided to HIV-infected persons, and several specific steps that could be taken to build on existing work and develop a national, standardized approach to quality assessment. Such refinements in the approach to distributing and evaluating the impact of RWCA resources could help the CARE Act remain a pathbreaking approach to providing care to some of the nation's most vulnerable citizens.

REFERENCES

Ball JK, Turner BJ. 1991. *AIDS in U.S. Hospitals in 1986–1987: A National Perspective.* Rockville, MD: Agency for Health Care Policy and Research. DHHS publication (PH) 91–0015.

Barre-Sinoussi F, Chermann JC, Rey F, Nugeyre MT, Chamaret S, Gruest J, Dauguet C, Axler-Blin C, Vezinet-Brun F, Rouzioux C, Rozenbaum W, Montagnier L. 1983. Isolation of a T-lymphotropic retrovirus from a patient at risk for acquired immune deficiency syndrome (AIDS). *Science* 220:868–71.

Bennett CL, Garfinkle JB, Greenfield S, Draper D, Rogers W, Mathews C, Kanouse DE. 1989. The relation between hospital experience and in-hospital mortality for patients with AIDS-related PCP. *Journal of the American Medical Association* 261:2975–9.

CDC (Centers for Disease Control and Prevention). 1981. Pneumocycstis Pneumonia–Los Angeles. *Morbidity and Mortality Weekly Report* 30:250–2. Atlanta, GA: CDC.

CDC. 1992. 1993 Revised classification system for HIV infection and expanded surveillance case definition for AIDS among adolescents and adults. *Morbidity and Mortality Weekly Report* 41(RR–17):1–19. Atlanta, GA: CDC.

CDC. 1999. Guidelines for national human immunodeficiency virus case surveillance, including monitoring for human immunodeficiency virus infection and acquired immunodeficiency syndrome. *Morbidity and Mortality Weekly Report* 48(13):1–28. Atlanta, GA: CDC.

CDC. 2003. Update on the Evaluation of the Performance of Integrated Human Immunodeficiency Virus (HIV)/Acquired Immunodeficiency Syndrome (AIDS) Surveillance Systems. (Email communication, Patricia Sweeney, CDC, March 4, 2003).

Colfax GN, Bindman AB. 1998. Health benefits and risks of reporting HIV-infected individuals by name. *American Journal of Public Health* 88(6):876–9.

Donabedian A. 1966. Evaluating the quality of medical care. *Milbank Memorial Fund Quarterly* 44(3 (Supp)):166–206.

Fauci AS, Pantaleo G, Stanley S, Weissman D. 1996. Immunopathogenic mechanisms of HIV infection. *Annals of Internal Medicine* 124(7):654–63.

Gallo RC, Salahuddin SZ, Popovic M, Shearer GM, Kaplan M, Haynes BF, Palker TJ, Redfield R, Oleske J, Safai B, et al. 1984. Frequent detection and isolation of cytopathic retroviruses (HTLV-III) from patients with AIDS and at risk for AIDS. *Science* 224:500–3.

Georgia Division of Public Health, Epidemiology Branch, HIV/STD Epidemiology Section. 2003. Proposal for HIV Infection Reporting in Georgia. [Online]. Available: http://www.ph.dhr.state.ga.us/epi/hivreporting.shtml [accessed September 25, 2003].

GAO (General Accounting Office). 1995. *Ryan White CARE Act of 1990: Opportunities Are Available to Improve Funding Equity.* GAO/T-HEHS-95-91. Washington, DC: GAO.

GAO. 2000. *Ryan White CARE Act: Opportunities to Enhance Funding Equity.* GAO/T-HEHS-00-150. Washington, DC: GAO.

Hecht FM, Chesney MA, Lehman JS, Osmond D, Vranizan K, Colman S, Keane D, Reingold A, Bindman AB. 2000. Does HIV reporting by name deter testing? MESH Study Group. *AIDS* 14(12):1801–8.

HRSA (Health Resources and Services Administration). 2001. A Primer on Title I and Title II Formula Allocation Calculations. Unpublished document. (Email communication, Steven Young, HRSA, November 21, 2001).

HRSA. 2002a. Title I: Grants to Eligible Metropolitan Areas. [Online]. Available: http://ftp.hrsa.gov/hab/titleifact.pdf [accessed May 22, 2003].

HRSA. 2002b. Title II: AIDS Drug Assistance Program. [Online]. Available: ftp://ftp.hrsa.gov/hab/adap1.pdf [accessed May 22, 2003].

HRSA. 2002c. Title III: Early Intervention Services. [Online]. Available: ftp://ftp.hrsa.gov/hab/titleiiifact.pdf [accessed May 22, 2003].

HRSA. 2002d. Title IV: Services for Women, Infants, Children, Youth, and Their Families. [Online]. Available: ftp://ftp.hrsa.gov/hab/titleiv.htm [accessed May 22, 2003].

HRSA. 2003. CARE Act Overview and Funding History. [Online]. Available: ftp://ftp.hrsa.gov/hab/fundinghis03.xls [accessed October 9, 2003].

IOM (Institute of Medicine). 2000. *To Err Is Human: Building a Safer Health System.* Washington, DC: National Academy Press.

IOM. 2001a. *Coverage Matters: Insurance and Health Care.* Washington, DC: National Academy Press.

IOM. 2001b. *Envisioning the National Health Care Quality Report.* Hurtado MP, Swift EK, Corrigan JM, Eds. Washington, DC: National Academy Press.

IOM/NAS (Institute of Medicine and the National Academy of Sciences). 1988. *Confronting AIDS, Update 1988.* Washington, DC: National Academy Press.

Kaiser Family Foundation. 2000. Financing HIV/AIDS Care: A Quilt with Many Holes. *Capital Hill Briefing Series on HIV/AIDS.*

Kates J, Ruiz S. 2002. *Sources of Coverage and Care for People with HIV/AIDS in the United States: Assessing Coverage in Southern States.* Southern States Summit on HIV/AIDS and STDs. Menlo Park, CA: Kaiser Family Foundation.

Kessler RC. 1998. A methodology for estimating 12-month prevalence of serious mental illness. *Mental Health, United States 1998.* DHHS Pub. No. (SMA) 99-3285 ed. Washington, DC: Government Printing Office.

Kitahata MM, Koepsell TD, Deyo RA, Maxwell CL, Dodge WT, Wagner EH. 1996. Physicians' experience with the acquired immunodeficiency syndrome as a factor in patients' survival. *New England Journal of Medicine* 334(11):701–6.

Mills R, Bhandari S. 2003. Health insurance coverage, 2002. *Current Population Reports.* Washington, DC: U.S. Census Bureau. Pp. 60–223.

Osmond DH, Bindman AB, Vranizan K, Lehman JS, Hecht FM, Keane D, Reingold A. 1999. Name-based surveillance and public health interventions for persons with HIV infection. Multistate Evaluation of Surveillance for HIV Study Group. *Annals of Internal Medicine* 131(10):775–9.

Pantaleo G, Graziosi C, Fauci AS. 1993. New concepts in the immunopathogenesis of human immunodeficiency virus infection. *New England Journal of Medicine* 328(5):327–35.

Pittman J, Andrews H, Struening E. 1986. The use of zip-coded population data in social area studies of service utilization. *Evaluation and Program Planning* 9(4):309–17.

Shevky E, Bell W. 1955. *Social Area Analysis.* Stanford, CA: Stanford University Press.

Thacker SB. 2000. Historical development. *Principles and Practice of Public Health Surveillance.* 2nd ed. Teutsch SM, Churchill RE, eds. New York: Oxford University Press.

Turner B, Markson L, Cocroft J, Cosler L, Hauck WW. 1998. Clinic HIV-focused features and prevention of *Pneumocystis carinii* pneumonia. *Journal of General Internal Medicine* 13(1):16–23.

U.S. Congress, House of Representatives. Committee on Commerce. 2000a. *Report on Ryan White CARE Act Amendments of 2000 (106-788).* 106th Cong., 2d Sess. July 25, 2000. Pp. 24–6.

U.S. Congress, House of Representatives. Committee on Commerce. 2000b. *Report on Ryan White CARE Act Amendments of 2000 (106-788).* 106th Cong., 2d Sess. July 25, 2000. P. 30.

U.S. Congress. 2000c. *Congressional Record.* 146(123): S10032.

U.S. Congress, Senate. 2000d. *Ryan White CARE Act Amendments of 2000—Managers' Statement of Explanation.* October 5, 2000.

Yeni P, Hammer SM, Carpenter CC, Cooper DA, Fischl MA, Gatell JM, Gazzard BG, Hirsch MS, Jacobsen DM, Katzenstein DA, Montaner JS, Richman DD, Saag MS, Schechter M, Schooley RT, Thompson MA, Vella S, Volberding PA. 2002. Antiretroviral treatment for adult HIV infection in 2002: Updated recommendations of the International AIDS Society-USA Panel. *The Journal of the American Medical Association* 288(2):222–35.

1

Introduction

The Ryan White Comprehensive AIDS Resources Emergency (CARE) Act (RWCA) provides funding to cities, states, and other public and private entities to provide care and support services to medically underserved individuals with HIV disease (Ryan White CARE Act. 42 U.S.C. § 300ff [2003]). Congress established the CARE Act in 1990 as the "payer of last resort": the act funds care for uninsured or underinsured individuals who have no other resources to pay for care (Ryan White CARE Act. 42 U.S.C. § 300ff-11 [2003]). While RWCA remains a safety-net program, funding has grown substantially over time and has helped create a major infrastructure for HIV/AIDS care. In fiscal year 2003 (FY2003) federal spending on RWCA totaled $2 billion (HRSA, 2003a), making it the third largest payer for HIV care behind Medicaid and Medicare (Foster et al., 2002). The CARE Act serves an estimated 533,000 individuals (HRSA, 2003b).[1] It is impossible to know the exact number of clients served, however, because individuals may receive care under several parts of the CARE Act and most areas do not report unduplicated client-level data.

The Health Resources and Services Administration's HIV/AIDS Bureau (HRSA/HAB), within the U.S. Department of Health and Human Services (HHS), has lead responsibility for implementing the CARE Act.

[1]This estimate includes those receiving support services, not just those in medical care, plus services to uninfected family members (HRSA, 2003c).

The RWCA is composed of four major program titles and several other components:

- Title I provides grants to Eligible Metropolitan Areas (EMAs—currently 51) that have been disproportionately affected by the HIV/AIDS epidemic. Title I funds a variety of medical care and support services for people living with HIV disease. To qualify as an EMA, a metropolitan area must have a population of 500,000 or more and more than 2,000 reported AIDS cases within the past five years. Half of Title I funding is distributed by a formula, while the other half is awarded through a competitive supplemental application process, based on severity of need and other criteria (HRSA, 2002a).
- Title II provides grants to states, the District of Columbia, Puerto Rico, and U.S. territories to improve the quality, availability, and delivery of health care and support services for individuals with HIV disease. Title II provides states with funds to provide access to HIV medications through the AIDS Drug Assistance Program (ADAP). In addition, Title II also provides funding for "Emerging Communities" that do not qualify as EMAs and are ineligible for Title I grants (HRSA, 2002b,c).
- Title III provides direct grants to nonprofit entities for primary care and early intervention services (such as testing, counseling, referrals, and case management), capacity-building, and planning (HRSA, 2002d).
- Title IV provides grants for family-centered care for infants, children, youth, women living with HIV disease, and their families. Title IV provides primary and specialty medical care, psychosocial services, and outreach and prevention services. Title IV also provides clients with increased access to HIV/AIDS clinical trials and research (HRSA, 2002e).

In addition, the RWCA supports AIDS Educational Training Centers, which provide clinical HIV training and education for providers, and the Dental Reimbursement Program, which covers uncompensated oral health care for individuals with HIV/AIDS (HRSA, 2002f,g). RWCA also funds the Special Projects of National Significance (SPNS) program, which establishes demonstration projects that address the challenge of providing care to underserved and vulnerable populations (HRSA, 2002h).

IMPETUS FOR THIS STUDY

Issues of equity have been at the heart of legislative and public debate over RWCA. That debate has often centered on the adequacy of the formulas and supporting data used to distribute Title I and II funds. A significant proportion of RWCA funds are allocated to EMAs and states using formulas based on information about the estimated number of persons living with AIDS in different areas. Many have raised concerns that such allocations are not equitable because the epidemic is not adequately reflected by AIDS cases alone, and that areas with emerging HIV epidemics are underfunded because cases of HIV (non-AIDS) are not included in the formulas (U.S. Congress, 2000a,b). A related concern with basing allocations on AIDS cases is that jurisdictions are not compensated for providing early access to care and treatment (U.S. Congress, 2000b). There is a widely held perception that incorporating HIV data in the formulas would increase the equity of RWCA allocations by targeting funds according to need (U.S. Congress, 2000a,b).

The hold-harmless floors, which prevent an area's funding from dropping drastically from one year to the next, also triggered debate about equity (U.S. Congress, 2000a). In the 2000 reauthorization, San Francisco was the only EMA to continue to benefit from this provision, leading to a significant difference between per-case allocations to San Francisco and other EMAs (GAO, 2000).

Concerns about equity have also centered on the quality of care. Since the first reauthorization in 1996, significant advances have been made in diagnosing and treating HIV disease. At the same time, research has shown that a large proportion of HIV-infected persons were not in care, and that others were not receiving appropriate treatment or support services (Bozzette et al., 1998; Shapiro et al., 1999). Inequalities were identified in access to and use of HIV services, and in overall health outcomes for minorities and women (Shapiro et al., 1999). Disparities in quality of care were also reported for persons with public or no health insurance compared with those with private insurance (Bozzette et al., 1998; Shapiro et al., 1999).

This information raised questions in Congress about whether the formulas for calculating Titles I and II grants allocated RWCA resources equitably. Legislators and other stakeholders also expressed concern about the effectiveness of the local planning and allocation process, and about the possibility that the CARE Act was not meeting the needs of members of historically underserved communities. As a result, the 2000 reauthorization made significant changes in the CARE Act and directed that this study be conducted. Specifically, Congress requested that the Institute of Medicine (IOM) examine three issues: (1) the potential inclusion of data on HIV cases in the allocation formulas, (2) the data and analytic tools that could be used to estimate severity of need and related resource needs, and (3) the availability of health outcome and other measures to assess the quality of and access to RWCA-funded services.

STUDY CHARGE

In October 2001, HRSA and the Centers for Disease Control and Prevention (CDC) commissioned the IOM to study these issues. Box 1-1 contains the charge to the committee, as stated in the 2000 reauthorization of the CARE Act. Although this study addresses some long-range issues, it is intended to provide guidance on issues currently faced by Congress, HRSA, and grantees in the administration of the CARE Act. Each of the three components of the Committee's charge is discussed below.

Use of HIV Data in the Title I and II Allocation Formulas

As part of the 2000 reauthorization, Congress conditionally directed that the Title I and II formulas incorporate data on reported cases of HIV infection as well as AIDS in order to "target funding to more accurately reflect the HIV/AIDS epidemic" (U.S. Congress, 2000c). A recent General Accounting Office (GAO) study also concluded that reported HIV cases should provide a better indicator of need than the number of AIDS cases, and that Title I and II formulas should include these data once they are available in all jurisdictions (GAO, 2000). As of October 2003, all states, territories, and cities, except Georgia and Philadelphia, have initiated a system of HIV reporting (CDC, 2003).

The use of such data in Title I and II formulas could take effect as early as FY2005—provided that the Secretary of HHS determines that such data are "sufficiently accurate" for RWCA resource allocation purposes (Ryan White CARE Act. 42 U.S.C. § 300ff-13 [2003]). The legislation authorized the Secretary of HHS to provide grants for technical assistance to ensure that such data are available from all eligible areas as soon as practicable, but not later than the beginning of FY2007 (Ryan White CARE Act. 42 U.S.C. § 300ff-13 [2003]).[2] The legislation also authorized the IOM to assist the Secretary in assessing the readiness of states to produce adequate and reliable HIV case-reporting data, determine the accuracy of using HIV cases within the existing allocation formulas, and establish recommendations regarding how states could improve their HIV case-reporting systems ((Ryan White CARE Act. 42 U.S.C. § 300ff-11 [2003]).

In interpreting its charge, the Committee recognized the difficulty of defining such terms as "sufficiently accurate," "adequate," and "reliable" to characterize the quality of HIV surveillance data. No absolute standards of accuracy, adequacy, or reliability exist; rather these standards and their definition will vary according to the purposes and tasks for which the data are used. Thus, evaluating HIV reporting systems for use

---

[2]No funds have been appropriated yet for this purpose.

BOX 1-1
Charge to the Committee

In the Ryan White CARE Amendments of 2000, Congress directed the IOM to examine the following issues (Ryan White CARE Act. 42 U.S.C. § 300ff-11 [2003]):

Use of HIV Data in the Title I and II Allocation Formulas

- "whether the surveillance system of each of the States regarding [HIV] provides for the reporting of cases of infection with the virus in a manner that is sufficient to provide adequate and reliable information on the number of such cases and the demographic characteristics of such cases, both for the State in general and for specific geographic areas in the State."
- "whether such information is sufficiently accurate for purposes of formula grants under parts A and B of title XXVI of the Public Health Service Act" [i.e., Title I and II of the RWCA].
- "With respect to any State whose surveillance system does not provide adequate and reliable information on cases of infection with the virus, [provide] recommendations regarding the manner in which the State can improve the system."

Information for Estimating Severity of Need for Resources

- "Existing and needed epidemiological data and other analytic tools for resource planning and allocation decisions, specifically for estimating severity of need of a community and the relationship to the allocations process."

Quality-of-Care Measures

- "The availability and utility of health outcome measures and data for HIV primary care and support services and the extent to which those measures and data could be used to measure the quality of such funded services"; and
- "other factors determined to be relevant to assessing an individual's or community's ability to gain and sustain access to quality HIV services."

NOTE: The Ryan White CARE Act Amendments of 2000 also directed the IOM to study the public financing and delivery of HIV care. HRSA commissioned a separate IOM study to address those issues.

in resource allocation formulas requires a different set of performance criteria than evaluation of these data for public health purposes (e.g., epidemic surveillance, contact tracing, and partner notification). With regard to resource allocation decisions, the "sufficiency," "adequacy," and "reliability" of case-reporting data must be understood in terms of over-

and underfunding errors to RWCA grantees in different areas. That is, rather than focus on an absolute standard of accuracy, it is more important to consider differential bias.

Information for Estimating Severity of Need for Resources

The CARE Act attempts to direct funds to areas in the greatest need of financial assistance through several of its discretionary grant programs, including Title I supplemental awards, Title II ADAP supplemental awards, and Title III and IV awards. In contrast to formula awards, which are based exclusively on estimates of living AIDS cases, these grants attempt to take into account other factors affecting severity of need. HRSA/HAB defines "severity of need" as "the degree to which providing primary medical care to people with HIV disease in any given area is more complicated and costly than in other areas based on a combination of the adverse health and socio-economic circumstances of the populations to be served" (HRSA, 2003d).

In the 2000 reauthorization, Congress charged the IOM Committee to examine ". . . existing and needed epidemiological data and other analytic tools for resource planning and allocation decisions, specifically for estimating severity of need of a community and the relationship to the allocations process" (Ryan White CARE Act. 42 U.S.C. § 300ff-11 [2003]).

The Committee focused its analysis on the application of severity-of-need criteria in determining Title I supplemental awards, the largest of these discretionary grant awards, because of the specific requests for assistance by Congress and HRSA/HAB in this area. HRSA currently uses a qualitative assessment process to make Title I supplemental awards. In the 2000 reauthorization, Congress expressed its intention to make the process more explicit: ". . . [HRSA/HAB] should employ standard, quantitative measures to the maximum extent possible in lieu of narrative self-reporting when awarding supplemental awards" (U.S. Congress, 2000c). Difficulty in finding timely, relevant, standardized data for every jurisdiction has hindered HRSA's efforts to develop such measures, and helped motivate this study. Although the Committee does not focus on other discretionary grant programs that use severity of need criteria in allocating resources, the Committee's findings and recommendations may have relevance for these programs.

Quality-of-Care Measures

The reauthorized CARE Act mandates that all title programs establish a quality-management program to "assess the extent to which HIV health services . . . are consistent with the most recent Public Health Service (PHS) guidelines for the treatment of HIV disease and related opportunistic infections, and . . . to develop strategies for ensuring such services are consistent with the guidelines for improvement in the access to and quality of HIV services" (Ryan White CARE Act. 42 U.S.C. §. 300ff-64 [2003]).[3] To further that goal, Congress charged the Committee with examining:

- "The availability and utility of health outcome measures and data for HIV primary care and support services and the extent to which those measures and data could be used to measure the quality of such funded services"; and
- "other factors determined to be relevant to assessing an individual's or community's ability to gain and sustain access to quality HIV services" (Ryan White CARE Act. 42 U.S.C. §. 300ff-11 [2003]).

The focus on quality in the most recent reauthorization reflects several national trends. First, the health sector has seen growing interest in measuring and improving quality (IOM, 1999, 2001a,b).[4,5] In addition, numerous reports have identified a gap between care that should be provided based on available professional knowledge and technology and the care that patients actually receive (IOM, 1999, 2001a; IOM and NRC, 1999). Another trend is the increasing emphasis on accountability across federal government agencies, pursuant to the Government Performance Results Act (1993) and other legislation.[6] As a result, HRSA/HAB and RWCA grantees must document the impact of CARE Act funds on improving access to care and treatment and in addressing unmet needs.

Considering this context, the Committee interpreted this charge as a request to examine and make recommendations regarding the availability and usefulness of not only outcomes, but a broad continuum of measures for assessing and improving the quality of both primary care and support services funded through the CARE Act.

---

[3]This is a new requirement for Title I and II programs; Title III and IV grantees had such programs in place.

[4]Major groups with quality initiatives include the National Committee for Quality Assurance (NCQA), the Agency for Healthcare Research and Quality (AHRQ), the Foundation for Accountability (FACCT), the National Quality Forum, and the Leapfrog Group, among others.

[5]For a more comprehensive review of quality-of-care activities in health care, see IOM, 1999, 2001a,b.

[6]Government Performance Results Act. H.R. 826. 103d Cong., 1st Sess. (1993); Federal Management Improvement Act (FMIA) of 1996 (P.L. 104-208); Chief Financial Officers (CFO) Act of 1990.

STUDY METHODS

The Committee met six times over the course of the study. It began by reviewing the scientific literature and key reports relating to HIV and AIDS surveillance, severity of resource needs, and quality of care. The Committee reviewed RWCA programmatic efforts, as well as HIV/AIDS surveillance data collection and analysis. The Committee reviewed data from HRSA and CDC on Title I and II allocations and HIV and AIDS cases, and analyzed the potential impact of including HIV data and other changes in the formulas on allocations. It also reviewed the data sources and methods used by grantees in their Title I supplemental applications to document severity of need. The Committee also conducted a thorough review of quality measures used by RWCA grantees and other major HIV providers, recommended by authoritative groups, and contained in the research literature.

The Committee heard testimony and received comments from many different stakeholders (see Acknowledgements). The Committee held public information-gathering sessions at its first three meetings to hear from CDC, HRSA, state and local HIV/AIDS programs, and clients. The Committee also met with groups of Title I and II grantees at the 2002 annual conference of the National Alliance of State and Territorial AIDS Directors (NASTAD) and the 2002 RWCA All-Titles conference, respectively, and held a conference call with state surveillance coordinators. Members of the Committee conducted site visits to CDC, HRSA, and to rural RWCA clinics and the state health department in Alabama. The Committee also examined information on states' HIV surveillance funding. The Committee also commissioned papers on the history of public health surveillance and on the legislative history of RWCA.

GUIDING PRINCIPLES

The Committee agreed upon several guiding principles that could be used to assess alternative approaches to resource allocation and quality assessment. One overriding consideration for any CARE Act allocation strategy or quality assessment should be the extent to which it furthers the goal of equity in care for HIV-infected individuals. The CARE Act operates against a backdrop of significant inequalities in access to health care in the United States. More than 43 million Americans are uninsured (Mills and Bandhari, 2003), and millions more hold insurance policies that do not cover basic medications or treatments (IOM, 2001c). Congress enacted the CARE Act in 1990 at least in part to address this challenge regarding people with HIV infection.

The Committee recognizes that resources allocated to the RWCA have at the outset been insufficient to address the unmet needs of all individuals with HIV disease. In this context, a reasonable objective would be to assure that all individuals with HIV infection be provided with comparable levels of the highest possible quality of care. Pursuit of such an objective in the context of constrained resources inevitably leads to tradeoffs. The Committee recognizes that difficult choices are unavoidable and that competing views exist about what it means to manage such choices "fairly." Thus, the Committee began its deliberations by considering broad principles of equity that bear on the allocation of health care resources and their relevance to the RWCA program.

Measures of inequality usually focus on differential access to goods, services, and benefits. Not all inequalities or disparities, however, are inequities. Inequity refers to disparities in a given domain that are considered unfair or unjust. For example, disparities in income are measured by the extent to which individuals earn less or more than those who work an equivalent number of hours. A judgment of inequity would reflect an assessment that inequalities are not morally justifiable.

There has been considerable controversy about how to measure inequalities in health care and which disparities constitute inequities. Disagreements exist over which clinical conditions, which interventions, provided under what circumstances, and with what attendant burdens should be of concern. The resolution of these questions has critical implications, given widespread acceptance of the moral claim that all citizens should have access to basic medical care, that need should dictate access, and that disparities in access to clinical care by those with similar medical conditions represents an inequity (President's Commission for the Study of Ethical Problems in Medicine and Biomedical and Behavioral Research, 1983; Beauchamp and Childress, 2001).

From this perspective, both the quantity and quality of services matter: equal access to clinical interventions of differing quality would not represent an equitable distribution. Settings or conditions that inhibit the use of needed services would also constitute inequities. Extended waiting time in clinics, the absence of psychologically or culturally appropriate settings, and the time required for travel may not be critical if they do not affect utilization. Some, however, would consider these conditions inequities because they erode the dignity of the individuals who require health services (Caplan et al., 1999).

In the face of constrained resources, some rationing—either implicit or explicit—will occur, and such rationing may be more or less equitable (Churchill, 1987; Callahan, 1995; Epstein and Gutmann, 1997; Hall, 1997). The Committee recognizes that difficult choices and tradeoffs are unavoidable, and that stakeholders may hold diverse, ambiguous, and mutually incompatible conceptions of what is fair when facing difficult rationing decisions.

Competing Views of Fairness

Need-based allocation is perhaps the most intuitively powerful conception of equity or fairness. Humans are naturally predisposed to focus on identifiable lives in imminent peril, and to allocate whatever resources are required to sustain them. According to this view, individuals with the worst prognoses should receive the most vigorous interventions even if the outcomes fall short of those attained by individuals with less demanding needs. Allocations based on need often result in unequal spending per case. Perhaps more important, meeting the needs of selected individuals may limit resources available to others.

A very different conception of fairness finds its roots in the philosophy of utilitarianism. In this view, society should allocate available resources to confer the greatest total good and the least amount of harm. According to this view, some segments of the population may justifiably receive limited services if they would derive little benefit, or if by withholding such services the system enables many others to enjoy a small incremental benefit. Such an efficiency-driven approach allocates health care resources to those for whom they will produce the greatest net improvement per unit spent. This view underpins cost-effectiveness analysis.

Tension among these and other conceptions of equity is unavoidable (NRC, 2001). The Committee did not see its role as adjudicating among philosophies of justice. These are political decisions that should be made by Congress when determining how RWCA funds should be allocated. Although Congress has emphasized different priorities in reauthorization debates and language, standards of equity are usually implied. Public decision making must be transparent to be legitimate. Transparency requires that when rationing occurs it must be explicit and the grounds for decisions fully stated. In this report, the Committee highlights the pros, cons, and tradeoffs implicit in any allocation process, given that RCWA resources have from the outset been insufficient to address the unmet needs of all individuals with HIV and AIDS. Within the context of constrained resources, and cognizant of competing conceptions of equity, the Committee's work was informed by the belief that all individuals with HIV infection should receive the highest-quality care possible regardless of where they live and their personal circumstances.

Equity and the Undiagnosed

A health care system that assures access only to those who are aware of their condition and of available services would fail some tests of equity. For clinical conditions that remain asymptomatic for long periods but for which early medical intervention can have a significant impact, such as HIV, this is an important matter. With the advent of highly active antiretroviral therapy, or HAART, in the mid-1990s, early diagnosis of HIV infection has become even more critical.

Persons living with HIV/AIDS comprise three groups: those who are not yet diagnosed with HIV or AIDS and therefore are not receiving care; those who are diagnosed with HIV or AIDS but who are not in regular care; and those who are diagnosed with HIV or AIDS and are receiving regular care. RWCA is intended to serve a subset of all people with HIV/AIDS: those who are uninsured or underinsured. State HIV and AIDS reporting systems capture only individuals who have been diagnosed with HIV or AIDS, regardless of insurance status. Because RWCA primarily focuses on the diagnosed population, it does not address the extraordinary unmet needs of unidentified HIV-positive individuals. National estimates postulate that 850,000–950,000 individuals in the United States have HIV disease (Fleming et al., 2002). Of those, approximately 75 percent, or 670,000, know they are infected, and an estimated 450,000 are in care (Fleming et al., 2002).

With the advent of HAART and the availability of a wide array of other support services and prevention efforts for HIV-infected individuals, it is essential to promote efforts to make individuals aware of their status and to facilitate their entry into care. Significant and continued improvements in long-term morbidity and mortality related to HIV will not occur unless these individuals are under appropriate care.

Fiscal Federalism

Fiscal federalism is another important issue that creates a moral quandary for funders. RWCA is funded and implemented with a complex local–state–federal partnership of HIV/AIDS care. The details of federal RWCA funding allocation impose important incentives on other government actors (NRC, 2003).

One important concern is that federal RWCA policies may reduce incentives for states and localities to offer important medications, medical, and social services. While federal policy makers may wish to establish proper incentives for states and localities to fund HIV/AIDS care, some also want to ensure high-quality care even when states and localities fail to provide adequate resources. Knowing these preferences, state and local policy makers may limit funding for basic HIV medications, services, and care because federal funders will cover all or some of the resulting shortfall. If a state can attract greater federal subsidies by offering very limited services to people with AIDS, it may reduce the total pool of resources available for HIV/AIDS care. It may also take unfair advantage of the commitment, honored by other states, to provide adequate HIV/AIDS care.

The Committee was mindful of the potential adverse incentives associated with current and potential alternative federal RWCA funding allocations. For example, potentially important incentive effects are created by including (or excluding) estimates of undiagnosed cases in determining resource allocation. Differences in the proportion of undiagnosed HIV cases are not an exogenous source of bias. They result from policy decisions about the aggressiveness of case finding and screening, and they are influenced by the availability of funds. If estimates of undiagnosed cases are included, there could be a perverse incentive for states and EMAs to avoid identifying cases in order to be able to provide more intensive services to cases already identified. By contrast, if estimates of undiagnosed cases are excluded, states and EMAs have an incentive to identify cases in order to maximize their funding. Under either scenario, quality measurements are required to monitor the rate at which new cases are identified, referred, and retained in care. The committee lacked specific data to measure the magnitude of these incentive effects.

ORGANIZATION OF THE REPORT

Chapter 2 provides an overview of the HIV/AIDS epidemic, financing of HIV/AIDS care, legislative history of RWCA, and its current structure. Chapter 3 provides background on public health and HIV/AIDS surveillance and provides context for how surveillance data are used in the allocation formulas. The ensuing chapters address the three components of the Committee's charge. Chapter 4 evaluates the potential for data on HIV cases to be incorporated into the Title I and II allocation formulas. Chapter 5 examines data and methods for estimating severity of need and related resource needs, with particular attention to Title I supplemental grants. Chapter 6 reviews measures that can be used to assess the quality of HIV/AIDS care provided by the RWCA. Chapter 7 summarizes the Committee's findings and recommendations.

REFERENCES

Beauchamp TL, Childress JF. 2001. *Principles of Biomedical Ethics.* 5th ed. New York: Oxford University Press.

Bozzette S, Berry SH, Duan N, Frankel MR, Leibowitz AA, Lefkowitz D, Emmons CA, Senterfitt JW, Berk ML, Morton SC, Shapiro MF. 1998. The care of HIV-infected adults in the United States. HIV Cost and Services Utilization Study Consortium. *New England Journal of Medicine* 339(26):1897–904.

Callahan D. 1995. *Setting Limits: Medical Goals in an Aging Society.* Washington, DC: Georgetown University Press.

Caplan RL, Light DW, Daniels N. 1999. Benchmarks of fairness: A moral framework for assessing equity. *International Journal of Health Services* 29(4):853–69.

CDC (Centers for Disease Control and Prevention). 2003. Current Status of HIV Infection Surveillance—April 2003. (Email communication, Patricia Sweeney, CDC, April 28, 2003).

Churchill LR. 1987. *Rationing Health Care: Perceptions and Principles of Justice.* Notre Dame, IN: Notre Dame University Press.

Epstein RA, Gutmann H, Eds. 1997. *Mortal Peril: Our Inalienable Right to Health Care?* Reading, MA: Addison-Wesley.

Fleming P, Byers R, Sweeney P, Daniels D, Karon J, Janssen R. 2002. HIV Prevalence in the United States, 2000. Presented at the 9th Conference on Retroviruses and Opportunistic Infections, Seattle, WA. Abstract 11.

Foster S, Niederhausen P, Westmoreland T. 2002. *Federal HIV/AIDS Spending: A Budget Chartbook, Fiscal Year 2001.* Washington, DC: Kaiser Family Foundation.

GAO (General Accounting Office). 2000. *Ryan White CARE Act: Opportunities to Enhance Funding Equity.* Washington, DC: GAO.

Hall MA. 1997. *Making Medical Spending Decisions: The Law, Ethics, and Economics of Rationing Decisions.* New York: Oxford University Press.

HRSA (Health Resources and Services Administration). 2002a. Title I: Grants to Eligible Metropolitan Areas. [Online]. Available: http://ftp.hrsa.gov/hab/titleifact.pdf [accessed May 22, 2003].

HRSA. 2002b. Title II: AIDS Drug Assistance Program. [Online]. Available: ftp://ftp.hrsa.gov/hab/adap1.pdf [accessed May 22, 2003].

HRSA. 2002c. Title II: Grants to States and Territories. [Online]. Available: http://htp.hrsa.gov/hab/titleiifact.pdf [accessed May 22, 2003].

HRSA. 2002d. Title III: Capacity Building Grant Program. [Online]. Available: http://ftp.hrsa.gov/hab/titleiiicap.pdf [accessed May 22, 2003].

HRSA. 2002e. Title IV: Services for Women, Infants, Children, Youth, and Their Families. [Online]. Available: http://ftp.hrsa.gov/hab/titleiv.htm [accessed May 22, 2003].

HRSA 2002f. AIDS Education and Training Centers Program. [Online]. Available: ftp://ftp.hrsa.gov/hab/aetcfact.pdf [accessed May 22, 2003].

HRSA. 2002g. HIV/AIDS Dental Programs. [Online]. Available: http://ftp.hrsa.gov/hab/drpfact.pdf [accessed May 22, 2003].

HRSA. 2002h. Special Projects of National Significance Program. [Online] Available: ftp://ftp.hrsa.gov/hab/spnsfact1.pdf [accessed May 22, 2003].

HRSA. 2003a. CARE Act Overview and Funding History. [Online] Available: ftp://ftp.hrsa.gov/hab/fundinghis03.xls [accessed October 9, 2003].

HRSA. 2003b. The AIDS Epidemic and the Ryan White CARE Act Past Progress, Future Challenges 2002-2003. [Online]. Available: http://hab.hrsa.gov/tools/progressreport/ [accessed September, 2003].

HRSA. 2003c. Individuals served by the CARE Act. (Email communication, Steven Young, HRSA, June 2, 2003).

HRSA. 2003d. Appendix 1: Glossary of Terms. *Ryan White Comprehensive AIDS Resources Emergency (CARE) Act: Needs Assessment Guide 2003 Version*. Rockville, MD: HRSA.

IOM (Institute of Medicine). 1999. *To Err Is Human: Building a Safer Health System*. Washington, DC: National Academy Press.

IOM. 2001a. *Crossing the Quality Chasm: A New Health System for the 21st Century*. Washington, DC: National Academy Press.

IOM. 2001b. *Envisioning the National Health Care Quality Report*. Hurtado MP, Swift EK, Corrigan JM, Eds. Washington, DC: National Academy Press.

IOM and NRC (Institute of Medicine and National Research Council). 1999. Hewitt M, Simone JV, Eds. *Ensuring Quality Cancer Care*. Washington, DC: National Academy Press.

Mills RJ, Bhandari S. 2003. Health Insurance Coverage, 2002. *Current Population Reports*. Washington, DC: U.S. Census Bureau. Pp. 60–223.

NRC (National Research Council). 2001. *Choosing the Right Formula Initial Report*. Washington, DC: National Academy Press.

NRC. 2003. *Statistical Issues in Allocating Funds by Formulas*. Louis TA, Jabine TB, Gerstein MA, Eds. Washington, DC: National Academy Press.

President's Commission for the Study of Ethical Problems in Medicine and Biomedical and Behavioral Research. 1983. *Securing Access to Health Care: A Report on the Ethical Implications of Differences in the Availability of Health Services*. Washington DC: U.S. Government Printing Office.

Shapiro MF, Morton SC, McCaffrey DF, Senterfitt JW, Fleishman JA, Perlman JF, Athey LA, Keesey JW, Goldman DP, Berry SH, Bozzette SA. 1999. Variations in the care of HIV-infected adults in the United States: Results from the HIV Cost and Services Utilization Study. *Journal of the American Medical Association* 281(24):2305–15.

U.S. Congress, House of Representatives. Committee on Commerce. 2000a. *Report on Ryan White CARE Act Amendments of 2000 (106-788)*. 106th Cong., 2d Sess. July 25, 2000. Pp. 24–6.

U.S. Congress, House of Representatives. Committee on Commerce. 2000b. *Report on Ryan White CARE Act Amendments of 2000 (106-788)*. 106th Cong., 2d Sess. July 25, 2000. P. 30.

U.S. Congress. 2000c. *Congressional Record*. 146(123):S10031.

2

Overview of the HIV/AIDS Epidemic and the Ryan White CARE Act

This chapter provides a brief overview of the HIV/AIDS epidemic, the Ryan White Comprehensive AIDS Resources Emergency (CARE) Act (RWCA) in the context of other federal spending programs for HIV/AIDS care, and the history and current structure of the CARE Act and its allocation formulas.

OVERVIEW OF THE HIV/AIDS EPIDEMIC

Natural History of HIV Infection

The AIDS epidemic was first recognized in June of 1981, when the Centers for Disease Control and Prevention (CDC) received reports of clusters of diseases that are not seen in persons with normally functioning immune systems (*Pneumocystis carinii* pneumonia and Kaposi's sarcoma) among mostly young, otherwise healthy gay men (CDC, 1981). Epidemiologic studies showed that the virus was transmitted from infected persons through sexual contact, exposure to infected blood or blood products, sharing of contaminated needles and syringes, transplantation of infected organs or tissue, and from mother to child during pregnancy, at delivery or through breastfeeding (IOM/NAS, 1988). In 1983 and 1984, two groups of investigators identified a retrovirus, now known as human immunodeficiency virus (HIV), as the etiologic agent of AIDS (Barre-Sinoussi et al., 1983; Gallo et al., 1984).

Most people have no symptoms at the time of HIV infection. Some people experience the acute retroviral syndrome, which is flu-like illness characterized by nonspecific symptoms such as fever, fatigue, rash, musculoskeletal pain, sore throat, swollen lymph nodes, arthralgias or myalgias, pharyngitis, and lymphadenopathy (Fauci et al., 1996). During this time, test for HIV antibody tests are usually negative and infection can only be diagnosed by testing the blood for viral products such as HIV RNA (viral load) or proteins (P24 antigen) (Pantaleo et al., 1993; Fauci et al., 1996). After the acute phase of infection, the amount of viral products in the blood is reduced, and tests for HIV antibody become positive. Patients then enter a prolonged period, usually 10 or more years, during which they have no (or perhaps few) symptoms despite the fact that HIV continues to actively multiply. Because of this, persons can still transmit the virus to others during the asymptomatic phase, allowing HIV to spread unnoticed (IOM/NAS, 1988; Pantaleo et al., 1993).

The ongoing multiplication of HIV causes progressive damage to a person's immune system through destruction of specific white blood cells known as CD4+ T-lymphocytes. With the progressive decline in CD4+ cell count, most infected persons eventually begin to develop symptoms which can include syndromes such as fever, unexplained weight loss, diarrhea, and dementia (Pantaleo et al., 1993). The damage to their immune system predisposes them to a wide range of unusual diseases. These so-called opportunistic conditions include infections with nonaggressive microorganisms and certain cancers. When these conditions occur in the presence of HIV infection or when the CD4+ cell count drops below 200 cells/μL, the patient is said to have developed AIDS. In the absence of treatment, the disease is nearly always fatal with the median time from a CD4+ count < 200 cells/μL to death of 3.7 years in an untreated patient (Pantaleo et al., 1993). To date, no cure or vaccine has been developed for HIV disease, although recent treatment advances in combination antiretroviral therapy have resulted in slowing of the progression of the disease, and often temporary restoration of immune functioning, in infected individuals.

Current Trends

The AIDS epidemic, now entering its third decade, has had an enormous impact in terms of morbidity and mortality. By the end of 2001, 816,149 AIDS cases and 467,910 deaths had been reported in the United States to the CDC (CDC, 2002). AIDS prevalence has increased steadily over time; at the end of 2001, an estimated 362,827 people were living with AIDS (CDC, 2002). Globally, an estimated 40 million people are living with HIV/AIDS and three million people have now died from AIDS (CDC, 2002).

Following the introduction of combination antiretroviral therapy in the 1990s, the number of deaths and new AIDS cases in the United States began to decline for the first time in the history of the epidemic (Karon et al., 2001). Between 1995 and 1998, the annual number of new AIDS cases fell by 38 percent (from 69,242 to 42,832) and deaths by 63 percent (from 51,760 to 18,823). These declines in morbidity and mortality have stabilized in more recent years (CDC, 2003a).

HIV incidence and total HIV prevalence cannot be measured directly because many newly infected persons either do not seek or are not offered an HIV test. CDC estimates, however, that approximately 40,000 new HIV infections occur per year and that between 850,000 and 950,000 people are infected with HIV (Fleming et al., 2002). An estimated 25 percent of individuals infected with HIV do not know their status (Fleming et al., 2002).

Racial and ethnic minorities, particularly African Americans and Hispanics, have been disproportionately affected by the HIV/AIDS epidemic. In 2001, more than 70 percent of newly diagnosed AIDS cases in the United States were among racial/ethnic minority groups (CDC, 2002) and 63 percent of all persons living with AIDS were among racial/ethnic groups (CDC, 2003a). Women have also been disproportionately affected by HIV/AIDS. From 1986 to 2002, the proportion of AIDS cases in women and adolescent girls increased from 8 to 26 percent (CDC, 2003b). HIV disease is also increasingly affecting people who are poor, unemployed, and confront a variety of barriers to care (Bozzette et al., 1998; Kaiser Family Foundation, 2000). The HIV Costs and Services Utilization Study (HCSUS), a nationally representative study of people with HIV/AIDS in care, found that in 1996, 46 percent of adults under medical supervision for HIV infection reported incomes of less than $10,000 per year and 63 percent were unemployed (Bozzette et al., 1998).

Providing treatment and care for people with HIV has become increasingly costly and complex. Combination antiretroviral therapy typically costs $10,000–$12,000 per individual per year (Kahn et al., 2001). The recently FDA-approved drug, Fuzeon (enfuvirtide), or T-20, the first in a new class of anti-HIV drugs known as fusion inhibitors, offers options to those who have failed other treatments.[1] However, the new drug costs $20,000 for each person annually—over and above the cost of other antiretroviral treatments (Brown, 2003). The presence of comorbid conditions, such as substance abuse, mental illness, or hepatitis, adds another layer of

[1]The drug has shown some success in treating drug-resistant strains of HIV (Brown, 2003). Recent studies estimate that a sizable proportion of recently infected individuals (11–27 percent in the years 1999-2001) have some resistance to antiretroviral drugs (Weinstock et al., 2000; Grant et al., 2002; Little et al., 2002; Simon et al., 2002).

complexity to the care of HIV-infected patients, as they can be paths to infection and/or barriers to care (IOM, 2001).

PAYING FOR HIV/AIDS CARE

The HCSUS estimated about one-half and as many as two-thirds of all people with HIV/AIDS were not in regular care (Bozzette et al., 1998). More recent estimates suggest that range may be between 42 and 59 percent (Fleming et al., 2002). Some of these people are not aware of their status; others do not have access to insurance programs, are underinsured, or face other barriers in accessing care.

There are multiple sources of insurance coverage and care for people living with HIV/AIDS in the United States. Most individuals with HIV/AIDS who have insurance and are in the care system, are covered by public-sector programs, namely Medicaid and Medicare. HIV-infected individuals without insurance or adequate coverage rely on a variety of safety-net programs, such as CARE Act providers, community and migrant health centers, free clinics, and public hospitals. CARE Act funds may also be used to fill gaps for individuals with inadequate private or public insurance. These sources of coverage are poorly coordinated and constitute a substantial barrier for people with HIV/AIDS to obtaining appropriate care (Kaiser Family Foundation, 2000).

Medicaid accounts for the largest amount of federal spending on health care for people with HIV/AIDS (48 percent, or $4.2 billion in fiscal year [FY]2002), followed by Medicare (24 percent, or $2.1 billion in FY2002), and the CARE Act (22 percent, or $1.9 billion in FY2002). The Department of Veterans Affairs, other programs in the Department of Health and Human Services (HHS), Department of Defense, and the Department of Justice account for the remainder (Kaiser Family Foundation, 2002) (Figure 2-1).

Medicaid and Medicare are entitlement programs which means that spending automatically expands or contracts with the need for benefits. Individuals who meet eligibility requirements are legally entitled to services, and federal and state budgets automatically appropriate funds to pay for them. Discretionary spending programs, in contrast, such as RWCA, are capped; each year Congress sets the overall level of spending through the appropriation process. Eligibility for or coverage of services may be limited if the costs of their care exceed the appropriated funds (Foster et al., 2002).

Sources of insurance coverage vary substantially by state contributing to differential access across geographic areas. Considerable differences in coverage by race, ethnicity, and sex also exist (Kaiser Family Foundation, 2000). The HCSUS found that African Americans and Latinos

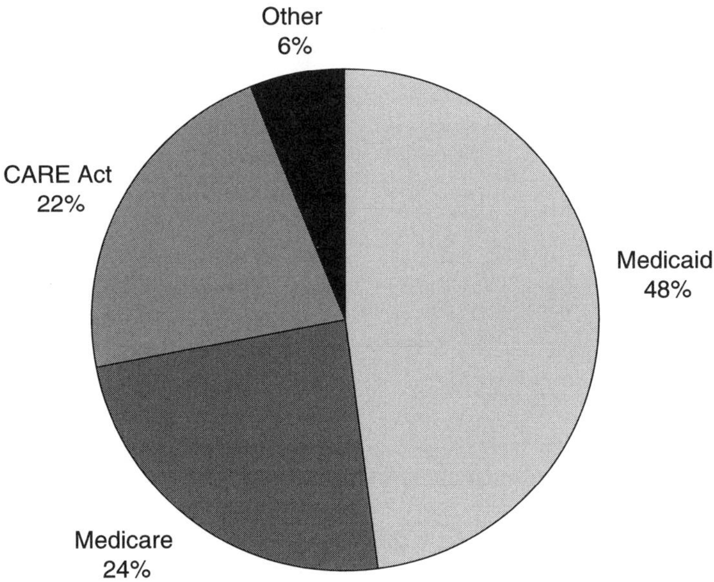

FIGURE 2-1 Federal spending on HIV/AIDS care by program, FY2002 (Total = $8.7 billion).
SOURCE: Kaiser Family Foundation, 2002.

were more likely to depend on Medicaid and to be uninsured than whites. Whites were more likely to have private insurance than other racial and ethnic groups. Women were also more likely to rely on public insurance, especially Medicaid, than men. HCSUS also found disparities in access to care according to type of insurance coverage and other demographic characteristics. Individuals with HIV who were on Medicaid or uninsured, along with women and racial/ethnic minority groups, did more poorly on a variety of access measures than individuals who were privately insured, male, and white (Bozzette et al., 1998; Shapiro et al., 1999; Kaiser Family Foundation, 2000).

HISTORY OF THE CARE ACT

The CARE Act was authorized by Congress and signed into law on August 18, 1990 as Title XXVI of the Public Health Service Act (Ryan White CARE Act of 1990. P.L. 101-381). Since the initial authorization, the bill has been reauthorized and amended in 1996 (Ryan White CARE Act Amendments of 1996. P.L. 104-146) and 2000 (Ryan White CARE Act

Amendments of 2000. P.L. 106-345). The purpose of the Act is "to provide emergency assistance to localities disproportionately affected by the HIV epidemic and to make financial assistance to States and other public and private nonprofit entities to provide for the development, organization, coordination, and operations of more effective and cost-efficient systems for the delivery of essential services to individuals and families with HIV disease" (Ryan White CARE Act of 1990. P.L. 101-381 § 2 Purpose). Numerous grant programs were included in the structure of the Act to address the varying effect of HIV disease on government agencies, health care providers and institutions, and persons and family members with HIV disease. Although modifications have been made to the Act as a result of reauthorization bills, the original structure and function have remained relatively intact.

Authorization of the Ryan White CARE Act (1990)

Several efforts within Congress and the Administration to assist localities and states in addressing the rapidly escalating cost of HIV care preceded the authorization of the Act. Congress had previously provided federal grant relief for highly affected areas and to states through various demonstration projects funded via appropriations bills, such as those under the Health Omnibus Programs of 1988 (P.L. 100-607) and HIV treatment demonstration projects.[2] These projects provided funds to highly affected communities in order to establish home and community-based health care services as an alternative to more expensive inpatient hospital care. Several other discretionary grant programs provided support to states for the purchase of HIV medications and to provide access to research and care among HIV-infected pregnant women and children. Although these efforts were effective, these federal grants had a limited authorization and were unable to provide support to the growing number of localities being affected by the epidemic.

In 1987, Congress began discussion toward developing a comprehensive federal relief program. Relieving the disproportionate effect of HIV/AIDS on specific urban settings and providers became one of the primary objectives for the development and implementation of the initial federal CARE Act program. Congressional hearings in the late 1980s highlighted the need for a stable long-term federal assistance program. Public health officials, health care providers (primarily representatives from public hospital systems), and persons with HIV disease provided testimony on the economic and personal burdens of the HIV epidemic (U.S. Congress,

[2]Funds for grants to states to provide therapeutics appropriated to the Public Health Emergency Fund authorized by section 319 of the Public Health Services Act.

1990). Public hospitals located in highly affected urban centers, such as New York, Miami, and San Francisco, reported being overwhelmed with the costs of providing medical care for under- and uninsured persons with complex medical problems related to AIDS (U.S. Congress, 1990). Persons with AIDS were reported as having lost access to private insurance coverage because of poor health, termination of employment, and ineligibility for Medicaid. After extensive debate, Congress finally supported the idea of a federal program to address the disproportionate nature of the epidemic. The authorized CARE Act established a discretionary program based on a multigrant structure designed to address the needs of state and local communities, health care providers, and persons and family members with HIV disease. The CARE Act was organized into four title programs.

Title I grants were targeted to highly affected urban centers, known as Eligible Metropolitan Areas (EMAs), for purposes of providing "emergency relief" to highly affected communities. EMAs were defined in the statute as any metropolitan area with a cumulative total of more than 2,000 AIDS cases or a per capita incidence of cumulative cases of AIDS equal to or greater than 25 cases per 100,000 persons reported to the CDC. Congress intended for the greatest proportion of funding to be directed to EMAs with the greatest HIV epidemic and economic and social burdens related to the epidemic. Congress created two distinct Title I grant awards, the base grant and the supplemental grant. The base grant award provided EMAs with direct and immediate access to federal support based on the cumulative AIDS cases. The base grant federal allocation formula included the cumulative number of AIDS cases in the EMA divided by the sum of all cumulative cases in all eligible areas for the base award. A per capita incidence rate of cumulative cases was included in the formula to adjust for the demand for services within the local community (Ryan White CARE Act 1990. P.L. 101-381. § 2603[a][3]).

The Title I supplemental grant provided funds through a separate application process. Congress provided the Secretary of HHS, through the supplemental award process, the authority to direct one-half of the total appropriation to eligible Title I grantees based on the following: the number of persons with AIDS who needed care, demographic data such as poverty levels, the average cost of providing each category of services and the extent to which third-party payer coverage is available, and the aggregate amounts expended on services (Ryan White CARE Act 1990. P.L. 101-381. § 2603[b][3] and § 2605[b]).

Title II grants were provided to all 50 states, the District of Columbia, and U.S. territories. These awards established the role of the state or territory as the primary entity responsible for the development and operation of a "comprehensive service delivery system." This included the establishment and support of provider networks (consortia), giving assistance for private health insurance coverage (but not to replace state Medicaid programs), and directing the purchase and distribution of HIV treatments. Grant awards were authorized to states and territories based on a defined distributional factor. This factor was the product of the cumulative AIDS cases reported to CDC during the two most recent years and the relation between average per capita income in the United States compared to that of the state.

Finally, the Act established various direct federal grant programs, Title III and IV, to support community-based providers and institutions delivering direct early intervention services, primary care, women's and family health, and social services. Title III(a) provided grants to states for early intervention service programs, such as HIV counseling, testing, referral, and treatment. Title III(b) provided grants directly to public and nonprofit eligible entities to provide early intervention services. Preference for such awards was given to providers experiencing an increase in burden in providing HIV services or lacking availability of primary health services. Title IV allowed for grants directed to a wide range of research and demonstration activities. This included the Demonstration Grants for Research and Services for Pediatric Patients with AIDS (Ryan White CARE Act 1990. P.L. 101-381. § 2671). Title IV continued previously funded federal grants, and provided support for clinical care and research on pediatric patients and pregnant women with HIV disease.

First Reauthorization of the CARE Act (1996)

When preparing for the first reauthorization, Congress had received input from key constituent groups regarding several apparent limitations to the existing federal allocation formula (U.S. Congress, 1995). One primary issue of concern was the significant interlocal or intergrantee variations in amount of awards per case. Given this input, Congress requested in 1995 a General Accounting Office (GAO) investigation of the equity of distributions in federal funding through CARE Act Title I and II.

In April 1995, GAO testified to Congressional committees on the results of its study. This testimony, and a report released later in the year, identified several problems in the federal allocation formulas methodology that contributed to inequities between inter-local funding levels. In addition, the GAO identified several issues of equitable distribution of federal funding based on criteria of "beneficiary equity" and "tax equity" (GAO, 1995a,b).

The GAO found that significant differences existed between grantees in the per AIDS case award amounts. These existed for two reasons. First, the use of cumulative AIDS case counts included those who were deceased. This resulted in an overestimation of the numbers of persons in need of services in certain EMAs, particularly, those that were heavily affected during early periods of the epidemic. As a result, the 1996 reauthorization instituted new formulas based on estimated living cases (ELCs). Second, AIDS cases were included in both Title I and Title II formulas, resulting in a double counting of EMA cases in states with EMAs. This resulted in an inflation of the numbers of cases within states (GAO, 1995a,b).

A second set of issues, "beneficiary equity" and "tax equity,"[3] was identified in the report. Neither Title I nor Title II formulas accounted for the variations in the cost of services or economic levels in the community. Regarding this, the GAO recommended the use of the Medicare Hospital Wage Index to adjust for labor costs and the cubed root of per capita personal income to adjust for the local tax base. The GAO recommended that both adjustments be applied simultaneously to Titles I and II formulas.

Based on the GAO's recommendations, Congress made several modifications to the Title I and II allocation formulas in 1996 to adjust for identified inequities. Changes were made to both base and supplemental grant awards, and provisions were enacted to protect Title I and II grantees against significant losses in federal CARE Act funds. In order to better estimate the numbers of persons living with AIDS, Title I and II allocation formulas were amended to include only AIDS case counts reported to CDC for the most recent ten years. The data were further weighted for the likelihood of deaths based on nationally devised mortality rates. Although the Senate bill included an adjustment for service costs (U.S. Congress, 1995), Congress could not reach final agreement on the use of cost data or funding capacity with regard to the base formula award. Thus, Congress did not reauthorize the use of average per capita income for the states in the Title II allocation formula. Neither the Title I nor Title II base formulas were amended to adjust for costs of services or the funding capacity of the local jurisdiction.

The process for allocating the Title I supplemental award was amended by Congress in 1996 to include new factors related to the additional severity of need in the community. Costs and demands for services were included as a component in the supplemental award. The Secretary of HHS was directed to consider the ability of the qualified applicant to expend funds efficiently, and the effect on the cost and complexity of delivering health care and support to individuals with HIV disease in the eligible areas (Ryan White CARE Act Amendments of 1996. P.L. 104-146.

[3]Defined as an absence of cost measures and an inappropriate fiscal capacity measure.

§ 2602[b][2][B]). No specific statutory language was included to indicate the types of cost data that would be included as part of the supplemental application.

The reauthorized Title II base formula included the allocation formula as indicated for Title I base awards, but was adjusted to address the funding differences between states because of EMAs. Congress adopted a formula with two separate components. The first component was the number of persons living with AIDS in the state respective of all states, and this constituted 80 percent of the award. The second component was the number of persons living with AIDS in non-EMA areas, and constituted 20 percent of the award.

The 1996 reauthorization also included several provisions to limit the loss of Title I funding to eligible EMAs. A hold-harmless provision was established to assure that no entity received less than 92.5 percent of its 1995 base award amount. This provision was phased in over five years "to avoid disruption of services to beneficiaries, while still allowing for the redistribution on funds" (U.S. Congress, 1995). In addition, Title I eligibility criteria were modified to exclude the case rate factor and to specify the size of the metropolitan area as those with more than 500,000 people.

The Second Reauthorization of the CARE Act (2000)

When preparing for the second reauthorization in 2000, Congress revisited the issue of interlocal equity but expanded its inquiry to include local planning activities. In doing so, it requested a series of GAO studies to assess the use of CARE Act funds for the coverage of HIV services (GAO, 1995c) as well as the opportunities to enhance funding equity (GAO, 2000), as previously examined. In addition to these studies, Congress examined several other research studies on the access and use of HIV services in the United States (Bozzette et al., 1998; Shapiro et al., 1999).

Congress continued to investigate the federal allocation formula and the influence of the hold-harmless provisions on resolving the inequities in per-case funding levels between Title grantees. GAO reported that minorities and women had used CARE Act services in proportion to the effect of AIDS within these populations. Yet, the GAO (2000) found, similar to the previous study (GAO, 1995c), that wide disparities continued to exist in the per-case funding levels between Title grantees. GAO explained this was most likely occurring because of two factors: a lack of appropriate data, specifically HIV surveillance data, to estimate numbers of HIV-infected persons in eligible areas, and the application of the hold-harmless provisions to EMA grant awards. However, the GAO reported that only 60 percent of states had operative HIV surveillance data available, as reported by the CDC. Some of those without such data were states that had been heavily affected by HIV, namely California and New York (GAO, 2000).

Based on the outcome of these studies and input from the Administration, grantees, and consumer representatives, Congress pursued a strategy to enhance the use of HIV surveillance data in the Title I and II allocation formulas, as well as in local planning activities. This was based on the perception that HIV data were becoming available in most areas and that HIV case reporting could be a more accurate measure of the number and unmet needs of persons with HIV disease (U.S. Congress, 2000). (Ryan White CARE Act Amendments of 2000. P.L. 106-345. § 2603[a][D]).

Legislative changes related to the equitable distribution of resources were not limited to the federal allocation formulas. Such changes were applied to the local level in planning and allocating CARE Act funds within communities. Congress established an extensive list of duties to be incorporated in the planning and allocation processes for EMAs and states. The aim of these provisions was to develop a comprehensive plan for all HIV-infected persons in the local community. Congress also intended to enhance the ability of the existing local planning process to establish and support services for newly infected persons and persons from historically underserved communities (Ryan White CARE Act Amendments of 2000. P.L. 106-345. § 2602 [a][B][4][C][v] and [D][i]). The chief vehicle for accomplishing these planning changes was to be a comprehensive plan developed by EMA and state grantees. The plan was expected to be based on the epidemiologic profile of the community, the unmet needs of persons eligible for CARE Act services, and the service capacity needs of local providers. Congress established duties related to determining "unmet needs" of communities, particularly for HIV-infected persons not in care and historically underserved communities and affected subpopulations. Additionally, such data were to be used in the "severity of needs" profiles of the competitive Title I supplemental grant program. Within the supplemental application, the "severity of need" measure was expanded to include one-third of the grant award. Grantees were required to assess and plan for capacity development activities related to services for historically underserved communities (e.g., minorities and women) and affected subpopulations (e.g., persons with substance abuse and mental health problems). Acknowledging that the availability of demographic and unmet needs information would be determined by the existence and reliability of the state and local HIV surveillance system, Congress allowed for a phase-in of the use of such data for states and EMAs without active HIV surveillance systems.

In summary, during the second reauthorization Congress moved the discussion of interlocal equity to local issues of distributional equity within the planning and allocation of CARE Act funds. In doing so, Congress reinforced the need to establish HIV case-reporting systems as the basis of understanding and planning in accordance with the local epidemic. In addition, Congress recognized the importance of linking case-reporting data to other data sources to determine issues related to access, service needs and use, and the quality of health services, including health outcomes. Within these efforts, Congress identified specific populations as requiring particular consideration when establishing service priorities; specifically, minorities, women, children, and persons with substance abuse or mental health problems.

CURRENT STRUCTURE OF THE ACT

Since its original authorization in 1990, CARE Act funding has grown from $220 million in FY1991 to $2.0 billion in FY2003 (Figure 2-2) (HRSA,

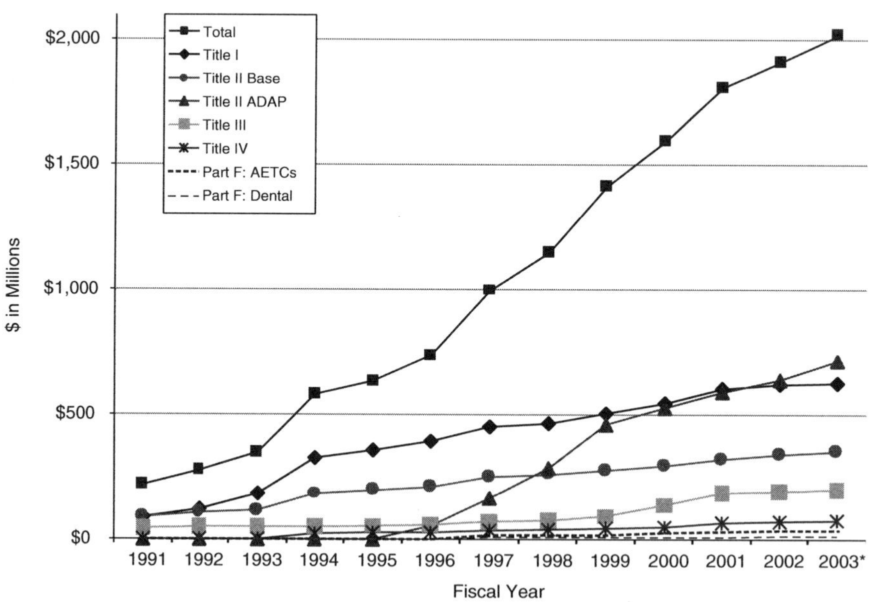

FIGURE 2-2 Ryan White CARE Act funding FY1991 to FY2003.
SOURCE: HRSA, 2003a.

2003a). The structure of the CARE Act has remained largely the same since its original enactment, although modifications were made over time. Today, the Act is composed of four major Title programs and several additional components.

Title I—Grants to Eligible Metropolitan Areas

Title I provides funding to EMAs with a population of at least 500,000 and more than 2,000 reported AIDS cases within the past five years. The geographic boundaries of these EMAs are based on Metropolitan Statistical Areas (MSA) of the U.S. Census Bureau. MSAs may range in size from one city or county to multiple counties that may cross state boundaries. The number of EMAs grew from 16 in FY1991 to 51 (in 21 states) in FY2003 (HRSA, 2002d) (Box 2-1).

Title I appropriations totaled $626.7 million in FY2003 (HRSA, 2003a). These funds may be used for inpatient case management (but not inpatient hospital care), outpatient and ambulatory health services (including substance abuse and mental health treatment), and outpatient support services (such as case management and early intervention). Figure 2-3 shows the Title I resource allocations by service category for FY2000.[4] A large proportion is spent on health care services, followed by support services and case management (HRSA, 2002i).

Title I funding includes two primary grants: formula grants and supplemental grants (HRSA, 2002d). An EMA's formula grant is based on its proportion of ELCs relative to the total ELCs among all EMAs (HRSA, 2002d). Congress intends to incorporate data on HIV cases into the formula for awarding these grants as early as FY2005 but no later than FY2007, provided that the Secretary of HHS determines that such data are "sufficiently accurate" and reliable for use in the formulas (Ryan White CARE Act. 42 U.S.C. § 300ff-28 [2003]). HRSA awards the remaining Title I funds through a competitive supplemental grant process based on severity of need and other criteria (HRSA, 2002d).

In 1998 the Department of HSS, in collaboration with the Congressional Black Caucus, created the Minority AIDS Initiative (MAI) to address the crisis in racial and ethnic minority communities. After targeting African-American and Hispanic communities in FY1999, the initiative expanded to encompass all racial and ethnic minority communities the following year. Congress appropriated $42 million in supplemental Title I funds to MAI in FY2002 (HRSA, 2003b).

Figure 2-4 shows the breakdown of the Title I allocations in FY2002

---

[4]FY2000 is the most recent year for which data were compiled.

BOX 2-1
CARE Act Eligible Metropolitan Areas (FY2003)

Atlanta, GA
Austin, TX
Baltimore, MD
Bergen-Passaic, NJ
Boston, MA
Caguas, PR
Chicago, IL
Cleveland-Lorain-Elyria, OH
Dallas, TX
Denver, CO
Detroit, MI
Dutchess Co., NY
Ft. Lauderdale, FL
Ft. Worth, TX
Hartford, CT
Houston, TX
Jacksonville, FL
Jersey City, NJ
Kansas City, MO
Las Vegas, NV
Los Angeles, CA
Miami, FL
Middlesex-Somerset-Hunterdon, NJ
Minneapolis-St. Paul, MN
Nassau-Suffolk, NY
Newark, NJ
New Haven, CT
New Orleans, LA
New York, NY
Norfolk, VA
Oakland, CA
Orange County, CA
Orlando, FL
Philadelphia, PA
Phoenix, AZ
Ponce, PR
Portland, OR
Riverside-San Bernardino, CA
Sacramento, CA
St. Louis, MO
San Antonio, TX
San Diego, CA
San Francisco, CA
San Jose, CA
San Juan, PR
Santa Rosa-Petaluma, CA
Seattle WA
Tampa-St. Petersburg. FL
Vineland-Millville-Bridgeton, NJ
Washington, DC
West Palm Beach, FL

SOURCE: HRSA, 2002d.

according to formula award, supplemental award, MAI, and hold-harmless funds (discussed in the next section).[5]

The Health Resources and Services Administration (HRSA) awards Title I grants to the chief elected official of the city or county that provides services to the greatest number of people living with AIDS in the EMA. A

[5]These numbers reflect funding available for distribution rather than the appropriations. FY2002 Title I appropriations were $619.5 million. Appropriations differ from the amount of funding available for awards, as the appropriation is subject to required set-asides for evaluation, the Special Projects of National Significance (SPNS) program, and technical assistance (Personal communication, S. Young, Deputy Director, Office of Science and Epidemiology, HIV/AIDS Bureau, HRSA, May 30, 2003).

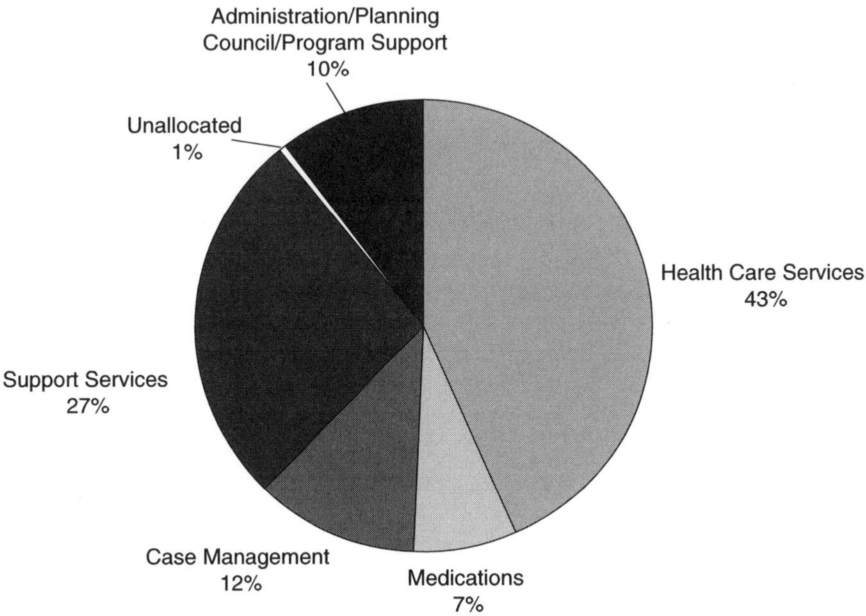

FIGURE 2-3 Ryan White CARE Act Title I resource allocations by service category in 49 EMAs, FY2000 (Total: $527,324,044).
NOTE: 2000 is the most recent year that data for service category are available.
SOURCE: HRSA, 2002j.

local Planning Council appointed by that official establishes funding priorities based on the size and demographics of the HIV population and the needs of this population with particular attention to those who know their HIV status but are not in care (Ryan White CARE Act. 42 U.S.C. § 300ff-12). Planning Councils are also responsible for developing a comprehensive plan that includes strategies for identifying HIV-positive persons not in care and strategies for coordinating services to be funded with existing prevention and substance abuse treatment services (Ryan White CARE Act. Sec. 42 U.S.C. § 300ff-12 [2003]). Although Planning Councils set funding priorities, the chief elected official or a designee (generally the health department) contracts with service providers.

The 2000 reauthorization requires that 33 percent of the Planning Council's members are people living with HIV/AIDS who use CARE Act services (Ryan White CARE Act. 42 U.S.C. § 300ff-12 [2003]). Planning councils must also include representatives with relevant expertise in areas such as substance abuse and mental health treatment, health care planning, and services for homeless and incarcerated populations.

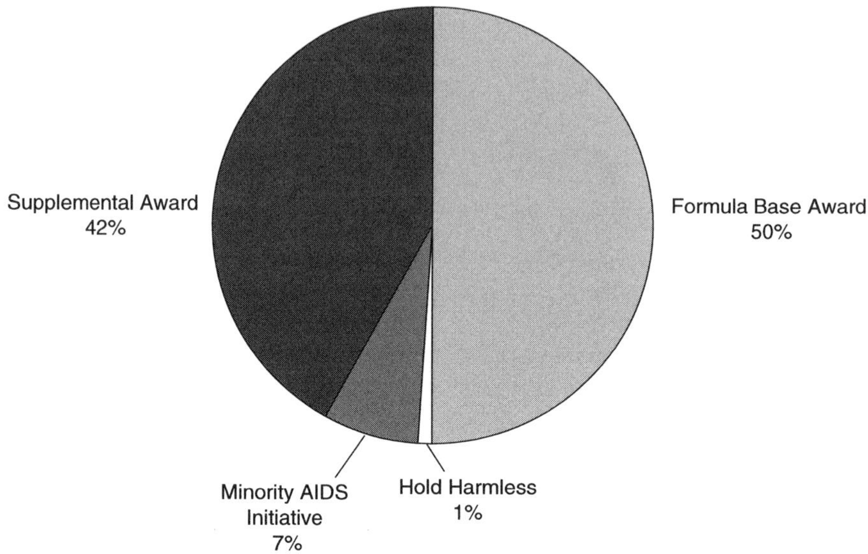

FIGURE 2-4 FY2002 Title I allocations (Total $597,256,000).
SOURCE: HRSA, 2002j.

Title II—Grants to States and Territories

Title II provides grants to all 50 states, the District of Columbia, Puerto Rico, Guam, the U.S. Virgin Islands, and five newly eligible Pacific territories (HRSA, 2002f). Title II funds totaled $977.4 million in FY2002 (HRSA, 2002f). Title II funds may be used for a number of services including ambulatory and home-based health care, purchase of insurance coverage, medications, support services, early intervention services, and outreach services to people who know their status (HRSA, 2002f). Many states provide these services directly, while others subcontract with Title II HIV care consortia. Consortia are networks composed of public, nonprofit health care and support service providers, and community-based organizations that provide for the delivery of services to people with HIV disease (HRSA, 2002f). Figure 2-5 shows the Title II resource allocations by service category for FY2000.[6]

[6]FY2000 is the most recent year for which these data were compiled.

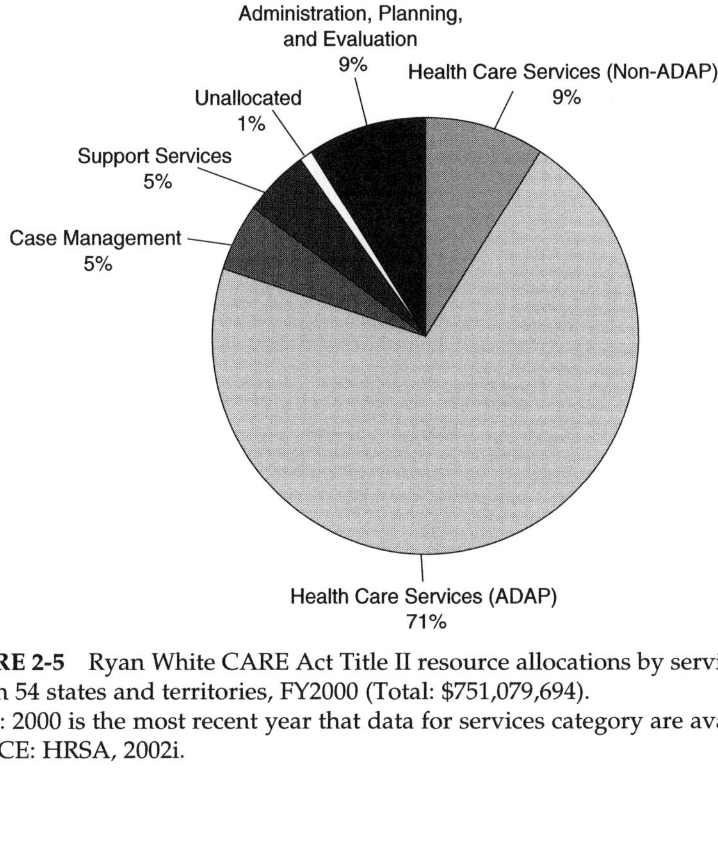

FIGURE 2-5 Ryan White CARE Act Title II resource allocations by service category in 54 states and territories, FY2000 (Total: $751,079,694).
NOTE: 2000 is the most recent year that data for services category are available.
SOURCE: HRSA, 2002i.

Title II awards are composed of base grants, the AIDS Drug Assistance Program, MAI awards and grants to Emerging Communities (ECs)—those communities reporting between 500 and 1,999 cases in the previous 5 years.

Title II base awards are determined using a formula that is based on ELCs. States with greater than 1 percent of the total number of AIDS cases reported nationwide during the previous two years must match a portion of the base award in a schedule outlined in the legislation (HRSA, 2002f). In FY2003, base grant awards totaled $353 million (HRSA, 2003a).

Additional Title II funds are earmarked for state AIDS Drug Assistance Programs (ADAPs), which primarily provide medications, but can also be used for treatment adherence and support efforts, and to purchase private insurance with drug coverage benefits. The ADAP earmark was $714 million in FY2003. ADAP accounts for the largest proportion of Title II funding and nearly one-third of overall CARE Act funding (HRSA, 2002e). Since FY2001, 3 percent of ADAP funds have been reserved for a supplemental grant program for states exhibiting severe need. In FY2002, 13 states received ADAP supplemental awards. States and territories need only meet one of the following criteria to qualify for the ADAP supplemental award:

- Inability of any individual at or below 200 percent of the federal poverty level to access the program.
- Ability of any individual to meet state-specific medical eligibility restrictions (for example, CD4+ T-cell count less than or equal to 500, specific viral load, etc.).
- Formulary limits on antiretrovirals and medications to treat opportunistic infections.
- Fewer than 10 medications to treat opportunistic infections (HRSA/HAB, 2001).

Financial eligibility criteria as well as drug coverage varies substantially by state. Although the ADAP budget has increased by 366 percent from 1996 to 2002, the per capita costs have also increased due to increasing treatment costs. Despite the budget increases, 16 states had more restrictions due to budget shortfalls in February 2003 and other states had limited enrollment in ADAPs (NASTAD, KFF, ATDN, 2003).[7]

In the 2000 reauthorization, Congress established a new category of grants for ECs—cities reporting 500–1,999 AIDS cases in the most recent 5-year period (HRSA, 2002f). Unlike EMAs, the eligibility of ECs is determined every year, with no guarantee of future funding. Title II also includes $7 million for the MAI to increase participation of minorities in ADAPs.

Figure 2-6 shows the breakdown of Title II allocations by the base award, ADAP award, MAI, and EC award.[8]

---

[7]The ADAP budget includes funding from the Ryan White CARE Act (ADAP earmark, Title I, Title II, ADAP supplemental), state funding, and other federal funding (NASTAD, KFF, ATDN, 2003).

[8]These numbers reflect funding available for distribution rather than the appropriations. FY2002 Title II appropriations were $977 million. Appropriations differ from the amount of funding available for awards, as the appropriation is subject to required set-asides for evaluation, the SPNS program, and technical assistance (Personal communication, S. Young, HRSA, HIV/AIDS Bureau, Office of Science and Epidemiology, May 30, 2003).

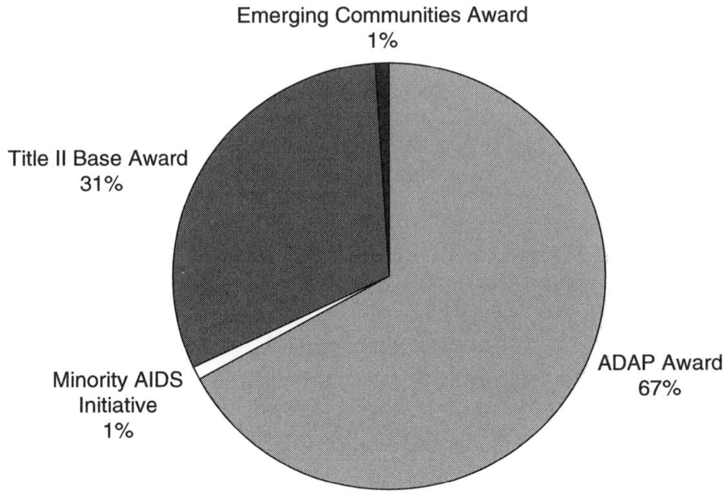

FIGURE 2-6 FY2002 Title II allocations (Total: $923,088,000).
SOURCE: HRSA, 2002k.

Title III—Early Intervention Services, and Planning and Capacity Grants

Title III of the CARE Act funds early intervention HIV services provided by public and nonprofit groups.[9] Early intervention services include counseling, testing, medical evaluation, primary care, antiretroviral therapies, medical and mental health care, case management, and other services. A smaller proportion of Title III funds helps such groups "plan for the development of HIV early-intervention services" (1-year $50,000 grants) or build their capacity to provide services (up to $150,000 over a 3-year period) (HRSA, 2002g). The Title III appropriation totaled $200.9 million in FY2003 (HRSA, 2003a).

Title IV—Women, Children, Infants, and Youth

Title IV funding addresses the specific needs of women, infants, children, and youth living with HIV. Title IV evolved from the Pediatric

[9]For-profit entities are eligible only if they are the sole provider of "quality HIV care" in an area.

AIDS Demonstration Program, which was established in 1988. The funds cover primary and specialty medical care, psychosocial services, logistical support and coordination, and outreach and case management (HRSA, 2002h). Title IV also provides clients with increased access to HIV/AIDS clinical trials and research. Congress appropriated $74.5 million for Title IV programs in FY2003 (HRSA, 2003a).

Other RWCA Funded Programs

RWCA also funds the Special Projects of National Significance (SPNS), AIDS Education and Training Centers, and the Dental Reimbursement Program.

Special Projects of National Significance

The SPNS program was established to advance the knowledge and skills needed to deliver health and support services to underserved populations with HIV infection. SPNS projects evaluate the effectiveness of models of care, support the design of innovative care programs, and help replicate effective models. SPNS is funded through a set-aside (not to exceed $25 million annually) from Title I–IV (HRSA, 2002c).

AIDS Education and Training Centers

The AIDS Education and Training Centers (AETC) program funds a network of 10 regional centers and more than 70 associated sites that conduct multidisciplinary education and training programs for providers who care for persons with HIV/AIDS. The program is designed to expand the number of providers who can counsel, diagnose, treat, and medically manage individuals with HIV, and who can help prevent high-risk behaviors that transmit HIV (HRSA, 2002a). The AETC program disbursed $35.6 million in FY2003 (HRSA, 2003a).

HIV/AIDS Dental Reimbursement Program

Congress added the Dental Reimbursement Program in 1996. The program provides funding to improve access to oral health care for people with HIV/AIDS, to help ensure that dental students are trained to care for people living with HIV, and to offset the cost of uncompensated dental HIV care provided by teaching institutions (HRSA, 2002b). Congress appropriated $13.4 million for these programs in FY2003 (HRSA, 2003a).

OVERVIEW OF CARE ACT ALLOCATION FORMULAS

Most allocation formulas include a measure of need, while some include measures of costs, fiscal capacity, and effort (Box 2-2). Some formulas also contain special features such as floors and ceilings (minimum and maximum awards), "hold-harmless" provisions that prevent an area's funding from declining too rapidly from year to year, or eligibility thresholds (NRC, 2001, 2003).

Formulas for Titles I and II of RWCA are described in Table 2-1. Most of these formulas allocate funds based on a jurisdiction's disease burden, often defined as ELCs. ELCs are calculated by applying annual national survival weights to 10 years of reported AIDS cases and summing the totals.[10] Most of these formulas also contain one or more features like hold-harmless provisions or thresholds.

Title I Awards to Eligible Metropolitan Areas

As noted, a metropolitan area becomes eligible for Title I if it has a population of 500,000 or more and has reported a cumulative total of more than 2,000 cases of AIDS during the most recent five calendar years for which data are available from the CDC (HRSA, 2002d). A type of hold-harmless provision applies to EMAs in that once a metropolitan area's eligibility is established, the area remains eligible even if the number of cases drops below the threshold in later years.

Base Award

An EMA's base award is determined by a formula based on its proportion of the total number of ELCs in all EMAs. The formula also includes a hold-harmless provision that limits the amount an EMA's funding can fall from year to year, according to a schedule specified in the legislation.[11] San Francisco is the only EMA that now benefits from the hold-harmless provision (HRSA, 2002j).

---

[10]Both the survival weights and the most recent 10 years of reported AIDS cases are sent from CDC to HRSA (see Chapter 4). The survival weights are updated and recalculated every 2 years.

[11]The hold-harmless award is subtracted from the total Title I supplemental funds before the latter are divided.

BOX 2-2
Overview of Formula Features

The National Research Council (NRC) Panel on Formula Allocations released two reports that provide an overview of the features of the formulas (NRC, 2001, 2003). Many of these features apply to RWCA formulas. The NRC panel identified four elements commonly used in the formulas:

Need: The resources a jurisdiction needs will depend, in part, on the number of individuals eligible for service. Need measures might include the number of individuals with HIV/AIDS who are uninsured or underinsured, or the changing rates of infection. Generally, different conceptions of need for resources have different implications for the allocation of those resources. Under any conception, the true level of need must be estimated (NRC, 2001, 2003).

Cost: Resources needed by a jurisdiction will also depend on the cost of providing services to eligible individuals. If possible, formulas should account for cross-jurisdictional variations in the costs of care stemming from factors such as differences in prevailing wages. Costs may also vary with the severity of cases and the complexity of providing services. Many public programs do not account for cost variations because of the difficulty of developing reliable estimates. Including cost measures in a formula may also create perverse incentives if recipients can influence allocations by overstating their costs (NRC, 2001, 2003).

Fiscal Capacity: Fiscal capacity is the ability of a jurisdiction to meet an identified need. Per capita income and total taxable resources are examples of common fiscal capacity measures (Tannenwald, 1999; NRC, 2001; Downes and Pogue, 2002). Measures of capacity require estimation (NRC, 2003).

Effort: Effort reflects the amount of available resources actually devoted to meeting the need. Total eligible medical expenditures is an example measure of effort (NRC, 2001). Including such measures in grant formulas may provide an incentive for recipients to overstate their effort. Although they vary widely among programs, most formulas combine two or more of these elements of need, cost, fiscal capacity, and effort. The NRC panel provides examples of how various measures are combined and discusses how errors

Supplemental Award[12]

Supplemental awards are determined by a competitive application process, rather than by a formula. Reviewers score the application according to criteria laid out by HRSA. Either HRSA staff or external reviewers score applications. The supplemental award is divided among all EMAs

[12]The process for awarding Title I supplemental funds is discussed in Chapter 5.

in the measurement or estimation of various formula elements may interact and lead to discrepancy between actual and desired allocations (NRC, 2003).

Special Features of Formulas

Formulas may also include special features such as hold-harmless provisions, thresholds, and limits that prompt funding allocations to depart from basic formulas (NRC, 2003).

Hold harmless: Hold-harmless provisions curtail the extent to which grants can decline from one period to the next, usually according to fiscal years. Hold-harmless provisions limit unpredictable changes in funding or service delivery within jurisdictions, but they also diminish a program's ability to respond to changing needs (NRC, 2003). The influence of hold-harmless provisions on funding depends on two factors: the allowed rate of reduction from year to year, and annual changes in total appropriations. A program with a 100 percent hold-harmless provision combined with no change in appropriation will result in no adjustment to the previous year's allocations, regardless of whether a jurisdiction's needs or other factors in the formulas have changed (NRC, 2003).

Thresholds: Some allocation formulas include eligibility thresholds that require jurisdictions to demonstrate some minimum level of need in order to qualify for the grant (NRC, 2001). With a threshold, a small change in estimated need—whether owing to a statistical error or a change in true need—can significantly affect a jurisdiction's funding (Zaslavsky and Schirm, 2002). The NRC panel recommends that evaluations explore how errors in estimated need affect jurisdictions' funding, and how variations in estimated need over time affect the allocations over time. Eligibility thresholds may also raise the potential for gaming by grant recipients (NRC, 2003).

Limits—minimums and caps: Some formula-based allocations ensure that no jurisdiction will receive less than a specified dollar amount or share of the total allocation. Other programs, however, impose a cap on individual awards. These upper and lower limits constrain the outcomes that would result if an allocation were determined solely by a basic formula or need (NRC, 2003).

taking into account the score as well as the proportion of all ELCs that an EMA has. Three different "smoothing" algorithms are applied to see which distributes the money most appropriately. In general, no grantee is given less than 80 percent of their base formula award (HRSA, 2001).

Title I Minority AIDS Initiative Award

MAI grant awards are divided among all EMAs according to a formula based on their proportion of racial and ethnic minorities AIDS

TABLE 2-1 Description of Formula Grants for Titles I and II of the Ryan White CARE Act

Title	Formula Grant	Description	Input Data
Title I	Base Award	Base award is divided among all EMAs based on the EMA's proportion of the total ELCs in all EMAs.	10 most recent years of ELCs
Title I	Minority AIDS Initiative (MAI)	MAI award is divided among all EMAs based on the EMA's proportion of non-white[1] reported AIDS cases in the most recent 2-year period.	Cumulative reported nonwhite AIDS cases for most recent 2 years (adjusted for reporting delays)
Title II	Base Award	80% of the base award is divided among states/territories based upon each state/territory's proportion of the total ELC in all states territories. 20% is based on each state's proportion of ELCs in all states and territories that are located outside the EMAs within a state.	10 most recent years of ELCs
Title II	AIDS Drug Assistance Program (ADAP) Base	ADAP award is divided among all states/territories based upon the state/territory's proportion of the total ELCs in all states and territories. There is no 80-20 split like base award.	10 most recent years of ELCs
Title II	AIDS Drug Assistance Program (ADAP) Supplemental	ADAP supplemental award is divided among qualifying** states/territories based upon the qualifying state/territory's proportion of the total ELCs in qualifying states and territories.	10 most recent years of ELCs

Threshold	Minimum Award	Hold-Harmless	Match Requirement
MSAs with a population ≥500,000 and with 2000 reported AIDS cases in most recent 5 years	No	Base year is FY2000 appropriation. FY2001 = 98%; FY2002 = 95%; FY2003 = 92%; FY2004 = 89%; FY2005+ = 85%	No
For jurisdictions with >0 reported AIDS cases among racial and ethnic minorities	No	No	No
No	$200,000 for states with <90 cases; $500,000 for states with ≥90 cases; $50,000 for territories	Base year is FY2000 appropriation. FY2001 = 99%; FY2002 = 98%; FY2003 = 97%; FY2004 = 96%; FY2005+ = 95%	For states[2] with >1% of national total reported AIDS cases in most recent 2 years. Match rate schedule: FY1: $1 state: $5 federal FY2: $1 state: $4 federal FY3: $1 state: $3 federal FY4+: $1 state: $2 federal
No	No	Base year is FY2000 appropriation. FY2001 = 99%; FY2002 = 98%; FY2003 = 97%; FY2004 = 96%; FY2005+ = 95%	No
To qualify, states must meet specified criteria.**	No	No	$1 state: $4 federal

Continued

TABLE 2-1 Continued

Title	Formula Grant	Description	Input Data
Title II	Emerging Communities	Funding for the EC award is divided in half. Half of the money is divided among MSAs[2] with 1000–1999 AIDS cases. The other half is divided among MSAs with 500–999 AIDS cases. Each half is divided among qualifying MSAs, based upon the MSA's proportion of the total AIDS cases for all qualifying MSAs.	Cumulative reported AIDS cases for most recent 5 years
Title II	Minority AIDS Initiative (MAI)	MAI award is divided among all states based on the state's proportion of reported AIDS cases in the most recent 2 year period among racial and ethnic minorities.	Cumulative reported nonwhite AIDS cases for most recent 2 years (adjusted for reporting delays)

SOURCE: HRSA, 2001.

Special formula features:
Threshold: A minimum level of need required before an area is eligible for any funds under the program.
Minimum: A minimum amount to be received by each state or jurisdiction.
Hold-harmless: A provision which limits decrease in amounts received by areas from one time period (generally fiscal year) to the next.
Match requirement: The minimum amount or rate a state must provide in non-federal funds on in-kind contributions according to the schedule established in the CARE Act.
SOURCE: NRC, 2003.

cases—including African Americans, Hispanics, Asian/Pacific Islanders, and Native Americans/Alaska Natives—diagnosed during the most recent two years for which data are available, and adjusted for reporting delays. For instance, data from 1998 and 1999 were used to calculate the FY2001 MAI award (HRSA, 2001).

Title II Awards to States and Territories

Base Award

Title II base awards are determined by a formula. Eighty percent of the base grant is based on each state's proportion of the total number of

Threshold	Minimum Award	Hold-Harmless	Match Requirement
For MSAs (areas with >50,000 population) not eligible for Title I AND that have 500–1,999 cumulative reported AIDS cases in most recent 5 years	Minimum of \$5 million for each tier	No	No
For jurisdictions with >0 reported AIDS cases among racial and ethnic minorities	No	No	No

**Qualifying Criteria for ADAP Supplemental Award:
A state or territory must meet one of the following "severe need" criteria, as defined by the Secretary of HHS:
(1) Financial eligibility requirement (number of eligible individuals at or below 200% of the official poverty line to whom the state is unable to provide therapeutics);
(2) Medical eligibility restrictions (e.g., CD4 T-cell count ≤500; specific viral load);
(3) Limited formula compositions for antiretrovirals;
(4) < 10 medications to treat opportunistic infections.
SOURCE: National Alliance of State and Territorial AIDS Directories, Kaiser Family Foundation, AIDS Treatment Data Network (2003).

NOTES:
[1]Metropolitan Statistical Areas (MSAs) include all communities in the U.S. with a population of 50,000 or greater.
[2]Puerto Rico is legislatively exempt from this requirement.
ELCs = Estimated Living AIDS Cases

ELCs. The remaining 20 percent is based on the number of ELCs in each state outside any EMAs, in proportion to the total number of such cases nationwide[13] (HRSA, 2001). The base award also includes a minimum award: \$200,000 for states with fewer than 90 ELCs, \$500,000 for states with more than 90 ELCs, and \$50,000 for all U.S. territories, regardless of the number of AIDS cases (HRSA, 2001). The base award formula includes a hold-harmless provision that declines annually according to a schedule established in the legislation.

[13]This provision was enacted under the 1996 reauthorization to provide an extra boost to states without EMAs.

States must match a portion of the Title II base award if they report more than 1 percent of the total number of AIDS cases for the two preceding fiscal years. The number of years that a state has been matching determines the percentage that it must match (20 percent the first year, 25 percent the second year, 33 percent the third year, and 50 percent in the fourth year and thereafter). Puerto Rico is exempt from this requirement (HRSA, 2001).

AIDS Drug Assistance Program Award

The ADAP award is based on a state's proportion of the total ELCs in all states and territories. Unlike the Title II base award, this award does not include an 80–20 split. The formula includes a hold-harmless provision that declines annually according to a schedule established in the legislation (HRSA, 2001).

ADAP Supplemental Award

Before the ADAP award is calculated, 3 percent of the appropriated earmark is set aside for the ADAP Supplemental Award, given to states in severe need (HRSA, 2002e). A state's supplemental ADAP award is based on its proportion of the total ELCs in qualifying states and territories. A state must match 25 percent of these federal funds to receive the award. If a qualifying state does not agree to do so, HRSA runs the formula again after deleting the nonparticipating states (HRSA, 2001).

Title II Minority AIDS Initiative Award

This award is based on each state's proportion of all African Americans, Hispanics, Asian/Pacific Islanders, and Native Americans/Alaska Natives diagnosed during the previous two calendar years, adjusted for reporting delays. If a state or territory has no diagnosed nonwhite AIDS cases during the past two years, it does not receive an award (HRSA, 2001). Montana, North Dakota, American Samoa, Marshall Islands, Northern Marianas, Republic of Palau, and the Federated States of Micronesia did not qualify for this award in FY2002 (HRSA, 2002k).

Emerging Communities Award

ECs are MSAs—a community with a population greater than 50,000—that do not meet the eligibility criteria to qualify as a Title I EMA, but that have 500–1,999 reported AIDS cases in the most recent five-year period.

Half the available funding goes to MSAs with 1,000–1,999 AIDS cases, while the other half is divided among MSAs with 500–999 AIDS cases. Each award is based on the area's proportion of the total number of AIDS cases among all qualifying MSAs (HRSA, 2001).

REFERENCES

Barre-Sinoussi F, Chermann JC, Rey F, Nugeyre MT, Chamaret S, Gruest J, Dauguet C, Axler-Blin C, Vezinet-Brun F, Rouzioux C, Rozenbaum W, Montagnier L. 1983. Isolation of a T-lymphotropic retrovirus from a patient at risk for acquired immune deficiency syndrome (AIDS). *Science* 220:868–71.

Bozzette S, Berry SH, Duan N, Frankel MR, Leibowitz AA, Lefkowitz D, Emmons CA, Senterfitt JW, Berk ML, Morton SC, Shapiro MF. 1998. The care of HIV-infected adults in the United States. HIV Cost and Services Utilization Study Consortium. *New England Journal of Medicine* 339(26):1897–904.

Brown D. 2003, March 14. FDA Approves First in Class of AIDS Drugs; 'Fusion Inhibitor' Will Help People Whose Bodies Resist Current Medications. *The Washington Post.* P. A2.

CDC (Centers for Disease Control and Prevention). 1981. Pneumocycstis Pneumonia–Los Angeles. *Morbidity and Mortality Weekly Report* 30:250–2. Atlanta, GA: CDC.

CDC. 2002. HIV/AIDS Surveillance Report, Year-End Edition. 13(2). Atlanta, GA: CDC.

CDC. 2003a. HIV/AIDS Surveillance in Women. L264 slide series through 2001. Slide 1 of 8. [Online]. Available: http://www.cdc.gov/hiv/graphics/images/l264/l264-1.htm [accessed August 2, 2003].

CDC. 2003b. Advancing HIV Prevention: New Strategies for a Changing Epidemic—United States, 2003. *Morbidity and Mortality Weekly Report* 52(15):329–32. Atlanta, GA: CDC.

Downes T, Pogue T. 2002. How Best to Hand Out Money: Issues in the Design and Structure of Intergovernmental Aid Formulas. *Journal of Official Statistics* 18(3):329-52.

Fauci AS, Pantaleo G, Stanley S, Weissman D. 1996. Immunopathogenic mechanisms of HIV infection. *Annals of Internal Medicine* 124(7):654–63.

Fleming P, Byers R, Sweeney P, Daniels D, Karon J, Janssen R. 2002. HIV Prevalence in the United States, 2000. Presented at the 9th Conference on Retroviruses and Opportunistic Infections, Seattle, WA. Abstract 11.

Foster S, Niederhausen P, Westmoreland T. 2002. *Federal HIV/AIDS Spending: A Budget Chartbook, Fiscal Year 2001.* Kaiser Family Foundation.

Gallo RC, Salahuddin SZ, Popovic M, Shearer GM, Kaplan M, Haynes BF, Palker TJ, Redfield R, Oleske J, Safai B, et al. 1984. Frequent detection and isolation of cytopathic retroviruses (HTLV-III) from patients with AIDS and at risk for AIDS. *Science* 224:500–3.

GAO (General Accounting Office). 1995a. Statement of William Scanlon, GAO. Testimony before the Subcommittee on Health and Environment, Committee on Commerce, House of Representatives. April 5, 1995. GAO/T-HEHS-95-126. Washington, DC: GAO.

GAO. 1995b. *Ryan White CARE Act of 1990: Opportunities Are Available to Improve Funding Equity.* GAO/T-HEHS-95-91. Washington, DC: GAO.

GAO. 1995c. *Ryan White CARE Act of 1990: Opportunities to Enhance Funding Equity.* GAO/HEHS-96-26. Washington, DC: GAO.

GAO. 2000. *Ryan White CARE Act: Opportunities to Enhance Funding Equity.* GAO/T-HEHS-00-150. Washington, DC: GAO.

Grant RM, Hecht FM, Warmerdam M, Liu L, Liegler T, Petropoulos CJ, Hellmann NS, Chesney M, Busch MP, Kahn JO. 2002. Time trends in primary HIV-1 drug resistance among recently infected persons. *Journal of American Medical Association* 288(2):181–8.

HRSA (Health Resources and Services Administration). 2001. A Primer on Title I and Title II Formula Allocation Calculations. 2001. (Email communication, Steven Young, HRSA, November 11, 2001).

HRSA. 2002a. AIDS Education and Training Centers Program. [Online]. Available: ftp://ftp.hrsa.gov/hab/aetcfact.pdf [accessed May 22, 2003].

HRSA. 2002b. HIV/AIDS Dental Programs [Online]. Available: http://ftp.hrsa.gov/hab/drpfact.pdf [accessed May 22, 2003].

HRSA. 2002c. Special Projects of National Significance Program. [Online]. Available: ftp://ftp.hrsa.gov/hab/spnsfact1.pdf [accessed May 22, 2003].

HRSA. 2002d. Title I: Grants to Eligible Metropolitan Areas. [Online]. Available: http://ftp.hrsa.gov/hab/titleifact.pdf [accessed May 22, 2003].

HRSA. 2002e. Title II: AIDS Drug Assistance Program. [Online]. Available: ftp://ftp.hrsa.gov/hab/adap1.pdf [accessed May 22, 2003].

HRSA. 2002f. Title II: Grants to States and Territories. [Online]. Available: http://ftp.hrsa.gov/hab/titleiifact.pdf [accessed May 22, 2003].

HRSA. 2002g. Title III: Planning Grant Program. [Online]. Available: ftp://ftp.hrsa.gov/hab/titleiiiplan.pdf [accessed May 22, 2003].

HRSA. 2002h. Title IV: Services for Women, Infants, Children, Youth, and Their Families. [Online]. Available: ftp://ftp.hrsa.gov/hab/titleiv.htm [accessed May 22, 2003].

HRSA. 2002i. National HIV CARE Program Resource Allocations. [Online]. Available: ftp://ftp.hrsa.gov/hab/allfigures.pdf [accessed July 14, 2003].

HRSA. 2002j. FY2002 Ryan White CARE Act Title I Emergency Relief Grants. (Email communication, Steven Young, HRSA, July 22, 2002).

HRSA. 2002k. FY2002 Ryan White CARE Act Title II Emergency Relief Grants. (Email communication, Steven Young, HRSA, July 22, 2002).

HRSA. 2003a. CARE Act Overview and Funding History. [Online]. Available: ftp://ftp.hrsa.gov/hab/fundinghis03.xls [accessed October 9, 2003].

HRSA. 2003b. Special Initiatives: Minority HIV/AIDS Initiatives (MAI). [Online]. Available: http://www.hab.hrsa.gov/special/mai.htm [accessed August 4, 2003].

HRSA/HAB (Health Resources and Services Administration/ HIV/AIDS Bureau). 2001. The Ryan White Comprehensive AIDS Resources Emergency (CARE) Act: Title II HIV Emergency Relief Program. Division of Service Systems. *FY 2001 Supplemental Treatment Drug Grants For AIDS Drug Assistance Programs (ADAP) Application Guidance.* Rockville, MD: HRSA.

IOM (Institute of Medicine). 2001. *No Time To Lose.* Ruiz MS, Gable AR, Kaplan EH, Stoto MA, Fineberg HV, Trussell J, Eds. Washington, DC: National Academy Press.

IOM/NAS (Institute of Medicine and the National Academy of Sciences). 1988. *Confronting AIDS, Update 1988.* Washington, DC: National Academy Press.

Kahn JG, Haile B, Kates J, Chang S. 2001. Health and federal budgetary effects of increasing access to antiretroviral medications for HIV by expanding Medicaid. *American Journal of Public Health* 91(9):1464–73.

Kaiser Family Foundation. 2000. Financing HIV/AIDS Care: A Quilt with Many Holes. *Capital Hill Briefing Series on HIV/AIDS.* Kaiser Family Foundation.

Kaiser Family Foundation. 2002. *Trends in U.S. Spending on HIV/AIDS.* A Three Part Series: Spending on the HIV/AIDS Epidemic.

Karon JM, Fleming PL, Steketee RW, De Cock KM. 2001. HIV in the United States at the turn of the century: An epidemic in transition. *American Journal of Public Health* 91(7):1060–8.

Little S, Holte S, Routy JP, Daar ES, Markowitz M, Collier AC, Koup RA, Mellors JW, Connick E, Conway B, Kilby M, Wang L, Whitcomb JM, Hellmann NS, Richman DD. 2002. Antiretroviral drug resistance among patients recently infected with HIV. *New England Journal of Medicine* 347(6):385.

National Alliance of State and Territorial AIDS Directors (NASTAD), Kaiser Family Foundation (KFF), AIDS Treatment Data Network (ATDN). 2003. National ADAP Monitoring Project. *Annual Report: April 2003.*

NRC (National Research Council). 2001. *Choosing the Right Formula.* Washington, DC: National Academy Press.

NRC. 2003. *Statistical Issues in Allocating Funds by Formulas.* Louis TA, Jabine TB, Gerstein MA, Eds. Washington, DC: The National Academies Press.

Pantaleo G, Graziosi C, Fauci AS. 1993. New concepts in the immunopathogenesis of human immunodeficiency virus infection. *New England Journal of Medicine* 328(5):327–35.

Shapiro MF, Morton SC, McCaffrey DF, Senterfitt JW, Fleishman JA, Perlman JF, Athey LA, Keesey JW, Goldman DP, Berry SH, Bozzette SA. 1999. Variations in the care of HIV-infected adults in the United States: Results from the HIV Cost and Services Utilization Study. *Journal of the American Medical Association* 281(24):2305–15.

Simon V, Vanderhoeven J, Hurley A, Remratnam B, Louie N, Dawson K, Parkin N, Boden D, Markowitz M. 2002. Evolving patterns of HIV-1 resistance to antiretroviral agents in newly infected individuals. *AIDS* 16:1511–9.

Tannenwald R. 1999. Fiscal disparity among the states revisited. *New England Economic Review* July/August:3–25.

U.S. Congress, House of Representatives. Committee on Commerce. 2000. *Report on Ryan White CARE Act Amendments of 2000 (106-788).* 106th Cong., 2d Sess. July 25, 2000.

U.S. Congress, Senate. Committee on Labor and Human Resources. 1990. *Report on HIV Emergency Relief Grant Program (101-273).* 101st Cong., 1st Sess. April 24, 1990.

U.S. Congress, Senate. Committee on Labor and Human Resources. 1995. *Report on Ryan White CARE Reauthorization Act of 1995 (104-25).* 104th Cong., 1st Sess. April 3, 1995.

Weinstock J, Respess R, Heneine W, Petropoulos CJ, Hellmann NS, Luo CC, Pau CP, Woods T, Gwinn M, Kaplan J. 2000. Prevalence of mutations associated with reduced antiretroviral drug susceptibility among human immunodeficiency virus type 1 seroconverters in the United States, 1993-1998. *Journal of Infectious Diseases* 182:330–3.

Zaslavsky A, Schirm A. 2002. Interactions between survey estimates and federal funding formulas. *Journal of Official Statistics* 18(3):371–91.

3

Public Health and HIV/AIDS Surveillance

This chapter reviews public health surveillance, and HIV and AIDS case reporting, to provide context for the use of such information in Ryan White CARE Act (RWCA) funding formulas. In this report, the Committee distinguishes between the terms "surveillance" and "case reporting." Surveillance is a more comprehensive term for data collection that can include case reporting, as well as other methods, such as population-based surveys, seroprevalence surveys, and behavioral risk factor surveillance. Case reporting is a subset of surveillance activities in which individuals who are diagnosed with specific diseases or conditions are reported to public health authorities (state or local health departments), typically by medical practitioners and laboratories and pursuant to requirements imposed by state statutes or regulations. This chapter focuses its discussion of HIV/AIDS surveillance on HIV/AIDS case reporting, because it is the predominant method of surveillance used by states to collect information about HIV infection and because it is the most relevant to the RWCA formulas.

PUBLIC HEALTH SURVEILLANCE

Public health surveillance has been defined as the ongoing, systematic collection of public health data, with analysis and dissemination of results and interpretation of these data to those who contributed to them and "all who need to know" (Langmuir, 1963). Public health surveillance was historically used to discover or identify and observe patients with contagious, infectious diseases and the people with whom they came in contact, to isolate and quarantine them, or take other measures to control the spread of disease (Birkhead and Maylahn, 2000). Since the 1950s, surveillance has gradually expanded to include monitoring disease trends in populations for the purpose of initiating population-based disease-control programs. More recently, traditional models for controlling communicable diseases have also been extended to noninfectious diseases, as well as occupational, environmental, behavioral, biological, and social factors that are believed to contribute to the onset and spread of disease (Thacker, 2000). Surveillance is a process that relies on increasingly sophisticated epidemiological and statistical techniques and requires a large and complex system that stretches from the individual practitioner to the World Health Organization.

In the United States, legal authority to require reporting of diseases resides primarily at the state level. In some states, legislation specifies reporting requirements for particular diseases; in others, legislation delegates authority to the state health department or local boards of health to designate reportable disease by regulation; and some states use both (Thacker, 2000).[1] Legislative authorization is necessary because health providers cannot lawfully release or disclose personal medical information about a patient without the patient's consent.[2] Health care facilities

[1]The state's sovereign police power, which authorizes it to adopt legislation to protect the public's health and safety, includes the power to protect the public from the spread of communicable diseases. The state legislature may authorize counties, cities, or towns to take action within their jurisdictions (Gostin, 2000; Hall et al., 2003). The federal government also has constitutional authority to enact legislation to prevent the spread of communicable diseases introduced by immigration, commerce with foreign nations, domestic interstate commerce, acts of war, or threats to national security (U.S. Constitution, article 1, sec. 8).

[2]Health care providers have a general common law (and, in some cases, statutory) duty to refrain from disclosing such information without the patient's consent (e.g., Federal Privacy Act, Health Insurance Portability and Accountability Act (HIPAA) regulations). In addition, the U.S. Constitution (and some state constitutions) protect an individual's right to privacy in his or her personal medical information and from disclosure without the individual's consent. The Fourth Amendment to the Constitution prohibits unreasonable searches and seizures, which include the disclosure of medical information. The Due Process Clause of the Fifth and Fourteenth Amendments prohibits the federal and state governments from depriving any person of liberty without due process of law. Liberty interests are also implicated because statutes that make diseases reportable may also typically subject individuals who are reported to deprivations of liberty, such as isolation. (The Committee notes that some state AIDS or HIV reporting laws are distinct statutes in order to avoid subjecting people with HIV or AIDS to such controls.) Several federal courts of appeal have recognized that "individuals who are affected by the HIV virus clearly possess a constitutional right to privacy regarding their condition" (*Doe v City of New York*, 15 F3d 264, 267 [2d Cir 1994]). See also *Doe v SEPTA*, 72 F3d 1133 (3d Cir 1995). Such rights are not absolute,

and providers are restricted in their disclosure of medical information by state laws, federal laws, and by Health Insurance Portability and Accountability Act (HIPAA) regulations.[3] However, all states have statutes or regulations authorizing and requiring providers and laboratories to report notifiable diseases to the state or local health department (Roush et al., 1999). HIPAA allows covered entities to release this health information to state health departments in compliance with state disease reporting laws (45 C.F.R. § 164.512 [2003]; CDC, 2003c).

States vary in the diseases they obligate physicians, other practitioners, and entities such as laboratories to report, and in the type and amount of information they require. Most systems for reporting infectious diseases require names because public health authorities often need to contact individuals to identify the source of infection, to identify others who may need treatment, and to possibly isolate individuals who pose a danger of infecting others. Name-based reporting has also been advocated as a way to facilitate the elimination of duplicate reports (CDC, 1999). States often require practitioners to report the source of exposure to infection, risk factors, and symptoms. Laboratories must often report a subset of diseases that can be diagnosed by laboratory tests, such as positive tests for measles antibody.

Although states and localities are responsible for collecting surveillance data, they broadly and voluntarily share such information with the federal government. In 1951, the Centers for Disease Control and Prevention (CDC) organized the Conference (now Council) of State and Territorial Epidemiologists to recommend diseases that states should voluntarily report to CDC, and to develop reporting procedures (Koo and

---

and some disclosures may be authorized by legislation designed to achieve a justifiable public health purpose. Laws requiring the disclosure of personally identifiable information, such as names and addresses, have been upheld where the law also required that the information be kept secure and confidential and not be disclosed to third parties and prescribed penalties for any violation of confidentiality (*Whalen v Roe*, 429 U.S. 5890 [1977]), but have been struck down when such protections were not part of the law. Reporting laws that do not include the collection of names or other personally identifiable information rarely raise privacy concerns. However, the Supreme Court has struck down a state law requiring physicians to report abortion procedures because, even though the law did not require reporting names, "the amount of information about [a patient] and the circumstances under which she had an abortion are so detailed that identification is likely," and the information sought went beyond the health-related interests that justified reporting (*Thornburgh v American College of Obstetricians & Gynecologist*, 476 U.S. 474 [1986]).

[3]"The U.S. Department of Health and Human Services (DHHS) issued the Privacy Rule to implement the requirement of the Health Insurance Portability and Accountability Act of 1996 (HIPAA). . . . A major goal of the Privacy Rule is to assure that individuals' health information is properly protected while allowing the flow of health information needed to provide and promote high quality health care and to protect the public's health and well being" (DHHS, 2003).

Wetterhall, 1996). The result—the National Notifiable Disease Surveillance System (NNDSS)—now recommends that states and territories voluntarily report 56 diseases and conditions to CDC (CDC, 2003b).[4] This list of nationally notifiable diseases is revised periodically.

Before transferring information on any of the diseases included in the NNDSS to CDC, states first strip the data of personal identifiers such as name, address, and social security number. For example, all states send AIDS and name-based HIV case reports to CDC using an alphanumeric code (Soundex code) derived from the person's last name and other identifying information (e.g., six-digit date of birth, and status of residence at diagnosis) (Schwarz et al., 2002; Nakashima and Fleming, 2003). CDC does not possess the names or other personal identifiers of reported cases (Nakashima and Fleming, 2003). CDC, in turn, analyzes the data and disseminates them on a national level and shares case counts for a much smaller group of communicable diseases with the World Health Organization. Data transfer from the state to national and international levels is computerized, while data transfer from practitioners and local health departments to state health departments occurs through mail, fax, phone, and computer.

Some categorical public health prevention programs funded primarily by CDC,[5] including childhood immunizations, tuberculosis, sexually transmitted diseases (STDs), and HIV/AIDS, make reporting a condition of federal funding. In these cases, CDC collects from states more detailed information on the disease, for example, on the probable route of exposure (for AIDS), treatment histories (for tuberculosis), or vaccine histories (for most vaccine-preventable diseases). Local health department staff usually complete these forms after reviewing patient records.

AIDS AND HIV CASE REPORTING

AIDS case reporting has been the cornerstone of efforts to monitor and track the HIV epidemic. Soon after the first cases of AIDS were reported by the CDC in June 1981 (CDC, 1981), state health departments began to require physicians and hospitals to report by name each newly diagnosed case. In the epidemic's early years, surveillance entailed not

---

[4]While reporting to the federal government is voluntary, states receive federal money for AIDS and HIV surveillance, unlike most other reportable diseases and conditions.

[5]CDC funds HIV/AIDS surveillance through cooperative agreements with 61 state and local health departments: 50 states; 6 cities (Chicago, Houston, Los Angeles, New York, Philadelphia, San Francisco), the District of Columbia, Puerto Rico, the U.S. Virgin Islands, American Samoa and the Federated States of Micronesia (Nakashima and Fleming, 2003).

only enumerating and mapping cases but also investigating commonalties for which there was no etiological explanation. By the end of 1983 most states required AIDS cases to be reported to public health officials (IOM and NAS, 1986). The system of AIDS reporting evolved over time, primarily through changes in the case definition to reflect growing clinical understanding of the disease and development of appropriate laboratory tests (CDC, 1985, 1987, 1992, 1999). All 50 states, the District of Columbia, and territories report AIDS cases by name using standardized data collection, case definitions, case reporting forms, and computer software (Nakashima and Fleming, 2003). (See sample Adult HIV/AIDS Confidential Case Report form, Annex 3-1.)

AIDS surveillance has been broadly accepted by the community of individuals living with HIV and AIDS. The relatively short time that existed in the past between diagnosis of AIDS and death and the need for health and medical services offset the risks of surveillance (Gostin et al., 1997).[6] Due in large part to federal investments in state and local surveillance and strong active surveillance efforts, AIDS case reporting is among the most complete of all reportable diseases and conditions (Doyle et al., 2002).

AIDS, the most advanced stage of HIV disease, develops in the absence of treatment an average of 10 years following initial infection (Pantaleo et al., 1993). Advances in treating HIV disease have extended that window even further and may prevent some people with HIV infection from ever developing AIDS. Thus, data from the AIDS case reporting system, while still important, have become less informative about current trends in HIV transmission (CDC, 1999).

Following the development of the first antibody test for HIV in 1985, states began to initiate reporting of HIV infection. The first successful efforts to mandate HIV case reporting occurred in Minnesota and Colorado in 1985. In contrast to the "relative ease" with which AIDS reporting was implemented (Bayer, 1989), HIV reporting "ignited a firestorm of community protest" (Gostin et al., 1997). Although very few breaches of security had occurred resulting in the release of unauthorized data from the AIDS surveillance system since 1981 (Nakashima and Fleming, 2003), many civil libertarians and gay-rights organizations were strongly opposed to name-based reporting of HIV infection because they did not trust the government to safeguard such information, and were concerned

[6]AIDS surveillance data, like other government-held health information in the United States, are subject to stringent legal protections of privacy. For example, in accordance with U.S. code, HIV/AIDS data are protected from subpoena or other disclosure without consent by an assurance of confidentiality (Nakashima and Fleming, 2003).

about invasion of personal privacy and discrimination in employment, housing, and insurance (Gostin et al., 1997).

Public health authorities justified reporting of HIV infection on several grounds. Reporting would alert public health officials to the presence of individuals with a lethal infection; would allow officials to counsel them about what they needed to do to prevent further transmission; would assure the linkage of infected persons with medical and other services; and would permit authorities to monitor the incidence and prevalence of infection. In the following years, CDC continued to press for name-based reporting of HIV cases, supported by a growing number of public health officials. Indeed, the Council of State and Territorial Epidemiologists adopted several resolutions between 1989 and 1995 recommending and encouraging that states consider the implementation of HIV case reporting by name (CSTE, 1997). Political resistance persisted however, and HIV cases typically became reportable by name only in states that did not have large cosmopolitan communities with effectively organized gay constituencies or high AIDS caseloads. By 1996, although 26 states had adopted HIV case reporting, they represented jurisdictions with only approximately a quarter of total reported AIDS cases (Bayer, 1989, 1991; CDC, 1996). By October 1998, name-based reporting had a stronger foothold with 32 states then reporting cases of HIV by name, although three states reported only pediatric cases (CDC, 1999).

As of October 2003, all states, territories, and cities except Georgia and Philadelphia[7] have implemented a confidential HIV case-reporting system (CDC, 2003a,d). Unlike AIDS case reporting, which uses a standardized name-based reporting system, states had adopted different procedures for reporting HIV cases (Figure 3-1, Table 3-1). As of October 2003, 34 states, the Virgin Islands, American Samoa, Puerto Rico, Northern Mariana Islands, and Guam had implemented the same confidential name-based reporting of HIV infection as is used for AIDS reporting and other reportable diseases and conditions. Eight states plus the District of Columbia use a coded identifier rather than the patient name to report HIV cases. Five states use a name-to-code system; initially, names are collected and then converted to codes by the local or state health department after any necessary public health follow-up. Connecticut conducts pediatric surveillance using name-based reporting but allows name or code reporting of adults/adolescents over 13 years of age. New Hampshire allows HIV cases to be reported with or without a name (CDC,

[7]Since the release of this report, Georgia implemented name-based reporting and Philadelphia adopted code-based reporting. All areas of the United States now have HIV reporting.

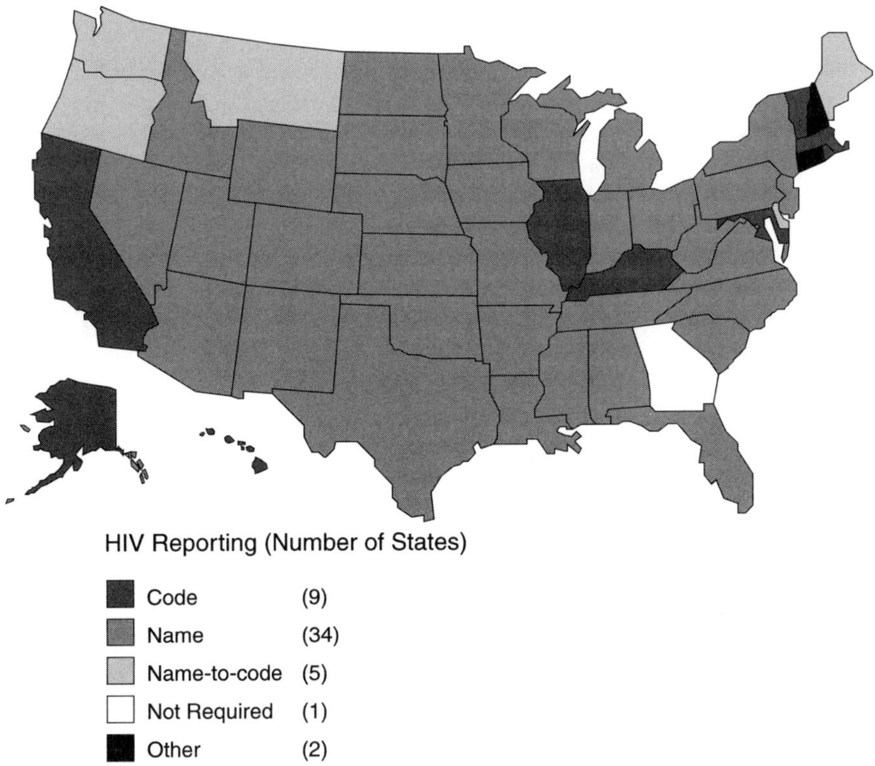

FIGURE 3-1 Status of HIV reporting in the United States as of October 2003.
SOURCES: CDC 2003a,d.

2003a,d). Of the 15 areas that use some form of code, only two use the same code. A brief case study of HIV reporting in San Francisco shows how the system works in practice (Box 3-1).

As with any surveillance system, HIV and AIDS case reporting fulfills a number of purposes. The allocation of resources appropriated through the RWCA is an example of how information collected from a case-reporting system has been used for different purposes. RWCA was structured to award grants to Eligible Metropolitan Areas (EMAs) and states that needed federal financial assistance to provide care and support services. States had enacted and implemented case-reporting systems for AIDS cases in the early 1980s and were voluntarily reporting data from those systems to CDC as part of their traditional disease-reporting activities. Therefore CDC was already receiving data on AIDS cases, albeit for a purpose independent of RWCA. Although the RWCA statute does not require that states adopt case reporting for the purpose of collecting data for the RWCA, data from such systems have been used for this purpose.

TABLE 3-1 Current Status of HIV Reporting, October 2003

Name-Based		Code-Based[a]
Alabama (1/88)	*North Dakota* (1/88)	California (7/02)
Alaska (2/99)	Northern Mariana Islands (10/01)	District of Columbia (12/01)
American Samoa (8/01)	Ohio (6/90)	Hawaii (10/01)
Arizona (1/87)	Oklahoma (6/88)	Illinois (7/99)
Arkansas (7/89)	Pennsylvania[g] (10/02)	Kentucky (7/00)
Colorado (11/85)	Puerto Rico (1/03)	Maryland (6/94)
Florida (7/97)	*South Carolina* (2/86)	Massachusetts (1/98)
Guam (3/00)	*South Dakota* (1/88)	Rhode Island (4/00)
Idaho (6/86)	*Tennessee* (1/92)	
Indiana (7/88)	Texas (1/99)	
Iowa (7/98)	*U.S. Virgin Islands* (12/98)	
Kansas (7/99)	Utah (4/89)	
Louisiana (2/93)	Virginia (7/89)	
Michigan (4/92)	West Virginia (1/89)	
Minnesota (10/85)	Wisconsin (11/85)	
Mississippi (8/88)	Wyoming (6/89)	
Missouri (10/87)		
Nebraska (9/85)	Pediatric Only:	
Nevada (2/92)	Connecticut[c] (1/01)	
New Jersey (1/92)		
New Mexico (1/98)	Symptomatic Infection:[f]	
New York (6/00)	Washington[h] (9/99)	
North Carolina (2/90)		

[a]These states conduct HIV case surveillance using coded identifiers. Each state conducts follow-up activities to fill in gaps in the information received and longitudinally updates information on clinical status using the code.

[b]HIV cases are initially reported by name. After public health follow-up and collection of epidemiological data, names are converted to codes.

[c]Requires name-based reports of HIV infection in children <13 years of age. Reports HIV infection in adults/adolescents 13 and older by name or code.

[d]As of October 2003, Georgia had anonymous HIV reporting only and did not conduct follow-up activities on this case information. Since the release of this report, however, Georgia has implemented a name-based HIV reporting system (Georgia Division of Public Health, 2003).

OTHER METHODS FOR ESTIMATING HIV PREVALENCE

Every case-reporting system has some degree of under-ascertainment. This can be due to failure of patients to present for diagnosis, failure of physicians to diagnose, failure of physicians to report, and failures within the health department itself to count cases owing to misclassification or other reasons. In addition to public health disease reporting, a number of different techniques have been designed to estimate the prevalence of disease and infections—both clinically apparent and subclinical—in a

Name-to-Code-Based[b]	Other	Not Required
Delaware (7/01)	Connecticut[c] (1/01)	Georgia[d]
Maine (7/99)	New Hampshire[e] (10/90)	
Montana (9/97)		
Oregon (9/88)		
Washington (9/99)		

[e]Allows HIV cases to be reported with or without a name.
[f]As defined in CDC classification of Group IV non-AIDS.
[g]Name-based HIV reporting was implemented in October 2002. However, HIV reporting had not been implemented in the city of Philadelphia as of October 2003.
[h]Requires name-based reports of symptomatic HIV infection and AIDS and has a name-to-code system for reporting asymptomatic HIV cases.
NOTE: States noted in italics do not have anonymous testing.
SOURCES: CDC, 2003a,d.

population.[8] Two approaches worth consideration are seroprevalence surveys and capture–recapture methods. Seroprevalence surveys are conducted in a sample of the population of interest, and the accuracy of the

[8]In this report, the Committee does not evaluate methods (e.g., Serologic Testing Algorithm for Recent HIV Seroconversion or STAHRS [Janssen et al., 1998]) for identifying incident, or new, HIV infections. Incidence is the ideal measure for understanding the dynamics, spread, and success of prevention programs. Prevalent, or known, HIV infection is appropriate for estimating the clinical burden to apportion care resources (see Chapter 5).

BOX 3-1
How HIV Reporting Works in San Francisco

Since 1981, California has required providers and laboratories to report by name individuals meeting the CDC's definition of an AIDS case to local health departments, which must participate in the surveillance system.

The San Francisco Department of Public Health—the local jurisdiction with the largest number of reported AIDS cases—relies on a number of activities and protocols to track the incidence of HIV and AIDS. Health care providers (or their designee, such as an office assistant or an infection control practitioner) forward a complete case report or other information that suggests that a person may have HIV or AIDS to the department. (When individuals reported with HIV progress to AIDS, providers must complete an AIDS case report form.)

Staff members at the San Francisco Department of Public Health determine if the information pertains to a previously reported person with AIDS. If it does, the department adds any new information to the record. If not, a staff member visits the health care facility to examine medical records to confirm that the person meets the definition of an AIDS case. To ensure that the department's information is as complete as possible, staff members collect information from all local health care facilities at which the patient was noted to have received care. The surveillance staff also conducts periodic reviews of medical charts to add information on subsequent opportunistic illnesses. The department actively follows up on 95 percent of notifications.

Staff members assign new cases a unique city and state number and convert the person's last name into a Soundex code before entering the data into CDC's HIV/AIDS database. The San Francisco Department of Public Health

results depends heavily on how representative survey participants are of the population being studied. For example, convenience samples of patients in sexually transmitted disease clinics will likely overestimate the prevalence of HIV in similar age and sex strata in the general population. Conversely, a careful random population sample, as has been done in selected geographical areas in the United States and in other countries, can provide a very accurate estimate of the overall prevalence of infection in a population.

In 1987 following pilot testing in two U.S. cities, CDC decided against attempting a random household survey of the United States to estimate HIV prevalence because of potential nonresponse bias. The agency decided instead to construct a composite estimate from various clinical populations at high risk of HIV infection, such as STD clinics, drug treatment centers, and women's health centers. These unlinked seropreva-

then forwards case report forms to the California Department of Health Services with all variables except the name of the individual, and the state forwards the reports to CDC.

California health and safety regulations specify that laboratories must report confirmed positive HIV tests and any HIV viral load tests to the local health department. The laboratory converts the patient's last name to a Soundex code and sends it to the local health department along with the date of birth, gender, date, type, test results, and the name and address of the provider. The laboratory also sends this information to the health care provider, who must report the case to the local health department after adding the last four digits of the person's Social Security number. Providers must retain a cross-reference log that links the Soundex to the patient's name to enable health department staff to follow up.

The Statistics and Epidemiology Section of the San Francisco Department of Public Health analyzes the data and presents the information to community groups and scientific meetings. The epidemiology section also publishes the results in peer-reviewed journals as well as quarterly and annual reports. Community groups, such as the RWCA Title I Planning Councils, Title II Consortia for the state of California, and HIV Prevention Community Planning Groups utilize these data for public health planning purposes. The section further augments HIV/AIDS case reporting with behavioral and other surveys among high-risk populations, with each approach using a distinct protocol and requiring staff training and monitoring. CDC and the California Department of Health Services fund the section's 25 staff members with a budget of $2.3 million.

SOURCE: San Francisco Department of Public Health, 2003.

lence surveys were conducted using residual serum from specimens collected for other purposes (e.g., syphilis testing) (Valdiserri et al., 2000). The one portion of this "family of surveys" that provided highly accurate and generalizable results, the Survey of Childbearing Women (Pappaioanou et al., 1990), was later discontinued because of political and ethical reasons.

Another approach that has been used successfully for chronic and some infectious diseases is the capture–recapture method. A technique adapted from wildlife biology, capture–recapture consecutively samples a population, and from the proportion of individuals found in more than one sample constructs an estimate of the overall population size (International Working Group for Disease Monitoring, 1995a,b). In clinical epidemiology capture–recapture surveys most often use different patient registers or clinical records as the "samples," and thus are largely limited to persons with diagnosed or at least symptomatic disease for which they are seeking medical care. In the context of HIV infection, a capture–recapture scheme would enumerate patients from a variety of clinical and social services lists, such as reportable disease registries, clinic records, pharmacy records, laboratory records, and social services agency records, and compare the proportion of patients who appear on one or more of the lists. This overlap can then be modeled to estimate the size of the entire population of persons with HIV infection. This technique has been used extensively for estimating the number of persons injecting drugs in a geographical area, and for estimating the size of various populations of persons with chronic diseases, such as diabetes and cancers. CDC is currently conducting one part of its HIV surveillance evaluation study using capture-recapture techniques. Methods that make use of information on AIDS incidence and on natural history, such as "back calculation," may also be of use; but application of such methods is more challenging than was the case earlier in the epidemic because of the impact of treatment on natural history of the disease.

An important consideration in evaluating alternative surveillance methods is the costs and benefits associated with acquiring data for use in allocating resources. The AIDS and HIV case-reporting systems have been substantially developed and are more or less in place. The primary source of funding for state HIV/AIDS case-reporting systems is from CDC, although many states, but not all, provide some additional funding (see Appendix B). For this reason, there may be a perception that the data from these systems are "free," or at least free in the sense of low marginal cost. However, adding more missions, such as resource allocation, to an already large, expensive, and complex enterprise may have additional costs. To the extent that additional data elements bearing on the specific needs of RWCA grantees are requested, additional resources will be required.

REFERENCES

Bayer R. 1989. *Private Acts, Social Consequences: AIDS and the Politics of Public Health.* New York: The Free Press.

Bayer R. 1991. Public health policy and the AIDS epidemic. An end to HIV exceptionalism? *New England Journal of Medicine* 324(21):1500–4.

Birkhead GS, Maylahn CM. 2000. State and local public health surveillance. *Principles and Practice of Public Health Surveillance.* Teutsch SM, Churchill RE, Eds. 2nd ed. New York: Oxford University Press.

CDC (Centers for Disease Control and Prevention). 1981. Pneumocycstis Pneumonia–Los Angeles. *Morbidity and Mortality Weekly Report* 30:250–2. Atlanta, GA: CDC.

CDC. 1985. Revision of the case definition of acquired immunodeficiency syndrome for national reporting—United States. *Morbidity and Mortality Weekly Report* 34:373–6. Atlanta, GA: CDC.
CDC. 1987. Revision of the CDC surveillance case definition of acquired immunodeficiency syndrome. *Morbidity and Mortality Weekly Report* 36(IS):1–15. Atlanta, GA: CDC.
CDC. 1992. 1993 Revised classification system for HIV infection and expanded surveillance case definition for AIDS among adolescents and adults. *Morbidity and Mortality Weekly Report* 41(RR–17):1–19. Atlanta, GA: CDC.
CDC. 1996. U.S. HIV and AIDS cases reported through December 1996. *HIV/AIDS Surveillance Report* 8(2). Atlanta, GA: CDC.
CDC. 1999. Guidelines for national human immunodeficiency virus case surveillance, including monitoring for human immunodeficiency virus infection and acquired immunodeficiency syndrome. *Morbidity and Mortality Weekly Report* 48(13):1–28. Atlanta, GA: CDC.
CDC. 2003a. Current Status of HIV Infection Surveillance: April, 2003. (Email communication, Patricia Sweeney, CDC, April 28, 2003).
CDC. 2003b. Nationally Notifiable Infectious Diseases: United States. [Online]. Available: http://www.cdc.gov/epo/dphsi/phs/infdis2003.htm [accessed October 15, 2003].
CDC. 2003c. HIPAA Privacy Rule and Public Health, Guidance from CDC and the U.S. Department of Health and Human Services. *Morbidity and Mortality Weekly Report* 52:1–12.
CDC. 2003d. Update on current status of HIV Infection Surveillance: April 2003. (Email communication, Patricia Sweeney, CDC, October 13, 2003).
CSTE (Council of State and Territorial Epidemiologists). 1997. National HIV Surveillance: Addition to the National Public Health Surveillance System. CSTE Position Statement 1997-ID-4.
DHHS (U.S. Department of Health and Human Services). 2003. OCR Privacy Brief. Summary of the HIPAA Privacy Rule. HIPAA Compliance Assistance. [Online]. Available: http://www.hhs.gov/privacysummary.pdf [accessed September 28, 2003].
Doyle T, Glynn K, Groseclose S. 2002. Completeness of notifiable infectious disease reporting in the United States: An analytical literature review. *American Journal of Epidemiology* 155(9):866–74.
Georgia Division of Public Health, Epidemiology Branch, HIV/STD Epidemiology Section. 2003. Proposal for HIV Infection Reporting in Georgia. [Online]. Available at: http://www.ph.dhr.state.ga.us/epi/hivreporting.shtml [accessed September 25, 2003].
Gostin LO. 2000. *Public Health Law: Power, Duty, Restraint.* Berkeley, CA: University of California Press.
Gostin LO, Ward JW, Baker AC. 1997. National HIV case reporting for the United States. A defining moment in the history of the epidemic. *New England Journal of Medicine* 337(16):1162–7.

Hall MA, Bobinski MA, Orentlicher D. 2003. *Health Care, Law, and Ethics.* 6th ed. Aspen Publishers.

International Working Group for Disease Monitoring and Forecasting. 1995a. Capture-recapture and multiple-record systems estimation I: History and theoretical development. *American Journal of Epidemiology* 142:1047–58.

International Working Group for Disease Monitoring and Forecasting. 1995b. Capture-recapture and multiple record systems estimation II: Applications in human disease. *American Journal of Epidemiology* 142:1059–68.

IOM and NAS (Institute of Medicine and the National Academy of Sciences). 1986. *Confronting AIDS: Directions for Public Health, Health Care, and Research.* Washington, DC: National Academy Press.

Janssen RS et al. 1998. New testing strategy to detect early HIV-1 infection for use in incidence estimates and for clinical and prevention purposes. *Journal of the American Medical Association* 280:42–8.

Koo D, Wetterhall S. 1996. History and current status of the National Notifiable Diseases Surveillance System. *Journal of Public Health Management and Practice* 2(4):4–10.

Langmuir AD. 1963. The surveillance of communicable diseases of national importance. *New England Journal of Medicine* 268:182–92.

Nakashima AK, Fleming PL. 2003. HIV/AIDS surveillance in the United States, 1981-2001. *Journal of Acquired Immune Deficiency Syndrome* 32(Suppl 1): S68–85.

Pantaleo G, Graziosi C, Fauci AS. 1993. New concepts in the immunopathogenesis of Human Immunodeficiency Virus infection. *New England Journal of Medicine* 328(5):327–35.

Pappaioanou M, George JR, Hannon WH, Gwinn M, Dondero TJ Jr, Grady GF, Hoff R, Willoughby AD, Wright A, Novello AC. 1990. HIV Seroprevalence surveys of childbearing women: Objectives, methods, and uses of the data. *Public Health Reports* 105:147–52.

Roush S, Birkhead G, Koo D, Cobb A, Fleming D. 1999. Mandatory reporting of diseases and conditions by health care professionals and laboratories. *Journal of the American Medical Association* 282(2):164–70.

San Francisco Department of Public Health. 2003. How HIV reporting works in San Francisco. (Email communication, Sandra Schwarcz, SFDPH, May 13, 2003).

Schwarcz S, Hsu L, Chu PL, Parisi MK, Bangsberg D, Hurley L, Pearlman J, Marsh K, Katz M. 2002. Evaluation of a non-name based HIV reporting system in San Francisco. *Journal of Acquired Immune Deficiency Syndrome* 29:504–10.

Thacker SB. 2000. Historical development. *Principles and Practice of Public Health Surveillance.* 2nd ed. Teutsch SM, Churchill RE, Eds. New York: Oxford University Press.

Valdiserri RO, Janssen RS, Buehler JW, Fleming PL. 2000. The context of HIV/AIDS surveillance. *Journal of Acquired Immune Deficiency Syndrome* 25(Suppl 2):S97–S104.

4

HIV Reporting Data and Title I and II Formulas

Seventy percent ($1.3 billion in fiscal year [FY] 2002) of all Ryan White CARE Act (RWCA) funds are distributed under Titles I and II through explicit numerical formulas. These formula allocations are based on estimated living AIDS cases (ELCs),[1] which are calculated using data from the AIDS case-reporting system[2] (HRSA, 2002). Discussions, testimony, and Congressional committee reports related to the 2000 reauthorization raised questions concerning inequity in the allocations resulting from these formulas (U.S. Congress, 2000a,b). By 2000, concerns about inequity arose from the perception that the epidemic was not truly reflected by AIDS cases alone, and that the effect of addressing HIV disease in areas with emerging epidemics had been underestimated (U.S. Congress, 2000a,b). Jurisdictions were also concerned that they were not compensated for providing early access to care and treatment and thus preventing persons from progressing to AIDS (U.S. Congress, 2000a). The hold-harmless provisions, which were added in the 1996 reauthorization, also raised concerns about equity. Some were concerned that the hold-harmless provisions, which prevent a jurisdiction's funding falling by

[1]ELCs are calculated by applying annual survival weights to the most recent 10 years of reported AIDS cases and summing the totals. The Centers for Disease Control and Prevention (CDC) updates the survival weights every two years. CDC provides both the survival weights and the most recent 10 years of reported AIDS cases to the Health Resources and Services Administration (HRSA), which performs the award calculations.

[2]See Chapter 3 for background on the AIDS and HIV case-reporting systems.

more than a set percent each year in order to help sustain needed health care infrastructure and continuity of services, seemed to accomplish their purpose at the expense of states and local areas believed to have younger epidemics and rising need (U.S. Congress, 2000a).

Congress asked the General Accounting Office (GAO) to examine opportunities to enhance the equity of funding to RWCA grantees prior to the 1996 and 2000 reauthorizations. The GAO's 1995 study found that CARE Act funding formulas led to disparities in per AIDS case funding that could not be completely explained by variations in service costs or the fiscal capacity of states and EMAs.

In a 2000 report, the GAO again found large disparities across Eligible Metropolitan Areas (EMAs) and states in allocations per ELC. The GAO concluded that two formula features in particular, the hold-harmless provision and the "double-counting" of EMA cases in Title I and II formulas,[3] contributed to these funding inequities. In particular, states with an EMA had up to 60 percent higher per case allocations than states without an EMA and the hold-harmless provision instituted in the 1996 reauthorization benefited only San Francisco (GAO, 2000).

The GAO report further concluded that the formulas, which were based on living AIDS cases, did not reflect the changing nature of the HIV/AIDS epidemic and recommended the inclusion of HIV case data in the Title I and II formulas to more effectively target and deliver funding to persons in need of care. The GAO noted that, at a minimum, all states would have to report HIV cases to provide an equitable distribution of funds. At the time, only 60 percent of states had HIV reporting systems in place (GAO, 2000).

Congress began the 2000 reauthorization with the expectation that HIV case-reporting data would be of value to the RWCA formula allocations, as well as to planning and evaluation efforts. The 2000 legislation specifies that, if appropriate, the Secretary of Health and Human Services (HHS) should incorporate cases of HIV disease in RWCA Title I and II funding formulas as early as FY2005 but no later than FY2007 (Ryan White CARE Act. 42 U.S.C. § 300ff-28 [2003]). The reauthorization legislation authorized the Institute of Medicine (IOM) to assist the Secretary of HHS in assessing the readiness of states to produce accurate and reliable HIV case-reporting data, determine the accuracy of using HIV cases within the existing allocation formulas, and establish recommendations regarding the manner in which states could improve their HIV case-reporting systems (Ryan White CARE Act. 42 U.S.C. § 300ff-11 [2003]).[4]

---

[3]EMA cases are counted in both Title I and II formulas.

[4]See Chapter 1 for legislative language relating to the Committee's charge.

At the outset, the Committee recognized the difficulty of defining such terms as "sufficiently accurate," "adequate," and "reliable" to characterize the quality of HIV surveillance data. No absolute standards of accuracy, adequacy, or reliability exist; rather these standards and their definition will vary according to the purposes and tasks for which the data are used. Thus, evaluating HIV reporting systems for use in resource allocation formulas requires a different set of performance criteria than evaluating these data for public health purposes (e.g., epidemic surveillance, contact tracing, and partner notification). While CDC (1999) has established performance criteria[5] for evaluating the latter functions, it was not the purpose of this Committee to assess these standards. Rather, the Committee defined criteria for "accuracy," "adequacy," and "reliability" in terms of over- and underfunding errors to RWCA grantees.

In assessing whether the current surveillance systems provide HIV data that are "sufficiently accurate" for the purpose of formula grants, the Committee focused on the primary argument for including HIV case data in the formulas: that doing so would provide a better representation of HIV disease-related resource needs across jurisdictions and would thus more fairly channel scarce RWCA resources. Four conditions would need to be met for this to occur:

- First, the HIV reporting systems of all states would need to be capable of providing data that are used for the formulas.
- Second, the quality of HIV data across jurisdictions would have to be comparable. This means that if there are biases in HIV reporting, those biases should be of similar direction and magnitude across areas.
- Third, incorporating HIV case-reporting data in the formula would need to produce different and more accurate assessments of "relative disease burden" and resource needs than AIDS data alone.
- Fourth, including HIV data in the RWCA allocation formulas would have to result in material variation in the relative size of awards to states and EMAs and more equitable allocations. If formula provisions, in

[5]CDC issued surveillance guidelines in December 1999 outlining the performance criteria for states' HIV/AIDS surveillance systems. The criteria outlined in the document stated that the system had to be timely (66 percent of HIV/AIDS cases reported to the health department within 6 months of diagnoses), provide accurate case counts (≤5 percent mismatched reports and ≤5 percent duplicate cases in the database), have complete ascertainment of mode of exposure to HIV (≥85 percent of reported cases, or representative sample, must have reported transmission mode after complete epidemiologic follow-up), and must include complete case reporting (≥85 percent of diagnosed cases reported to the health department). In addition, states must show that they can match to other databases of public health importance, follow up cases of public health importance, collect valid and reliable data for key data elements, and use data for public health planning (CDC, 2003i).

contrast, limit or dampen the influence of new HIV data, then the formulas may not result in more equitable allocations.

The Committee sought evidence to determine whether each of these conditions would be met if reported HIV cases were used in the formulas. Specifically, the Committee examined:

- Whether state HIV reporting systems are capable of providing data for the formulas;
- Whether the quality of HIV data across jurisdictions is comparable;
- Whether the relative ranking of need among states and EMAs varies depending on whether HIV case data or AIDS case data are employed to measure disease burden; and
- Whether the RWCA formulas are sensitive enough to translate changes in input data into more equitable allocations.

Each of these conditions proved difficult to verify. The evidence does not lead unequivocally to the conclusion that inclusion of HIV case-reporting data in the formulas would lead to a more equitable allocation of RWCA resources.

Finally, the Committee concluded that it was beyond its capacity to evaluate the HIV case-reporting system of each state and territory. The Committee's recommendations, however, could be used to make general improvements to HIV case reporting for allocating RWCA resources.

CAPABILITY OF STATE HIV REPORTING SYSTEMS TO PROVIDE DATA FOR THE FORMULAS

Three criteria are particularly relevant for evaluating the capability of HIV reporting systems to provide data for allocating resources under RWCA:

1. *Coverage:* Does each state have an HIV reporting system?
2. *Maturity:* Has the HIV reporting system of each state had sufficient time for full implementation?
3. *Full use of available data:* Would the formulas use HIV reporting data from every state with a system of HIV reporting?

Coverage

For HIV case-reporting data to be used in RWCA funding formulas, all states and territories would need to report HIV cases. As of October

2003, all states, territories, and cities except Georgia[6] and Philadelphia, had implemented a confidential HIV case-reporting system (CDC, 2003a,h) (see Chapter 3, Table 3-1). Unlike AIDS case reporting, which uses a standardized name-based reporting system, states have adopted different procedures for reporting HIV cases (Chapter 3, Figure 3-1). As of October 2003, 34 states, the Virgin Islands, American Samoa, Puerto Rico, Northern Mariana Islands, and Guam had implemented the same confidential name-based reporting of HIV infection as is used for AIDS reporting and other reportable diseases and conditions. Eight states plus the District of Columbia use a coded identifier rather than the patient name to report HIV cases. Five states use a name-to-code system; initially, names are collected and then converted to codes by the local or state health department after any necessary public health follow-up. Connecticut conducts pediatric surveillance using name-based reporting but allows name or code reporting of adults/adolescents over 13 years of age. New Hampshire allows HIV cases to be reported with or without a name (CDC, 2003a,h). Of the 15 areas that use some form of code, only two use the same code.

Maturity

Case-reporting systems for new diseases take time to mature and become fully operational. For a system to operate well, physicians and other practitioners need to be educated about the need for new requirements for disease reporting. The burden of new reporting obligations can be increased by complex data requirements, such as the creation of encryption codes for patients in states with code-based reporting. For a disease like HIV infection, where physicians may have followed patients prior to the initiation of an HIV reporting requirement, practitioners will need to report a backlog of existing patients when HIV reporting is first implemented. This takes time and clinician effort, particularly in high-morbidity states that have only recently implemented HIV reporting, such as California. Even laboratories, which rely more heavily on information automation, will still require some time to completely develop, refine, and implement reporting procedures. Further, health departments need time to design and pilot test their surveillance systems for capturing and analyzing newly reportable disease data.

While the Committee could not identify any standard criterion for

[6]Since the release of this report, Georgia implemented name-based reporting and Philadelphia adopted code-based reporting. All areas of the United States now have HIV reporting.

how much time is needed to ensure that state reporting systems are fully operational, it was clear from discussions with surveillance experts from multiple states that it takes at least 18 months to several years after a reporting system is introduced for it to reach a reasonable level of completeness and timeliness (Birkhead, 2002; Kopelman, 2002). In a previous assessment by the GAO, CDC officials estimated that it would take 1 to 3 years for the backlog of HIV cases to be entered into a new reporting system (GAO, 2000). The GAO study compared the experience of states that had been reporting HIV for different periods of time and found: "The potential for lags in reporting the older cases was clear when we compared the experience of states that had been reporting HIV cases for different lengths of time. States with long reporting histories had many more HIV cases compared with their number of AIDS cases than did newly reporting states" and that "states that begin reporting more recently may continue for some time into the future to have a larger proportion of previously diagnosed but not reported cases" (GAO, 2000).

Variations in the maturity of systems can create differential errors across states and EMAs. Immature systems capture a lower percentage of prevalent cases and are more likely to be missing key pieces of information. The HIV reporting systems of states are in various stages of maturity. Some, such as Minnesota and Colorado, implemented HIV reporting in the mid-1980s and have mature systems. Other states such as California and Pennsylvania adopted HIV reporting only recently and may require additional time to report the backlog of cases.

Several of the factors determining system accuracy, such as the ability to follow up on a backlog of cases, depend on the capacity to conduct surveillance. As one indicator of capacity, the Committee examined federal and state funding for HIV/AIDS case reporting (Appendix B). This review identified important issues. First, state HIV/AIDS surveillance programs are largely dependent upon federal financing (Appendix B). In addition, neither federal nor state sources of program funding have changed appreciably from 1999 to 2002 when many states were implementing HIV case reporting. Although the 2000 reauthorization of RWCA authorized limited additional funds to help states implement HIV reporting systems (Ryan White CARE Act. 42 U.S.C. § 300ff-13 [2003]), that funding has yet to be appropriated. Even though HIV and AIDS data may be perceived to be readily available for RWCA purposes at no additional cost, states must often include different or more-detailed data for RWCA planning than are provided in standard epidemiological reports. Such efforts can be costly, especially for states that have recently implemented HIV reporting and for states that lack adequate surveillance resources. States are facing financial crises, and state surveillance programs do not anticipate additional state contributions (see Appendix B). Thus, it is important for Congress, HRSA, and RWCA grantees to recognize the burden imposed upon the state surveillance programs as they strive to meet the information needs of RWCA. Additional funds will be required to accommodate the additional informational burdens placed on states by the RWCA.

Full Use of Available Data

Currently, CDC accepts only name-based HIV reports in the national HIV reporting database, largely because algorithms have not been developed to unduplicate HIV data from the 15 code-based states and territories. Duplicate case reporting can occur for several reasons: case reports are completed by different practitioners at several different times (HIV diagnosis, AIDS diagnosis, and death); laboratories may send results from diagnostic and staging laboratory tests (CD4+ cell count or viral load) independently to the health department; and people may move and be reported in both their original and new state of residence (CDC, 2003b). CDC estimates that approximately 5 percent of HIV cases (from name-based reporting states only) in the national dataset represent duplicate reports. CDC suggests the potential for greater duplication grows as state HIV reporting systems mature and as people remain healthier longer owing to antiretroviral therapy (CDC, 2003b).

Name-based reporting is cited as one way to facilitate elimination of duplicate reports (CDC, 1999). However, it is unclear if name-based reporting is intrinsically superior to code-based reporting for eliminating duplicate reports. Due to name variations, even name-based systems do not permit complete unduplication. In addition, code-based reporting systems were developed by some states after substantial political debate, and altering those systems would require significant legislative changes, time, and effort. For this reason, and because name-based reporting is not clearly superior to code-based reporting for the specific goal of accurately estimating the number of known cases for determining RWCA allocations, better methods for unduplicating reports for both code- and name-based reporting states need to be developed and implemented so allocation formulas can include data from all states. At the same time, the Committee recognizes that there are strong feelings, both pro and con, about the use of name-based reporting for other surveillance functions (Colfax and Bindman, 1998; Osmond et al., 1999; Hecht et al., 2000). The Committee did not take a position on these issues because its charge limits its scope of activity to reporting for allocation purposes.

Finding About States' Capability to Provide Data for the Formulas

Finding 4-1 While the Committee supports Congressional intent to incorporate data into the RWCA allocation formulas that reflect the evolving needs of the epidemic, the Committee finds that states' HIV reporting systems are neither ready nor adequate for purposes of RWCA resource allocation. One state and one city have yet to implement HIV case reporting, states' HIV reporting systems are in different stages of maturity across the United States, and the national HIV database does not include HIV cases from code-based reporting states.

COMPARABILITY OF DATA QUALITY ACROSS JURISDICTIONS

Even if states are capable of providing data on HIV cases, data would need to be of comparable quality across jurisdictions before they could be used in the RWCA formulas. Differences in the completeness and timeliness of data across jurisdictions have the potential to create significant biases in allocations. The greater the variability in the way HIV data are collected across states or EMAs, the greater are the chances for bias. The inclusion of data of varying quality across jurisdictions can decrease rather than increase the equity of resulting RWCA allocations.[7]

It is important to note that not all biases will adversely affect the fairness of resource allocation. Biases in prevalence that are consistent across states or EMAs will not affect allocations if the formulas depend only on the relative value of these measures across states or EMAs rather than the absolute value. For example, if all states underreported cases by 30 percent, then there would not necessarily be an effect on allocations, depending on the nature of the formula used (although such underreporting would be important for determining the gap between prevalent and diagnosed cases). By contrast, if variability across states in underreporting were large, such variability might have a major influence on allocations. Measuring or reducing biases may entail substantial cost. Such costs need to be weighed against the likely improvements in the allocation process. HIV data should be included in the formulas only if doing so enhances the equity of the resulting allocations.

To examine these potential biases, the Committee reviewed published evaluations of the completeness and timeliness of HIV and AIDS case-reporting systems. These studies are summarized in Table 4-1. The Committee found that most evaluations have focused on the completeness of reporting—the degree to which all individuals with these conditions are

[7]The concept of equity is discussed in Chapter 1.

reported to public health authorities. The accuracy of the elements of the report such as sex, primary risk factor, and place of residence has received less attention. To the extent that characteristics such as sex and primary risk factor are systematically misreported or underreported, estimates of the prevalence of HIV or AIDS based on those characteristics will also be biased. These types of biases would not necessarily affect allocations across states and EMAs if the proportion of such subgroups was similar across jurisdictions.

Given the more recent advent of HIV case reporting, most published evaluations have focused on AIDS rather than HIV case reporting. The Committee found little information from existing evaluations about the completeness, accuracy, and timeliness of HIV case reporting, and about the variation in these factors for HIV reporting across states and EMAs. Because of the inadequacy of available information, the Committee could not fully investigate the potential influence of possible patterns of underreporting or reporting delays on resulting formula allocations.

Completeness of AIDS and HIV Case Reporting

Studies of the completeness of reporting compare AIDS and HIV case reports with independent data on AIDS or HIV cases that should have been reported—typically medical or administrative records or death certificates. The external source may also be incomplete, so capture–recapture methods may be required.[8] Accuracy studies typically look at the correspondence between reported characteristics of cases that appear in both sources, so the results may not be representative of individuals who appear in only one or neither source. The Committee notes, however, that not all elements requested in case-reporting forms may be relevant to resource allocation. While certain data elements may be important in determining whether a state's reporting system serves the state's own case-finding purposes and identifies populations at risk, such information may not be relevant to resource allocation.

AIDS case reporting is the most complete and highest quality of nearly any disease surveillance system (Doyle et al., 2002). AIDS case reporting

[8]Capture–recapture methods can be used to adjust for incomplete ascertainment using information from two or more distinct sources. Capture–recapture estimates the size of a population (in this case, the number of cases) by making statistical assumptions about the proportion of individuals identified in various samples of the population (in the case of surveillance, reported from different sources) (Hook and Regal, 1995). The U.S. Census Bureau uses a similar method (dual-systems estimation) to estimate the U.S. population and population groups (NRC, 2001).

TABLE 4-1 Completeness and Timeliness of HIV and AIDS Case Reporting

Study	AIDS or HIV	Purpose	Methods
AIDS STUDIES			
Scheer et al. (2001)	AIDS	To determine whether AIDS surveillance misses a substantial number of persons who die with unreported AIDS.	Cross-sectional survey of decedents examined by San Francisco Medical Examiner. Decedents with positive or indeterminate HIV antibody test results were cross-referenced against the SF AIDS registry. Medical records of unreported cases reviewed to determine whether AIDS had been reported prior to death.
Klevens et al. (2001)	AIDS	To assess the completeness, validity, and timeliness of AIDS surveillance system after the 1993 surveillance case definition change.	In Louisiana and San Francisco, completeness was assessed by comparing the number of persons found in health facilities (hospitals, outpatient clinic, and private providers' offices) to the number of cases reported to the AIDS surveillance registry. In Massachusetts, completeness assessed using capture–recapture method. Validity was assessed by comparing agreement of case report with medical record for same sites. Timeliness calculated using median delay from time of diagnosis to case report for same sites.
Jara et al. (2000)	AIDS	To assess the completeness of AIDS case reporting in Massachusetts. To determine the effect of the 1993 AIDS case definition on the completeness of AIDS case reporting to the state registry and unreported case based on sex, race, and mode of transmission.	Multisource capture–recapture using 1994 Massachusetts Uniform Hospital Discharge Data Set (UHDDS) and Medicaid claims was used to evaluate completeness of Massachusetts state registry.

Setting	Results	Conclusions
San Francisco	Diagnosis and reporting of AIDS 93% complete. HIV-infected decedents were more likely than uninfected to be men and <45 years old, less likely to be Asian/Pacific Islander or Native American, and more likely to have died of suicide or drug abuse/overdose.	AIDS case reporting in San Francisco is highly complete. Current surveillance activities which identify cases from health care settings are appropriate.
Louisiana, Massachusetts, San Francisco	Completeness of case reporting in hospitals (≥93%) and outpatient clinics (≥90%); validity/concordance of info for sex was high (>98%), but lower for race/ethnicity (>83%) & mode of exposure to HIV (>67%); median reporting delay was 4 months, but varied by site from 3 to 6 months.	Completeness, validity, and timeliness of AIDS surveillance system remain high after 1993 change in case definition.
Massachusetts	92.6% (95% CI 91.6-93.5) complete using UHDDS; 94.5% (95% CI 93.7-95.3) complete using Medicaid claims dataset. Being unreported was significantly more likely in women than in men (OR = 1.72. 95% CI 1.20-2.46), and slightly more likely in IDU than in MSM (OR = 1.49, 95% CI 1.00-2.23).	Completeness of state AIDS registry is high, but there are differences by gender and mode of transmission of HIV.

Continued

TABLE 4-1 Continued

Study	AIDS or HIV	Purpose	Methods
Schwarcz et al. (1999)	AIDS	To assess the effect of the 1993 change in the AIDS case definition on the completeness and timeframe of AIDS case reporting in San Francisco.	Reporting completeness was calculated as the number of previously reported cases divided by the number of previously reported cases plus newly identified cases. Reporting delay was calculated as the difference between the case report and the date of AIDS diagnosis. AIDS cases were obtained through retrospective review of records at hospitals, public/community health clinics, and physician offices.
Klevens et al. (1997)	AIDS	To measure the effect of laboratory-initiated reporting of CD4+ results on timeliness of reporting of AIDS in the U.S.	States were categorized by whether CD4+ reporting was required. The study compared the number and percentage of AIDS cases reported through 12/31/1994 based on immunologic criteria, controlling for whether states also required HIV infection reporting.
Payne et al. (1995)	AIDS	To improve methods of identifying possible AIDS-related hospital discharges in administrative databases and to measure AIDS-reporting completeness in MA.	Fiscal year 1998 discharge data from the Massachusetts Rate Setting Commission and data from the MA AIDS Reporting System were reviewed for diagnosis codes which were HIV-specific or pertain to AIDS-defining illnesses. Medical records with HIV/AIDS diagnoses that were not reported to the reporting system were identified.
Greenberg et al. (1993)	AIDS	To assess the completeness of AIDS case reporting in NYC and to determine whether completeness of reporting differs in various populations.	Retrospective record review from 7/1988 to 11/1991 of hospital laboratory logs, death certificates, hospital discharge records, & patient registries at private physicians' offices and hospital outpatient clinics.

Setting	Results	Conclusions
San Francisco	Reporting completeness was 97%. The median reporting delay was 1 month and was shorter for persons who met the 1993 AIDS case definition (1 month) than for persons who met the 1987 case definition (3 months).	AIDS case reporting in San Francisco is highly complete, but less so for persons diagnosed at physician offices. The 1993 AIDS case definition has resulted in more timely reporting.
All 50 states and DC	States with lab-initiated CD4+ reporting were able to identify proportionately more AIDS cases and with less reporting delay than states without lab reporting.	CD4+ reporting may enable states to report AIDS cases earlier in the course of HIV disease.
Massachusetts	Of the 927 AIDS cases identified from the 3362 discharges, only 36 had not been reported. AIDS cases among women, IV drug users, and persons residing outside the Boston metropolitan area were more likely to be unreported than those among comparison groups.	Using HIV-specific ICD-9-CM codes are useful for identifying AIDS-related hospital discharges and previously unreported AIDS cases.
New York City	Overall completeness was 84%. Completeness ranged from 81 to 87% for all major gender, race, risk, borough of residence, and age subgroups. Outpatients at hospital clinics, out of state residents, persons with diagnosis other than PCP, and recently diagnosed persons less likely to be reported.	Findings indicate that NYC AIDS surveillance system functioned effectively during first decade of epidemic.

Continued

TABLE 4-1 Continued

Study	AIDS or HIV	Purpose	Methods
Elcock et al. (1993)	AIDS	To assess completeness of AIDS case reporting.	The authors initiated a validation study in seven hospitals. Cases were identified from medical discharge records with ICD-9 codes 042.0 through 042.9 for the period from 1/1989 through 12/1990. Unreported AIDS cases were identified by comparing cases in the San Mateo County AIDS registry. Based on the validation study, active surveillance efforts were initiated in one hospital, and active surveillance protocols were developed for the other hospitals. Underreporting rates were determined by comparing cases reported through the validation study or active surveillance with the total number of cases reported during the time period.
Rosenblum et al. (1992)	AIDS	To evaluate the completeness of AIDS case reporting.	Statewide or hospital-specific 1988 medical records were linked with AIDS surveillance in six sites. Medical records were reviewed for persons with diagnoses suggesting HIV or AIDS but who had not been reported to the registry.
Buehler et al. (1992)	AIDS	To describe the completeness of AIDS surveillance in specific state and local areas and to assess the completeness of reporting at a national level.	State/local completeness assessed by reviewing state and local health dept studies of completeness (conducted after 1987 and w/ ≥20 cases); most studies matched AIDS cases in registry with alternate data sources (death certificates, hospital discharge records, etc.). National completeness assessed by comparing estimate from vital records of HIV-related deaths among men 25–44 in 1988 to mortality data from AIDS case reporting in 1987.

Setting	Results	Conclusions
San Mateo County, CA	The validation study demonstrated that 24% of AIDS cases in all hospitals were not reported through passive surveillance in 1990.	The hospital-based case finding method developed by the authors may be needed to ensure that diagnosed AIDS cases from active surveillance are timely diagnosed, complete, and accurate.
Alabama, Georgia, Los Angeles, Maryland, New Jersey, Washington State	Overall completeness was 92% among 4500 hospitalized persons diagnosed with AIDS through 1988 in six sites. Completeness ranged from 89 to 97% across the sites.	Completeness of AIDS reporting was high, overall and in each major demographic and HIV exposure group. Surveillance data in these six sites were timely and accurate.
Various state and local health departments and at national level	> 80% completeness in most states and localities, but lower levels of reporting found in some outpatient settings. At national level, AIDS surveillance identified 70–90% of all HIV-related deaths in men 25–44 years of age.	Efforts to maintain levels of reporting are challenged by increasing role of outpatient diagnosis of AIDS.

Continued

TABLE 4-1 Continued

Study	AIDS or HIV	Purpose	Methods
Modesitt et al. (1990)	AIDS	To retrospectively determine the number and characteristics of AIDS cases that had gone unreported under the previous passive surveillance system.	The authors used four active surveillance methods (review of death certificate and medical records, and enhanced infection control practitioner and physician surveillance) to identify unreported cases diagnosed from 2/1/1986 to 1/31/1987, one year before active surveillance began. Cases were classified as reported by passive surveillance if the case was not reported by any reporting source after active surveillance began and more than 6 months after diagnosis.
Lindan et al. (1990)	AIDS	To examine the completeness of reporting of AIDS deaths to the California AIDS registry.	The authors compared death certificates for 1985–1986 where AIDS or an associated condition was listed as cause of death to cases reported to the California AIDS registry. Authors only examined death certificates with race classification of Hispanic, white, or black.

Setting	Results	Conclusions
Oregon	Active surveillance retrospectively identified 29 additional cases. 90% of these cases were diagnosed by a physician and cared for in hospitals that previously reported cases. Under the passive surveillance system, reporting completeness was 64%.	Passive AIDS surveillance is incomplete.
San Francisco	The proportion of deaths not reported to the California AIDS registry was similar among Hispanics, blacks, and whites (5–8%). Race misclassification varied in the AIDS registry. For Hispanics, 20% were misclassified as white, and for blacks, 4% were misclassified as white. On the other hand, only 1% of whites were misclassified as either black or Hispanic. The proportion of deaths still listed as living in the registry varied among the three different race groups. For Hispanics, blacks, and whites, 12%, 9%, and 5% were still considered living in the registry, respectively.	The findings suggest that overrepresentation of minorities among AIDS cases in the United States may be greater than indicated by current reporting data.

Continued

TABLE 4-1 Continued

Study	AIDS or HIV	Purpose	Methods
Brookmeyer and Liao (1990)	AIDS	To analyze delays in AIDS reporting in the United States.	The authors developed a simple method to analyze delays in AIDS reporting. Cases in the AIDS Public Information Dataset reported to CDC prior to 10/1/1989 were included in the analysis. Reporting delays were assessed by estimating the reporting delay distribution and determining the influence of geographic region of residence, risk group, and calendar year time of diagnosis on reporting.
Conway et al. (1989)	AIDS	To evaluate the completeness and accuracy of AIDS case reporting.	The authors identified hospital discharge records submitted from 1/1/1986 to 6/30/1987 with ICD-9 AIDS-related and AIDS-defining conditions. AIDS cases were compared to those reported in the South Carolina AIDS registry at time of their diagnosis.
Hardy et al. (1987)	AIDS	To assess the completeness of AIDS reporting.	Completeness was assessed by reviewing death certificates for period of 3 months during July through December 1985. Death certificates were selected and matched to the AIDS surveillance registries in each city. Medical records of those not in the AIDS registry were reviewed to determine if AIDS had been diagnosed.

Setting	Results	Conclusions
United States	In cases that met the pre-1987 AIDS surveillance definition, delays were shortest in regions in the Northeast and longest in the South. The influence of risk groups and calendar year of diagnosis was not consistent across each of the geographic regions. Most risk-group variation was due to longer reporting delays in the blood-transfusion and pediatric groups. An overall trend of longer delays with calendar time of diagnosis was attributed to a trend toward longer delays in the Northeast. Results were similar for cases that met the 1987 AIDS surveillance definition, except there was a trend toward shorter delays over calendar year, which was attributed to possible increased awareness of the new surveillance definition.	The results demonstrated variation in reporting delays by geographic region, risk factors, and calendar year time of diagnosis. Methods and results are useful for the evaluation of surveillance procedures to improve AIDS reporting.
South Carolina	Only 91 (59.5%) of identified AIDS cases were reported in the South Carolina AIDS registry. There was significant underreporting in blacks (53.1%) compared to whites (71.6%).	There was a degree of underreporting or under-recognition of AIDS that was considerably more extensive than previously reported.
DC, NYC, Boston, Chicago	The estimated completeness of AIDS case reporting in all four cities was 89%. In Boston and Chicago, completeness was 100%. In NYC, completeness was 87%, and in DC, completeness was 83%. Unreported cases were similar to reported cases with respect to sex, race, risk factor, and specific diagnosis.	AIDS case reporting in four participating cities was nearly complete. The study suggests that reviewing death certificates may be useful in evaluating AIDS surveillance efforts.

Continued

TABLE 4-1 Continued

Study	AIDS or HIV	Purpose	Methods
Chamberland et al. (1985)	AIDS	To evaluate the timeliness of AIDS case reporting in an active surveillance system.	The authors reviewed hospital laboratory and autopsy records in active and modified-active surveillance hospitals. Patients who had opportunistic diseases characteristic of AIDS diagnosed in 1982 (before active surveillance) and 1983 (after active surveillance) were compared to cases reported to the health department's AIDS surveillance.
HIV STUDIES			
Schwarcz et al. (2002)	HIV (Code)	To develop and evaluate the completeness, accuracy, and timeliness of a non-name-based HIV reporting system.	A population-based study of a set of nonname codes and a prospective study of a lab-initiated HIV surveillance system was conducted at San Francisco county hospital (site 1) and an HMO (site 2). Participants include persons reported with AIDS in San Francisco or patients with positive tests for HIV, p24 antigen, viral load or CD4+ cell count at the study sites.
Lee et al. (2002) (Note: Unpublished)	HIV (Name) and AIDS	To determine the proportion of adult HIV and AIDS cases reported within 6 months of diagnosis.	Used cases diagnosed from 1995–2000 reported through June 2001. Measured HIV timeliness and AIDS timeliness separately. Provided states with software program to ensure consistent measures.

Setting	Results	Conclusions
New York City	96% of AIDS patients in the active surveillance hospitals and 100% patients in the modified-active surveillance hospitals had been reported to the health department. Delays between diagnosis and reporting to health departments decreased between 1981 and during the first half of 1983 in all hospitals. During this period, the proportion of cases reported within one month of diagnosis increased from 45% to 69%.	The AIDS surveillance program in New York City was effective and that case reporting is complete for accurate analysis of disease trends.
San Francisco	*Completeness:* 89% at county hospital and 87% at HMO; *Accuracy:* proper match rate for 95% of records w/ complete codes & w/at least 50% of the codes; proper nonmatch rate for 99% of records w/complete codes & 96% w/ at least 50%; *Timeliness:* 82% completed reports from site 1 and 48% reports from site 2 were returned to the health department within 60 days; median days between test and receipt of test report: 9 (site 1), 7 (site 2); *Risk info* was present for 84% reports from hospital and on 71% reports from HMO.	A nonname-based laboratory reporting system for HIV is feasible.
For HIV: 27** states with name-based reporting systems. For AIDS: 52 states	HIV: 83.4% of cases reported within 6 months of diagnosis. AIDS: 71.1% of AIDS cases reported within 6 months.	26 of 27 states met timeliness standard for HIV reporting (>66% of HIV cases reported within 6 months of diagnosis). 45 of 52 states met timeliness standard for AIDS reporting (>66% of AIDS cases reported within 6 months of diagnosis).

Continued

TABLE 4-1 Continued

Study	AIDS or HIV	Purpose	Methods
Solomon et al. (1999)	HIV (Code)	To evaluate the uniqueness and completeness of the UI number, the accuracy of the reporting, and the completeness of HIV reporting in a statewide nonname-based HIV surveillance system.	Uniqueness of UI number was assessed by measuring the contribution of each component of the UI to the uniqueness of the number. Accuracy was assessed by examining the AIDS registry for multiples of identical UIs. Completeness of HIV reporting was assessed by matching the HIV counseling and testing (C&T) reports with AIDS registry data.
Marsh et al. (1999) (Note: Unpublished)	HIV (Code)	To evaluate the performance of non-name-coded identifiers to CDC's performance standards.	13 nonname codes were constructed using preliminary AIDS case reports collected in Los Angeles (from 9/97 to 12/97 and HIV and AIDS reports collected in New Jersey (from 3/98 to 1/99). Each code was then tested to assess proper match rate and proper nonmatch rate.
CDC (1998)	HIV (Code)	To evaluate UI surveillance for HIV for completeness, timeliness, potential for UI matching to other databases, and proportion of reports with full UI code.	The study evaluated cases reported from 1/1995 to 6/1996 in two states (Maryland and Texas) with UI-based HIV surveillance systems. Completeness was assessed by comparing UI-database reports w/AIDS surveillance registry data & HIV counseling/testing sites data. Timeliness was calculated by median delay from time of test to report. Ability for epidemiological follow-up was assessed by evaluating ability to follow UI reports back to patient record (in TX) and by provider compliance in maintain patient surveillance logs (in MD).

Setting	Results	Conclusions
Maryland	When complete, the 12-digit UI number provided unduplicated count that was 99.8% unique, 99.9% unique with only last 4 digits of SSN, DOB, and race, and 77.7% unique if last 4 digits of SSN were missing. Overall completeness of reporting for HIV tests was 87.8% (matching complete UI with HIV C&T reports) and 84.8% (matching UI w/AIDS registry data).	Findings demonstrate that a nonname-based system can provide accurate, timely, and valid data concerning the scope of the HIV epidemic, without the creation of statewide name-based registry.
Los Angeles County and New Jersey	In Los Angeles, the performance of codes ranged from 87.3% to 96.1% on subset of AIDS reports in which all data used to construct the codes were complete and in which codes matched exactly. In New Jersey, performance of the codes ranged from 74.3% to 90.8%.	Results from these two locations suggest that meeting CDC performance standards in nonname surveillance systems will be a challenge. It is critical for states implementing surveillance based on non-name identifiers to use standardized evaluation methods.
Maryland, Texas	*Maryland*—50% complete (UI data compared to AIDS cases), 52% complete (UI data compared to HIV counseling/testing site data); median time of HIV test to receipt of report by state health dept: 20 days (range 1–847); 71% of reports with full UI code; *Texas*—26% complete (UI data compared to AIDS cases); median time of HIV test to receipt of report by state health department: batched reports—173 days (range 26–974), individual reports—59 days (range 2–906); 62% of reports had full UI code; 60% of reports could be matched for follow-up.	Findings suggest some limitations to use of SSN-based UI for HIV surveillance, UIs limited the performance of an HIV surveillance system, and that UIs complicated efforts to collect risk-behavior information. Both systems demonstrated timely reporting.

Continued

TABLE 4-1 Continued

Study	AIDS or HIV	Purpose	Methods
Klevens et al. (1998)	HIV (Name)	To evaluate the completeness of name-based HIV reporting.	Medical records of potentially HIV-infected patients at a sample of health care facilities in Louisiana were reviewed and matched with HIV/AIDS surveillance registry.
Meyer et al. (1994)	HIV (Name)	To assess the completeness of HIV reporting among hospital inpatients whose records listed diagnostic codes for HIV infection but who did not meet the 1987 case definition.	Hospital discharge data for 1986 through 1990 were searched for patients with any HIV-related discharge codes who did not meet the AIDS case definition. These reports were compared to cases in the state HIV registry.

*All AIDS cases in the United States are reported using a confidential, name-based reporting system.
**Timeliness of reporting of HIV cases from states conducting alternatives to name-based reporting were not included.

completeness has increased over time. Earlier studies (Hardy et al., 1987; Conway et al., 1989; Modesitt et al., 1990; Buehler et al., 1992; Rosenblum et al., 1992; Elcock et al., 1993; Greenberg et al., 1993) demonstrate completeness rates ranging from 60 percent to 92 percent. More recent studies (Schwarcz et al., 1999; Jara et al., 2000; Klevens et al., 2001; Scheer et al., 2001) show completeness rates more consistently higher at 93 percent to 97 percent.

The Committee notes, however, that completeness rates may vary across these studies in part because some examine the completeness of passive reporting systems while others examine active reporting systems.

Setting	Results	Conclusions
Louisiana	Completeness of HIV reporting was 96.8% in hospitals, 98.9% in clinics, 95.6% in private physicians' offices.	Evaluation indicates that completeness of HIV reporting is comparable to that of AIDS reporting.
South Carolina	Of 396-HIV infected hospital inpatients, 313 (79%) had been reported to the state registry. This proportion varies from 81% in black women to 76% in white men. There are more substantial differences in mode of HIV exposure, varying from 85% in MSM and 81% in IDUs to 61% in blood product recipients. Temporal improvements were observed in completeness of HIV reporting among hospital patients and prior to their first admission. Women were more likely than men to be reported prior rather than during or after their first hospital admission (71% vs. 55%, $p<0.01$). Of the 155 HIV-infected patients with CD4 counts, 41 met the 1993 case definition but not the 1987 definition.	In SC, most diagnosed, hospitalized, HIV-infected patients had been reported to the state HIV registry, with improvements over time. Findings suggest that the 1993 AIDS case definition will improve the ability to monitor severe morbidity related to HIV.

Passive surveillance typically has lower rates of completeness because it relies on the cooperation of health care professionals to report AIDS cases (Elcock et al., 1993). Active reporting (which involves searching death records, hospital discharges, and other administrative data sources to identify cases that have not been reported to the system) tend to have much higher rates of completeness. All states are now funded by CDC to conduct active surveillance of AIDS (CDC, 1999).

Published studies that primarily examined the effect of the 1993 case definition expansion on completeness of AIDS surveillance in Louisiana, Massachusetts, and San Francisco found that completeness typically tops

90 percent and approaches 100 percent (Schwarcz et al., 1999; Jara et al., 2000; Klevens et al., 2001). Reporting completeness by race/ethnicity or risk factors, however, varied. In San Francisco, completeness of AIDS reporting did not differ significantly by race, gender, or age (Schwarcz et al., 1999). In contrast, unreported cases in Massachusetts were significantly more likely to be female (OR = 1.72, 95% CI 1.20-2.46), and injection drug users were slightly more likely to be unreported than cases of transmission between men who have sex with men (OR = 1.49, 95% CI 1.00-2.23) (Jara et al., 2000). These findings are in agreement with findings from earlier studies that demonstrated reporting completeness of around 90 percent (Hardy et al., 1987; Buehler et al., 1992; Rosenblum et al., 1992) and similar reporting variations by race/ethnicity or risk factor (Conway et al., 1989; Lindan et al., 1990). The greater the variability in the completeness of data across states or EMAs, the greater the chance for bias. Minimizing variation is more important for allocation decisions than a high average level of completeness.

Studies examining the completeness of HIV reporting (Meyer et al., 1994; CDC, 1998; Klevens et al., 1998; Marsh et al., 1999; Solomon et al., 1999; Schwarcz et al., 2002) compared reported HIV cases to the number of individuals in care for HIV-related illness. These studies show that HIV case reports are only slightly less complete than AIDS case reports. No published studies have directly scrutinized cross-state variability in HIV completeness rates. CDC is currently conducting an evaluation of cross-state completeness, but results were unavailable when this report was prepared. Cross-state variability is likely to be higher for HIV than for AIDS case reporting, however, because the HIV completeness rate is related to the use of health care services by HIV-infected persons. Persons with asymptomatic HIV infection and those who do not know they are infected may not present for care, while those with syndromic AIDS are more likely to present for care. The aggressiveness of HIV counseling and testing policies also varies greatly across states. It is therefore likely that estimates of HIV prevalence may be both more biased and more variable than are estimates of AIDS prevalence and incidence.

Timeliness of AIDS and HIV Case Reporting

Timing studies identify the lag between the first diagnosis of a case and its report to CDC by comparing reported cases to an external source. Variation in reporting delays across jurisdictions can result in systematic biases in estimates of HIV or AIDS prevalence and incidence. While statistical adjustments are routinely used to account for incompleteness and delays in AIDS reporting (Green, 1998), these adjustments often assume that patterns of delays in missing reports are constant over time and across geographic areas. Estimates of AIDS or HIV incidence or prevalence resulting from an AIDS or HIV case-reporting system will be biased if the assumptions made in correcting for reporting delays are not met, but such assumptions are usually difficult, if not impossible, to assess.

Studies of timeliness of AIDS case reporting (Chamberland et al., 1985; Brookmeyer and Liao, 1990; Schwarcz et al., 1999; Klevens et al., 2001) indicate important variability in reporting delays across state and local reporting systems. Median reporting delays vary from 1 month to 6 months. States with lab-initiated CD4+ cell reporting had less reporting delay than states without such reporting (Klevens et al., 1997).

Brookmeyer and Liao (1990) and Pagano and colleagues (1994) have developed statistical methods for estimating and adjusting for AIDS reporting delays. One earlier study by Brookmeyer and Liao (1990) found significant geographical variation in the timeliness of AIDS reports; delays were shortest in the Northeast and longest in the South. Pagano and colleagues (1994) found significant variation in time trends in AIDS reporting delays by region. From 1983 to 1990, reporting delays appeared to increase most in the Northeast and decrease most in the Central region.

More recent research (Klevens et al., 2001) examined the timeliness of reporting in three locations before and after the 1993 change in the CDC definition of AIDS.[9] California saw a substantial decrease in the median reporting delay, from 14 to 3 months. The change in the median reporting delay in Louisiana and Massachusetts was less. After 1993, however, the median reporting delay differed substantially across states, varying from 6 months in Massachusetts to 3 months in California and Louisiana.

At the time of this report, no published studies had examined the timeliness of HIV case reporting. However, CDC provided the Committee with results from an evaluation of the timeliness of HIV and AIDS reporting in 10 areas.[10] The CDC specified, as a minimum performance standard, that 66 percent or more of HIV and AIDS cases should be reported to the state within 6 months of diagnosis (CDC, 2003e). The evaluation was designed to determine the proportion of HIV and AIDS cases among adults and adolescents > 13 years of age reported within 6 months

---

[9]In 1993, CDC expanded the AIDS case definition to include individuals with CD4+ cell counts of ≤ 200 cells/μL, or less than 14 percent of total lymphocyte, and three additional conditions among HIV-infected persons (CDC, 1992).

[10]The evaluation uses standardized protocols to assess the performance of HIV reporting systems for eight attributes: timeliness, accuracy, ascertainment of transmission mode, completeness, validity of data elements, ability to match to other public health databases, ability to follow up on cases of public health importance, and use of data for public health planning. With the exception of the timeliness analyses, the results of this evaluation will not be available until after this report is issued.

of initial diagnosis of HIV or AIDS. Using the national HIV/AIDS Reporting System (HARS) as the data source for the evaluation, CDC examined HIV and AIDS cases diagnosed from 1995 to 1999.[11] HIV timeliness and AIDS timeliness were evaluated separately using an 18-month follow-up (CDC, 2003e). Results show that 88 percent of HIV cases were reported within six months of diagnosis, with all 27 states that reported HIV during this time period meeting the performance standard (CDC, 2003f). Approximately 78 percent of AIDS cases nationally were reported within 6 months of diagnosis, with 50 of 52 (96 percent) states (including the District of Columbia and Puerto Rico) meeting the standard (CDC, 2003f). The evaluation showed variation, however, in the timeliness of reported cases across states.[12] The percent of HIV cases reported within 6 months varied from 67 percent to 100 percent across states, while the percent of AIDS cases reported within 6 months varied from 64 percent to 96 percent (CDC, 2003e). The results did indicate that the timeliness of HIV reporting improved over time; in 1995, 86 percent of HIV cases were reported within 6 months of diagnosis, compared with 91 percent of cases in 1999 (Lee et al., 2002).

CDC's evaluation may shed light on the relative completeness and timeliness of HIV and AIDS case reporting in selected jurisdictions. However, the evaluation was not designed to specifically address the use of these data in RWCA resource allocation studies, and thus may not address key issues related to differential bias across jurisdictions. Additional studies are needed to examine the comparability of data from the HIV case-reporting system across jurisdictions for the purpose of allocating RWCA resources.

Methodological Consistency

The Committee noted three areas in which variation in methods (across states and EMAs) for finding and reporting cases of HIV might introduce differential biases in HIV cases. First, variation across jurisdictions in the rates of migration of people living with HIV or AIDS can affect allocations. The distribution of RWCA funds is based primarily on AIDS cases, which reflect the place of residence at time of the original AIDS diagnosis. Although individuals with AIDS may move to a new state or metropolitan area, the state or metropolitan area where the per-

---

[11]A timeliness measure for AIDS was calculated for each of the 5 years (1995, 1996, 1997, 1998, and 1999). In states with HIV reporting, an evaluation of the timeliness of HIV reporting was initiated 2 years after the implementation of the reporting system.

[12]Data were provided without state identifiers in this analysis.

son was originally diagnosed continues to receive funding for that person. As a result, immigration of persons with AIDS after diagnosis can lead to inequitable allocation because jurisdictions that now provide care for those persons do not receive funding for those cases. Many grantees have expressed concern about this issue (LaMendola, 2002). It is important to consider the rate of out-migration as well, as jurisdictions may receive funding for individuals that no longer live there. Individuals with HIV that have not progressed to AIDS may be even more mobile and likely to migrate to another state or EMA over the course of their lifetime than individuals with AIDS. Thus, the potential incorporation of data on HIV cases into the RWCA formulas raises concerns about the possible inequitable allocations that may result from increased migration of people with HIV.

The evidence regarding migration is limited. Early in the epidemic, the vast majority of individuals living with HIV were concentrated in several major urban areas. With time, HIV spread to other areas of the country and into nonmetropolitan areas. Studies concluded that the nonmetropolitan areas were the sites of greatest rate of increase in AIDS cases in the early 1990s (Lam and Liu, 1994). A number of early studies indicated that large numbers of persons who were infected with HIV in an urban area moved home to rural communities (Verghese et al., 1989; Davis and Stapleton, 1991; Ellis and Muschkin, 1996). Other studies documented that a sizable number of persons were diagnosed in one state or metropolitan area, but living in another area (Davis and Stapleton, 1991; Verghese et al., 1995; Beltrami et al., 1999). One study that examined migration of persons with AIDS across states (Buehler et al., 1995) found that approximately 1 in 10 persons with AIDS changed his or her place of residence between diagnosis and death, and half of these individuals moved to another state. The researchers concluded that place of residence at diagnosis was a reasonable measure of the impact of AIDS in large urban communities with heavy concentration of the epidemic, but that residence at time of diagnosis underestimated the impact of AIDS in rural communities. A more recent study (Berk et al., 2003) based on the national probability sample of persons with HIV in care found that only 8 percent of persons with HIV migrated from urban to rural areas. The researchers concluded that urban areas are drawing as many people with HIV as rural areas (Berk et al., 2003).

CDC is currently evaluating migration among people with HIV and the assignment of cases to jurisdictions as part of its interstate deduplication evaluation project (CDC, 2003b), but results were not available at the time of this report. An evaluation of such possible effects should be part of developing standard protocols that would be acceptable to CDC for reporting.

Second, states and territories vary in the procedures laboratories use to report HIV cases (Table 4-2). According to CDC data, in 40 of the 54 states and territories (74 percent), laboratories report CD4+ cell results, and 43 of 54 (80 percent) report plasma viral load results. Those states with laboratory CD4+ reporting vary in the reportable levels; for example, some states set the reportable level at <200 cells/μL, while others set it at <400 cells/μL, <500 cells/μL, or <800 cells/μL. In addition, not all states have viral load laboratory reporting. Twenty-nine (54 percent of) states, Puerto Rico, the U.S. Virgin Islands, American Samoa, and the District of Columbia had some form of electronic laboratory reporting for HIV (CDC, 2003c,d).

Those states without laboratory-based reporting will systematically underestimate the number of patients with diagnosed HIV infection, which may bias allocations. While electronic laboratory-based reporting improves the completeness of HIV reporting, it adds substantial workload because patients diagnosed with HIV infection require numerous laboratory tests to manage their antiretroviral therapy, and each test must be linked to a known case or determined to be a new case.

The third methodological phenomenon that might introduce differential estimates among states is the aggressiveness of case finding. Some states screen more people for HIV and conduct more follow-up investigations than other states. For example, states that have more aggressive screening programs (e.g., those that screen high proportions of pregnant women, arrestees and prisoners, and premarital couples) will likely report a greater percentage of cases than states that do not. States that make fuller use of anonymous testing will report a lower percentage of cases than those that make minimal use of this option or prohibit it by law.[13] Anonymous testing tends to decrease reporting because there is no identified person to report.

---

[13]HIV testing is conducted either confidentially or anonymously. With confidential testing, a person's name is recorded with the test result. Other health care personnel and the state and/or local health department may have access to this information. With anonymous testing, there is no link between the patient's name or other identifying information and the test result (Kaiser Family Foundation, 2003). All states offer confidential testing. As of October 2003, 10 states (Alabama, Idaho, Iowa, Mississippi, Nevada, North Carolina, North Dakota, South Carolina, South Dakota, Tennessee) and the U.S. Virgin Islands did not offer anonymous testing (See Table 4-1).

TABLE 4-2 Status of CD4+ Cell Count and HIV Viral Load Reporting (as of April 2003)

State/Area	CD4+ Reporting	Reportable Level (CD4+ Cell Count/μL)	HIV Viral Load
Alabama	No		No
Alaska	Yes	<200	Yes
American Samoa	No		No
Arizona	No		Yes
Arkansas	Yes	All	Yes
California	No		Yes
Colorado	Yes	<500	Yes
Connecticut	Yes	<200	No
Delaware	Yes	<200	Yes
District of Columbia	Yes	<200	No
Florida	No		No
Georgia	No		No
Hawaii	Yes	<200	Yes
Idaho	Yes	<500	Yes
Illinois	Yes	<200	Yes
Indiana	Yes	All	Yes
Iowa	Yes	<400	Yes
Kansas	Yes	<500	Yes
Kentucky	Yes	All	Yes
Louisiana	Yes	All	Yes
Maine	Yes	<200	Yes
Maryland	Yes	<200	Yes
Massachusetts	Yes	<200	No
Michigan	No		No
Minnesota	No		Yes
Mississippi	Yes	All	Yes
Missouri	Yes	All	Yes
Montana	No		Yes
Nebraska	Yes	<800	Yes
Nevada	Yes	<500	Yes
New Hampshire	Yes	All	Yes
New Jersey	Yes	<200	Yes
New Mexico	Yes	All	Yes
New York	Yes	<500	Yes
North Carolina	No		Yes
North Dakota	No		Yes
Ohio	Yes	<200	Yes
Oklahoma	Yes	<500	Yes
Oregon	Yes	<200	Yes
Pennsylvania	Yes	<200	Yes
Puerto Rico	Yes	<200	No
Rhode Island	Yes	<200	Yes
South Carolina	Yes	<200	Yes
South Dakota	No		No

Continued

TABLE 4-2 Continued

State/Area	CD4 Reporting	Reportable Level (CD4+ Cell Count/µL)	HIV Viral Load
Tennessee	Yes	<200	Yes
Texas	Yes	<200	Yes
Utah	Yes	All	Yes
Vermont	No		Yes
Virgin Islands	Yes	<200	No
Virginia	No		Yes
Washington	Yes	<200	Yes
West Virginia	Yes	<200	Yes
Wisconsin	Yes	<200	Yes
Wyoming	Yes	<200	Yes

SOURCE: CDC, 2003c.

Findings About Comparability of Data

Finding 4-2 Different rates of completeness and timeliness of HIV reports across states and EMAs have the potential to create significant biases in RWCA formula allocations. To date, studies have not answered key questions about the comparability of HIV case-reporting data for use in resource allocation formulas. Additional studies are needed to examine the comparability of data from the HIV case-reporting system across states and EMAs.

RELATIVE DISEASE BURDEN AND RANKING OF NEED ACROSS JURISDICTIONS

Many grantees, researchers, advocates, and policy makers assume that adding HIV reporting data will produce a fairer allocation of resources than will reliance on ELCs alone. One premise underlying this assumption is that the HIV epidemic is in different stages of "maturity" in different areas of the country. Here maturity refers to the length of time that the epidemic of HIV infection has been established in at-risk populations. Because the risk of AIDS is low in the first years after infection and then rises over time, one would expect the ratio of reported HIV to AIDS cases to be higher in more recently infected populations than in populations where the epidemic had been established for a longer period of time, and most infected individuals acquired HIV many years ago. Thus assuming very different stages of maturity of the epidemic would lead one to expect significant variation in this ratio across jurisdictions.[14] States that believe their HIV epidemic was established relatively recently suspect that the current measure (based on AIDS cases alone) places them at a disadvantage in RWCA formula allocations. If, however, the epidemic is at similar levels of maturity across jurisdictions, and therefore the ratio of reported AIDS cases to reported HIV cases is relatively constant, including data on HIV cases in the formula will, in fact, have little influence on the relative measure of disease burden, and hence little influence on the awards.

Although it seems reasonable to assume that the epidemic is in various stages of maturity in different jurisdictions, it is difficult to confirm this belief. Some data do suggest the possibility of regional variation—specifically that the epidemic may be growing more quickly in the southern region of the United States than elsewhere. The South is registering a growing share of newly reported AIDS cases, rising from 40 percent to 46 percent between 1996 and 2001 (Kates and Ruiz, 2002).[15] While estimated AIDS incidence (new AIDS cases) for the entire United States remained relatively flat (increasing only 1 percent) between 2000 and 2001, estimated AIDS incidence in the South rose by 9 percent during that period (Kates and Ruiz, 2002). AIDS incidence fell in the Northeast by 8 percent and in the West by 4 percent, but rose in the Midwest by 2 percent during the same time period (Kates and Ruiz, 2002).

Inspection of the cumulative distribution of AIDS cases (reported by year of diagnosis and adjusted for reporting delays) by state and EMA from 1981 to 2001[16] suggests that the AIDS incidence curves have fairly similar—though not identical—shape across states over time (Figures 4-1 and 4-2); similarity in shape implies roughly similar epidemic dynamics. These figures also illustrate shifts over time in these curves, implying that the stage of epidemic maturity differs somewhat from state to state (and from EMA to EMA). Each individual curve in the figure represents the cumulative reporting of AIDS cases in a given jurisdiction (EMA or state) from 1981 to 2001. Hence, all curves begin at 0 percent in 1981 and reach 100 percent by 2001.[17]

---

[14]HIV cases refers to reported cases of HIV that have not progressed to AIDS. Reported HIV cases are exclusive of reported AIDS cases.

[15]In Kates and Ruiz (2002), the southern region of the United States was defined as including the following states: Alabama, Arkansas, Delaware, District of Columbia, Florida, Georgia, Kentucky, Louisiana, Maryland, Mississippi, North Carolina, Oklahoma, South Carolina, Tennessee, Texas, Virginia, and West Virginia.

[16]These figures include cases reported through December 2002 but in which the diagnosis year was 2001 or earlier.

[17]There is an implicit assumption in the construction of these figures that all jurisdictions have attained the same "100 percent mature" level by 2001, artificially normalizing the distributions to 2001.

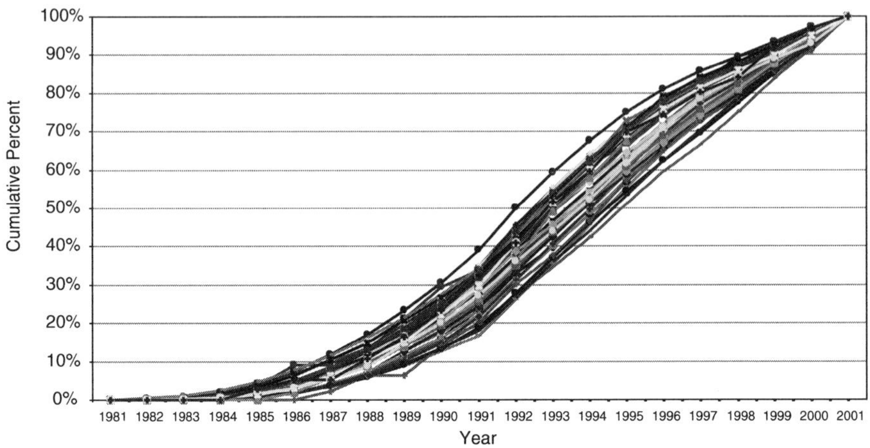

FIGURE 4-1 Cumulative AIDS cases by state and diagnosis year, adjusted for reporting delays, 1981 to 2001.
SOURCE: CDC, 2003g.

For any calendar year between these two anchors, curves denote the cumulative cases reported up to that point in time (as a percent of the eventual total cases reported by 2001). In Figure 4-1, for example, the topmost curve denotes cumulative AIDS cases in state A. This curve indicates that 50 percent of all AIDS cases reported to have occurred by 2001 in state A had been reported by 1992; 75 percent of these cases had been reported by 1995. At any given time, state A had reported a greater fraction of its 2001 cumulative total than any other state; in this sense, this state was at the leading edge of the epidemic. By contrast, the epidemic is least mature in state B (the bottom curve in the figure). More than half of state B's eventual total AIDS cases were reported after 1994; 75 percent of all cases had not been reported until 1998. The horizontal distance between any two curves represents the time lag between states in attaining the same cumulative proportion of reported AIDS cases—a measure of "epidemic maturity." Figures 4-1 and 4-2 illustrate the extensive overlap in the cumulative distribution cases over the course of the epidemic across jurisdictions, with the 50th percentile of all cases reached between the earliest and latest state being only 3 years. The conclusion is that while we might expect a higher ratio of HIV to AIDS cases in some jurisdictions than others, this effect is not likely to be particularly large.

Using the ratio of HIV to AIDS cases as a proxy for epidemic maturity has some limitations. Variation in the proportion of HIV to AIDS cases can be plausibly attributed to factors beyond differences in the maturity of the epidemic, such as regional variations in treatment practices that

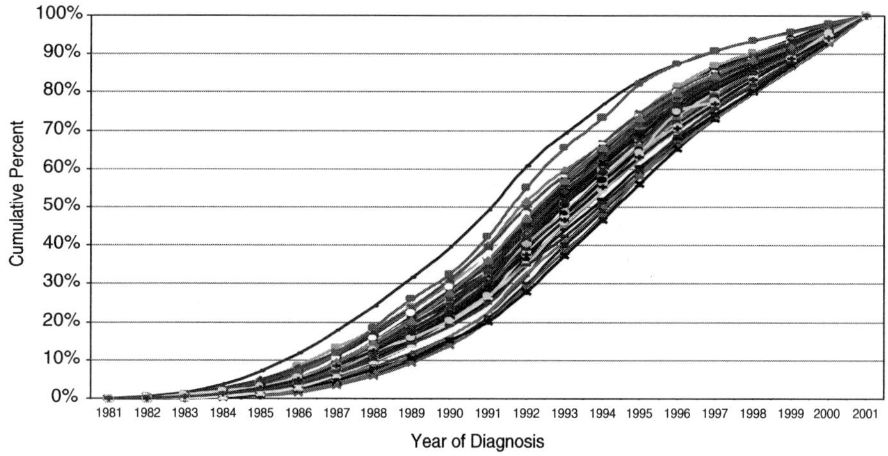

FIGURE 4-2 Cumulative AIDS cases by EMA and diagnosis year, adjusted for reporting delays, 1981 to 2001.
SOURCE: CDC, 2003g.

delay the onset of AIDS. States and EMAs may also differ in the aggressiveness and quality of HIV screening and case finding, with some identifying a higher proportion of new cases, thus increasing the ratio of HIV to AIDS cases.

Finding Regarding Relative Disease Burden and Ranking of Need

Finding 4-3 The Committee could not confirm the hypothesis that the maturity of the HIV epidemic varies significantly across regions. If the ratio of reported AIDS cases to HIV cases differs across states or EMAs, including data on HIV cases in the RWCA formulas could affect the relative measure of disease burden and the allocations. Data examined by the Committee suggest that the rate of new HIV infections is somewhat greater in the southeastern region of the United States. Due to the lack of HIV case data in all areas, however, assumptions regarding interregional variability in epidemic maturity need further assessment.

SENSITIVITY OF THE FORMULA ALLOCATIONS TO CHANGES IN THE UNDERLYING INPUT DATA

In this section, the Committee examines whether the allocation formula would be sensitive to changes in the underlying data, and whether variation across measures of the relative number of reported cases of HIV in a state or EMA changes the relative allocation of resources. The Committee originally intended to conduct extensive "what-if" policy simulations. That is, it intended to compare different factors in the funding formulas to examine the impact of including HIV cases on resource allocations across regions, and to compare the inclusion of HIV cases to other features, such as hold-harmless provisions, set-asides, minimum funding thresholds, and the potential addition of new EMAs based on a more inclusive definition of HIV burden. The Committee could not examine the effect of including HIV data in the formula because data on HIV cases were not available from all states, including several key states with a high disease burden. Since data from those states could have a large influence on results, any analyses based on partial data could be very misleading. Nevertheless, the analyses and policy assessment in Appendix C highlight the implications of current policies. These findings should allow policy makers to explore the implications of proposed changes in funding allocations.

Instead, the Committee chose to explore how assessments of the "fairness" of those awards might be influenced by including data on estimated HIV and AIDS prevalence.[18] In particular, the Committee examined what the current allocation is using the ELCs (the measure now used for RWCA resource allocation) and combined estimates of HIV prevalence and AIDS prevalence.[19]

The Committee also employed multiple linear regression analysis to identify predictors of RWCA Title I and Title II funding. The findings from these analyses are summarized in the following pages, but are discussed in detail in Appendix C.

In its analyses, the Committee examined total allocations per case (i.e., Title I and II funds) across states and EMAs as a point of departure. The Committee acknowledges that there are many reasons why an equitable system would depart from this standard, including unequal costs of care, unequal need, differences in the efficiency with which jurisdictions apply funds, differences in the quality and comprehensiveness of the

---

[18]For states with mature name-based HIV reporting systems, estimates of HIV prevalence were based on data from their individual case-reporting systems. For code-based states or states without mature name-based reporting systems, CDC used modeling to produce the HIV prevalence estimates. California and Massachusetts declined to release CDC's estimates of HIV prevalence, and thus no data were available for these two states.

[19]These data were provided by the CDC based on a data request to the states. The Committee also examined current allocations using AIDS prevalence alone. The differences in allocations using estimated AIDS prevalence and ELCs were not informative, suggesting that any methodological differences between the calculation of ELCs and the calculation of AIDS prevalence is not important for the purposes of identifying allocation variations.

existing resource base from one jurisdiction to another, and differences in economies of scale.

In some instances, deviations from the "equal dollars per case" standard will highlight disparities to be corrected; in other instances, they will confirm the view that the system is applying appropriate flexibility to its standards to reflect legitimate differences in need from one jurisdiction to another. Viewed in this light, the Committee's goal is not to hold up equal dollar allocation as an absolute standard, but rather to make explicit the consequences of allocation formulas that are the product of complex political negotiation, epidemiological evidence, and competing conceptions of fairness.

Findings About the Sensitivity of the Formula to Changes in the Underlying Data

Finding 4-4 When examining combined Title I and II funds, the Committee found that those awards depart from a nationwide standard of equivalent spending per unit of HIV burden. Although such departures may be appropriate, the justification for such departures was not clear. Such departures persist regardless of the measure of disease burden used, but they are most pronounced when using a combined measure of estimated HIV prevalence and AIDS prevalence.

Finding 4-5 With the exception of San Francisco, Title I formula allocations per ELC are quite uniform across EMAs. Because of hold-harmless provisions, the San Francisco EMA receives significantly greater resources per ELC than do other EMAs. Removal of this provision would reduce San Francisco's allocation to within the reported range for other EMAs. However, removing the hold-harmless protection would have a small influence on other EMAs, which would observe a 2.6 percent increase in their allocation if San Francisco's allocation were reduced. As noted by others (GAO, 2000), hold-harmless provisions have a small overall effect on allocations to EMAs, yet a large effect on a single EMA.

The Committee identified several structural features that dampen the effect of variation introduced by the addition of HIV cases, including:

- **Presence of an EMA in a state.** Disparities in funding per ELC across states and localities appear most pronounced between states that do and do not have an EMA. Although Title II funding formulas include adjustments for non-EMA states, the cumulative effect of these provisions is small compared with cross-state disparities in Title I funding. Moreover, states whose ELCs are concentrated within an EMA benefit from current allocation rules. This is because reported cases within an EMA contribute to both a state's Title I award and its Title II funding. States that lack an EMA face a corresponding disadvantage.

- **Explicit set-asides for non-EMA states under Title II.** Several features of the Title II award are designed to compensate jurisdictions that lack an EMA. These include the 20 percent of the Title II award that is reserved for non-EMA states and the minimum Title II base award of $500,000 per state. Both of these formula features would not be affected if HIV plus AIDS cases, instead of just AIDS cases, were used in the formulas.
- **Set-asides for emerging communities.** Title II Emerging Communities provisions, defined as cities with 500–1,999 reported AIDS cases in the most recent 5 years, expressly set funds aside for non-EMA localities. While the Emerging Communities provision may be an appropriate response to the geographic expansion of the epidemic, it will reduce the effect of including HIV data in allocation formulas.

Finding 4-6 Several structural features of the Title I and Title II funding formulas—most notably the counting of EMA cases in both Title I and II state formula allocations, but also such measures as hold-harmless provisions and set-asides for emerging communities—have a large influence on resulting allocations. Such structural features may dampen the effect of variation introduced by the addition of HIV cases, and could obviate the potential benefits of adding HIV cases to the CARE Act allocation formulas.

The Committee notes with concern that southeastern states appear to receive the smallest allocations per ELC under current allocation rules. Some of this disparity arises from the rurality of southeastern states. People living with AIDS in the Southeast are less likely to reside in EMAs than are their counterparts in other regions. Viewing combined Title I and Title II funding, southeastern states are thus less likely to benefit from counting of EMA cases in both the Title I and II formulas. Southeastern states might also benefit from changes in RWCA allocation formulas that consider HIV in addition to reported AIDS cases. However, the role of EMAs in RWCA formula allocations appears to matter more than alternative definitions of HIV burden in accounting for regional differences in per ELC funding.

The Committee also notes the discordance between the intent of the RWCA formulas and their structure. RWCA is statutorily limited to acting as a payer of last resort, as it precludes expenditures for anything covered by other public or private insurance or benefit programs. Funds are intended for services to individuals who are low income, and uninsured or underinsured. Yet formula allocations are made purely on the estimated number of living AIDS cases. Insofar as the current RWCA case-reporting–based formula counts patients that have other sources of insurance or funding, it overestimates the number of cases that qualify for RWCA services, just as it may underestimate the needs of a particular jurisdiction with greater proportions of patients with HIV who are not included in the formula but who would qualify for RWCA services. The current formulas also do not account for variations in the costs of care or fiscal capacity across Title I and II jurisdictions. A 1995 GAO report cited similar concerns with the formulas and concluded that the equity of the formulas could be improved through the use of more appropriate measures of services costs and funding capacity of jurisdictions. Other formula-based programs, including Medicaid and the Substance Abuse and Mental Health block grants, consider costs and/or fiscal capacity (NRC, 2003).

Finding 4-7 RWCA Title I and II formula allocations are determined by the ELC. Thus, they do not take into account factors defining those for whom such funds were intended, such as lack of insurance and special needs. That is, there are no provisions to estimate the number of persons in need of a "payer of last resort."

METHODS FOR IMPROVING DATA FOR THE FORMULAS

The Committee believes that there are several ways to improve the overall quality and completeness of the HIV case-reporting system for allocating resources under RWCA. First and foremost is the need to include all reported HIV cases in the national database rather than only those reported from states with name-based reporting. Other sources of data, particularly from laboratories, and potentially from pharmacies and other drug providers, can also be more fully utilized to improve the completeness and comparability of HIV reporting systems.[20] Twenty-nine states rely on electronic laboratory-based reporting of HIV test results as

---

[20]Most states specifically require laboratories (as well as medical providers) to report cases of HIV or AIDS to the state health department pursuant to their state disease reporting laws or regulations. The Health Insurance Portability and Accountability Act allows covered entities to release this health information to state health departments in compliance with state disease-reporting laws. States that do not expressly require laboratories to report would have to enact a statute or issue a regulation (depending on the state's statutory structure) to allow laboratories to report. An amendment to the state's reporting statute or regulation could accomplish this rather simply and ensure that the laboratory is subject to

part of their HIV reporting systems; comparability in the completeness and timeliness of reporting could be enhanced if all states adopted electronic laboratory reporting. States can also boost their completeness of reporting by including laboratory reporting of other tests unique to HIV infection, such as plasma viral load, CD4+ cell counts, and phenotypic and genotypic resistance testing, as well as pharmacy records for antiretroviral drugs unique to HIV infection. Integrating laboratory-based and pharmacy-based reporting with the National Electronic Disease Surveillance System (NEDSS)[21] may require additional research. Second, it is important to explore ways of accounting for differential bias in prevalence estimates due to migration.

In addition to these concerns, it is important to evaluate other approaches, such as survey- and modeling-based approaches, for estimating both the overall burden of HIV and the differential disease burden among states and EMAs and to compare these estimates to those produced by case reporting. Such approaches have the potential of providing estimates that are more accurate, more timely, and more consistent across jurisdictions than complete enumeration. One such approach may rely on statistical models and make use of information from a variety of sources. An example of the use of a statistical model is backcalculation of HIV incidence and prevalence from data on AIDS incidence using estimates of the distribution of time from HIV infection to onset of AIDS (Brookmeyer and Gail, 1994). The usefulness of this method, however, has declined over time since the distribution of time from infection to AIDS has become less predictable with the advent of improved therapies. Other attempts to estimate HIV prevalence in specific metropolitan areas have made use of information about sizes of populations at risk and prevalence of HIV infection in those populations from a wide variety of sources (Holmberg, 1996). Holmberg and colleagues suggested as useful sources:

---

the same requirements and privileges as other entities that are required to report, including the duty of the state health department to keep personally identifiable information, if any, confidential. This would allow the state health department to collect relevant data from laboratories in the same manner that it collects data from providers. Thus, statutes protecting the confidentiality of such information should not be a major impediment to collecting information from laboratories and pharmacies to improve the accuracy of HIV case data at the state level.

[21]NEDSS is a project to integrate surveillance systems so that appropriate public health, laboratory, and clinical data can be transferred efficiently and securely over the Internet. NEDSS is designed to integrate and replace several current CDC surveillance systems, including the National Electronic Telecommunications System for Surveillance (NETSS), the HIV/AIDS reporting system, the vaccine preventable diseases and systems for tuberculosis (TB) and infectious diseases. See http://www.cdc.gov/nedss/ for more information on NEDSS.

specific studies of prevalence and transmission among people at risk of infection; information from sexually transmitted disease (STD) clinics, counseling and testing sites, and drug treatment centers; and information from other sources of population testing, such as the Veterans Administration and other medical centers or household-based surveys. The addition of information from population-based surveys could greatly increase the usefulness of such approaches.

A previous IOM report (2001) recommended the use of sentinel surveillance in conjunction with population-based surveys as a way to estimate HIV incidence, but it could also be applied to obtain estimates of HIV prevalence. In this approach, one obtains prevalence data from targeted samples of special populations. For example, one might use information from blood donors, military recruits, and/or members of some special high-risk group. One then uses information from other, more representative samples, to estimate the prevalence of the characteristics that identify these special populations. For example, one could determine how likely different groups of people (defined by specific characteristics) in specific areas are to donate blood or join the military. Information from the targeted prevalence studies and representative surveys can then be used to develop estimates of the prevalence of HIV infection. Such an approach has the potential of providing estimates that are more accurate, more timely, and more consistent across jurisdictions than complete enumeration. However, there are also limitations to such approaches. For example, adequate data may not be available to produce accurate models and sampling can be both complex and expensive to implement. Many constituencies are also concerned about the confidentiality and ethics of surveillance surveys. Such a strategy should be reconsidered, with a review of the substantial technical, political, and ethical barriers to its implementation that were pointed out after the 2001 IOM report appeared.

Both modeling and survey methods can also be used to estimate cases of undiagnosed HIV infection. Although the primary reasons to have accurate surveillance of the number of persons with known HIV infection are epidemiological, the total number of people with HIV infection is relevant to assessing the size of the population that is likely to need health care services, either currently or in the future, especially if a goal is to encourage everyone to enter care. The resource requirements for treating people who are in care vary widely depending on disease stage, and other factors, such as the patient's own health insurance status. All HIV-infected persons—even those without clinical symptoms—require some services such as patient education and monitoring as well as treatment of primary infection and associated medical conditions. Most will require extensive medical intervention in the future even if they currently do not. Therefore, information on the total number of HIV infections is important. Although the RWCA now focuses on providing care to individuals who have been diagnosed, if policy shifts to include more outreach to individuals, allocation decisions will benefit from information on the total HIV-infected population.

Finding 4-8 The completeness of the data from existing HIV case-reporting systems can be improved by making changes, specifically counting all HIV cases that are reported to the national system rather than only those reported from states with name-based reporting, and more fully utilizing data from laboratories and other sources, such as pharmacies, to enhance the completeness of HIV reporting.

Finding 4-9 Techniques exist to estimate the prevalence of HIV infection independently of the HIV case-reporting systems. Sample-based surveys and modeling approaches permit estimates of the total HIV-infected population, regardless of diagnostic status.

Finding 4-10 A surveillance mechanism that provides information about the total population of persons with HIV infection, be they diagnosed or undiagnosed, is highly desirable. Knowing the size and distribution of the undiagnosed HIV-infected population is an important marker of success in providing care to all people with HIV.

RECOMMENDATIONS

The Committee's recommendations are listed below. These recommendations should be implemented in a timely manner to provide evidence to either (1) justify inclusion of reported HIV cases in RWCA allocations formulas by FY2007, as contemplated by Congress, or (2) conclude that reported HIV cases do not result in more equitable resource allocation so that Congress can reconsider its recommendation prior to implementation in FY2007. Additional resources may be required to implement some of these recommendations.

Recommendation 4-1 For at least the next four years, HRSA should continue to use ELCs in the RWCA Title I and II formulas. During that period, concerted effort should be devoted to improving the consistency, quality, and comparability of HIV case reporting. Specific attention should be paid to two, complementary approaches in this regard: (1) the attainment of coverage, maturity, and comparability standards and the development of de-duplication strategies that permit full use of all reported HIV cases; and (2) implementation of alternative strategies for estimating HIV cases, such as survey- or model-based estimation.

Recommendation 4-2 The following steps should be taken by states as quickly as possible to improve the consistency, quality, and comparability of HIV case reporting for RWCA allocation purposes.

a. The CDC should accept reported HIV cases from all states. Until this occurs, large numbers of HIV cases will not be included in the national HIV reporting system, and there will be no reliable centralized way to use reported HIV cases to apportion CARE Act funds. CDC should work with all states to develop and evaluate methods for unduplicating HIV cases regardless of whether such cases are code- or name-based. The Secretary should provide CDC with the funding to provide the technical assistance to states necessary to support the integration of code with name-based data into the national HIV reporting database. Because of the importance of obtaining consistent data from all jurisdictions, CDC should include HIV reporting data from code-based states and estimate the degree of overcounting due to duplication while procedures and infrastructure for definitive unduplication are developed.

b. CDC should collaborate with all states to periodically assess and compare the completeness and timeliness of their HIV reporting systems.

c. The Secretary of HHS should provide additional funds to CDC to assist states in improving the completeness and timeliness and overall comparability of their HIV reporting systems. Enhancing electronic laboratory reporting in all states is critical in achieving this goal. Pharmacy-based surveillance, with a focus on the AIDS Drug Assistance Program (ADAP), is another potential source of information for enhancing completeness.

Recommendation 4-3 CDC should obtain estimates of total HIV prevalence (including the undiagnosed population) and evaluate methods other than case reporting for use as an alternative or supplement in estimating HIV cases for RWCA Title I and II formula allocations, with advice and review by an independent body. This assessment should address the accuracy and costs of different strategies and should be repeated periodically.

Recommendation 4-4 Prior to future reauthorizations of the CARE Act, the Secretary of HSS should initiate studies to improve the evidence base for understanding how well HIV case reporting and other methods for estimating HIV cases reflect the relative burden of disease and the relative resources necessary to respond to those needs in different areas. The Secretary should engage an independent body to estimate the dollar allocations that would result for Title I and II grantees from alternative input data and alternative RWCA allocation formulas. Specifically:

a. "What-if" assessments should be reported every five years on the range of each EMA's and state's RWCA formula allocation, depending on whether ELCs or total HIV cases are used as the measure of disease burden.

b. Analyses should be conducted to estimate the dollar allocations that would result from modifying different structural elements of the formula, such as:
   - Hold-harmless provisions,
   - The eligibility requirements for becoming an EMA,
   - The percentage set-aside in the Title II base award for non-EMA states (currently 20 percent),
   - The minimum base Title II award (now $500,000 for states and $50,000 for territories),
   - The eligibility criteria for becoming a Tier 1 and Tier 2 Emerging Community.

c. Evaluate the extent of interregional variability in HIV epidemic maturity and its effect on relative resource needs.

These activities should be repeated periodically.

Recommendation 4-5 In keeping with the CARE Act's intent as a payer of last resort, Congress should reevaluate the RWCA formulas to determine whether they allocate resources in proportion to the estimated number of individuals with HIV/AIDS who are uninsured or underinsured in states and EMAs. Readily available data on the insurance coverage of the general population may mirror insurance coverage of people with HIV/AIDS, but additional estimation will likely be required.

REFERENCES

Beltrami JF, Vermund SH, Fawal HJ, Moon TD, Von Bargen JC, Holmberg SD. 1999. HIV/AIDS in nonurban Alabama: Risk activities and access to services among HIV-infected persons. *The Southern Medical Journal* 92(7):677–83.

Berk ML, Schur CL, Dunbar JL, Bozzette S, Shapiro M. 2003. Short report: Migration among persons living with HIV. *Social Science and Medicine* 57:1091–7.

Birkhead, G. Panel discussion with committee members during public committee meeting, Washington, DC. May 15, 2002.

Brookmeyer R, Gail MH. 1994. *AIDS Epidemiology: A Quantitative Approach.* New York: Oxford University Press.

Brookmeyer R, Liao J. 1990. The analysis of delays in disease reporting: Methods and results for the Acquired Immunodeficiency Syndrome. *American Journal of Epidemiology* 132(2):355–65.

Buehler J, Berkelman R, Stehr–Green J. 1992. The completeness of AIDS surveillance. *Journal of Acquired Immune Deficiency Syndromes* 5:257–64.

Buehler J, Frey R, Chu S. 1995. AIDS mortality project group. The migration of persons with AIDS: Data from 12 states, 1985 to 1992. *American Journal of Public Health* 85(11):1552–55.

CDC (Centers for Disease Control and Prevention). 1992. 1993 Revised classification system for HIV infection and expanded surveillance. *Morbidity and Mortality Weekly Report* 41(RR17;001). Atlanta, GA: CDC.

CDC. 1998. Evaluation of HIV case surveillance through the use of non–name unique identifies—Maryland and Texas, 1994–1996. *Morbidity and Mortality Weekly Report* 46(52 & 53):1254–72. Atlanta, GA: CDC.

CDC. 1999. Guidelines for national human immunodeficiency virus case surveillance, including monitoring for human immunodeficiency virus infection and acquired immunodeficiency syndrome. *Morbidity and Mortality Weekly Report* 48(13):1–28. Atlanta, GA: CDC.

CDC. 2003a. Current Status of HIV Infection Surveillance—April 2003. (Email communication, Patricia Sweeney, CDC, April 28, 2003).

CDC. 2003b. Evaluation of the Performance of Integrated Human Immunodeficiency Virus (HIV)/Acquired Immunodeficiency Syndrome (AIDS Surveillance Systems). Update: Interstate Duplication Evaluation Project, April 2003. (Email communication, Patricia Sweeney, CDC, April 25, 2003).

CDC. 2003c. Table 1—Status of CD4 and Viral Load Reporting—Draft April 2003 (Email communication, Patricia Sweeney, CDC, May 13, 2003).

CDC. 2003d. Laboratory Reporting Issues Discussed with HIV/AIDS Surveillance Coordinators. Summary of Preliminary Findings for IOM Committee—Draft April 2003. (Email communication, Patricia Sweeney, CDC, April 28, 2003).

CDC. 2003e. Preliminary Analysis: Timeliness of HIV/AIDS Reporting Among Adults/Adolescents. April 2002. (Email communication, Patricia Sweeney, CDC, June 26, 2002).

CDC. 2003f. State Timeliness Results. Percentage of HIV Cases Reported Within 6 Months; Percentage of AIDS Cases Reported Within 6 Months. (Email communication, Patricia Sweeney, CDC, April 18, 2003).

CDC. 2003g. Number of AIDS Cases by State and EMA and Diagnosis Year, Adjusted for Reporting Delay. Data reported as of December 2002. (Email communication, Patricia Sweeney, CDC, June 20, 2003).

CDC. 2003h. Update on current status of HIV Infection Surveillance: April 2003. (Email communication, Patricia Sweeney, CDC, October 13, 2003).

CDC. 2003i. Update on the Evaluation of the Performance of Integrated Human Immunodeficiency Virus (HIV)/Acquired Immunodeficiency Syndrome (AIDS) Surveillance Systems. (Email communication, Patricia Sweeney, CDC, March 4, 2003).

Chamberland ME, Allen JR, Monroe JM, Garcia N, Morgan C, Reiss R, Stephens H, Walker J, Friedman SM. 1985. Acquired Immunodeficiency Syndrome in New York City: Evaluation of an active surveillance system. *Journal of the American Medical Association* 254(3):383–7.

Colfax GN, Bindman AB. 1998. Health benefits and risks of reporting HIV-infected individuals by name. *American Journal of Public Health* 88(6):876–9.

Conway GA, Colley-Niemeyer B, Pursley C, Cruz C, Burt S, Rion P, Heath CW. 1989. Underreporting of AIDS cases in South Carolina, 1986 and 1987. *Journal of the American Medical Association* 262(20):2859–63.

Davis K, Stapleton J. 1991. Migration to rural areas by HIV patients: Impact on HIV-related healthcare use. *Infection Control and Hospital Epidemiology* 12(9): 540–3.

Doyle T, Glynn K, Groseclose S. 2002. Completeness of notifiable infectious disease reporting in the United States: An analytical literature review. *American Journal of Epidemiology* 155(9):866–74.

Elcock M, Simon T, Bradley GP, Copello AG, Klezer PJ. 1993. Active AIDS surveillance: Hospital-based case finding in a metropolitan California County. *American Journal of Public Health* 83(7):1002–5.

Ellis M, Muschkin C. 1996. Migration of persons with AIDS—A search for support from elderly parents? *Social Science and Medicine* 43(7):1109–18.

GAO (General Accounting Office). 1995. *Ryan White CARE Act of 1990: Opportunities Are Available to Improve Funding Equity*. GAO/T-HEHS-95-91. Washington, DC: GAO.

GAO. 2000. *Ryan White CARE Act: Opportunities to Enhance Funding Equity*. GAO/ T-HEHS-00-150. Washington, DC: GAO.

Georgia Division of Public Health, Epidemiology Branch, HIV/STD Epidemiology Section. 2003. Proposal for HIV Infection Reporting in Georgia. [Online]. Available: http://www.ph.dhr.state.ga.us/epi/hivreporting.shtml [accessed September 25, 2003].

Green TA. 1998. Using surveillance data to monitor trends in the AIDS epidemic. *Statistics in Medicine* 17(2):143–54.

Greenberg A, Hindin R, Nicholas AG, Bryan EL, Thomas PA. 1993. The completeness of AIDS case reporting in New York City. *Journal of the American Medical Association* 269(23):2995–3001.

Hardy A, Starcher T, Morgan W, Druker J, Kristal A, Day JKC, Ewing E, Curran J. 1987. Review of death certificates to assess completeness of AIDS reporting. *Public Health Reports* 102:386–9.

Hecht FM, Chesney MA, Lehman JS, Osmond D, Vranizan K, Colman S, Keane D, Reingold A, Bindman AB. 2000. Does HIV reporting by name deter testing? MESH Study Group. *AIDS* 14(12):1801–8.

Holmberg SD. 1996. The estimated prevalence and incidence of HIV in 96 large U.S. metropolitan areas. *American Journal of Public Health* 86(5):642–54.

Hook E, Regal RR. 1995. Capture-recapture methods in epidemiology: Methods and limitations. *Epidemiologic Reviews* 17:243–64.

HRSA (Health Resources and Services Administration). 2002. Ryan White Care Act overview. *HRSA Ryan White Care Act Information Sheets*:1–2. Rockville, MD: HRSA.

IOM (Institute of Medicine). 2001. *No Time to Lose: Getting More from HIV Prevention*. Washington, DC: National Academy Press.

Jara MM, Gallagher KM, Schieman S. 2000. Estimation of completeness of AIDS case reporting in Massachusetts. *Epidemiology* 11(2):209–13.

Kaiser Family Foundation. June 2003. Fact Sheet: HIV/AIDS Testing in the United States. [Online]. Available: http://www.kff.org/hivaids/6094-index.cfm.

Kates J, Ruiz S. 2002. Sources of coverage and care for people with HIV/AIDS in the United States: Assessing coverage in southern states. *Southern States Summit on HIV/AIDS and STDs*. Menlo Park, CA: Kaiser Family Foundation.

Klevens R, Fleming P, Li J, Karon J. 1997. Impact of laboratory-initiated reporting of CD4 T lymphocytes on U.S. AIDS surveillance. *Journal of Acquired Immune Deficiency Syndromes & Human Retrovirology* 14:56–60.

Klevens R, Fleming PL, Gaines CG, Troxler S. 1998. Completeness of HIV reporting in Louisiana, USA. *International Journal of Epidemiology* 27:1105.

Klevens RM, Fleming PL, Li J, Gaines CG, Gallagher K, Schwarcz S, Karon JM, Ward JW. 2001. The completeness, validity, and timeliness of AIDS surveillance data. *Annals of Epidemiology* 11(7):443–9.

Kopelman, J. Panel discussion with committee members during public committee meeting, Washington, DC. May 15, 2002.

Lam NS, Liu KB. 1994. Spread of AIDS in rural America, 1982-1990. *Journal of Acquired Immune Deficency Syndromes* 7(5):485–90.

LaMendola B. 2002, August 5. South Florida Losing Out on AIDS Funding as More Patients Move There. *South Florida Sun-Sentinel*. LOCAL. P. 1A.

Lee L, Harris N, Glynn K, Phelps R. 2002. Evaluating Integrated HIV/AIDS Surveillance: Part 1. *Presentation at the 2002 National HIV/AIDS Surveillance Workshop*.

Lindan CP, Hearst N, Singleton JA, Trachtenberg AI, Riordan NM, Tokagawa DA, Chu GS. 1990. Underreporting of minority AIDS deaths in San Francisco bay area, 1985-1986. *Public Health Reports* 105(4):400–4.

Marsh K, Morgan M, Bunch G, Costa S, Fleming P, Wortley P. 1999. Evaluation of Non-Name-Coded Identifiers in Los Angeles County and New Jersey. *1999 National HIV Prevention Conference*.

Meyer P, Jones J, Garrison C. 1994. Completeness of reporting of diagnosed HIV-infected hospital inpatients. *Journal of Acquired Immune Deficiency Syndromes & Human Retrovirology* 7(10):1067–73.

Modesitt SK, Hulman S, Fleming D. 1990. Evaluation of active versus passive AIDS surveillance in Oregon. *American Journal of Public Health* 80(4):463–4.

NRC (National Research Council). 2001. *The 2000 Census: Interim Assessment*. Washington, DC: National Academy Press.

NRC. 2003.*Statistical Issues in Allocating Funds by Formula.* Louis TA, Jabine TB, Gerstein MA, Eds. Washington, DC: The National Academies Press.

Osmond DH, Bindman AB, Vranizan K, Lehman JS, Hecht FM, Keane D, Reingold A. 1999. Name-based surveillance and public health interventions for persons with HIV infection. Multistate Evaluation of Surveillance for HIV Study Group. *Annals of Internal Medicine* 131(10):775–9.

Pagano M, Tu X, De Gruttola V, MaWhinney S. 1994. Regression analysis of censored and truncated data: Estimating reporting-delay distributions and AIDS incidence from surveillance data. *Biometrics* 50:1203–14.

Payne SM, Seage GR 3rd, Oddleifson S, Gallagher K, vanBeuzekom M, Losina H, Hertz T. 1995 Using administratively collected hospital discharge data for AIDS surveillance. *Annals of Epidemiology* 5(5):337–46.

Rosenblum L, Buehler JW, Morgan MW, Costa S, Hidalgo J, Holmes R, Lieb L, Shields A, Whyte BM. 1992. The completeness of AIDS case reporting, 1988: A multisite collaborative surveillance project. *American Journal of Public Health* 82(11):1495–99.

Scheer S, McQuitty M, Denning P, Hormel L, Stephens B, Katz M, Schwarcz S. 2001. Undiagnosed and unreported AIDS deaths: Results from the San Francisco medical examiner. *Journal of Acquired Immune Deficiency Syndromes & Human Retrovirology* 27(5):467–71.

Schwarcz SK, Hsu LC, Parisi MK, Katz MH. 1999. The impact of the 1993 AIDS case definition on the completeness and timeliness of AIDS surveillance. *AIDS* 13(9):1109–14.

Schwarcz S, Hsu L, Chu PL, Parisi MK, Bangsberg D, Hurley L, Pearlman J, Marsh K, Katz M. 2002. Evaluation of a non-name-based HIV reporting system in San Francisco. *Journal of Acquired Immune Deficiency Syndromes & Human Retrovirology* 29(5):504–10.

Solomon L, Flynn C, Eldred L, Caldeira E, Wasserman MP, Benjamin G. 1999. Evaluation of a statewide non-name–based HIV surveillance system. *Journal of Acquired Immune Deficiency Syndromes & Human Retrovirology* 22(3):272–9.

U.S. Congress, House of Representatives. Committee on Commerce. 2000a. *Report on Ryan White CARE Act Amendments of 2000 (106-788).* 106th Cong., 2d Sess. July 25, 2000.

U.S. Congress, Senate. 2000b. Committee on Health, Education, Labor, and Pensions. *Report on Ryan White CARE Act Amendments of 2000 (106-294).* 106th Cong., 2d Sess. May 15, 2000.

Verghese A, Berk SL, Sarubbi F. 1989. Urbs in rure: Human immunodeficiency virus infection in rural Tennessee. *The Journal of Infectious Diseases* 160(6):1051–5.

Verghese A, Nabhan D, Escobedo MA, Guardado J, Guerra LG, Ho H, Casner P, Berk ML. 1995. Profile of HIV disease in an American border city. *Southern Medical Journal* 88(4):429–32.

5

Estimating Resource Needs

The Ryan White Comprehensive AIDS Resources Emergency (CARE) Act (RWCA) attempts to direct funds to areas in the greatest need of financial assistance through several of its discretionary grant programs, including Title I supplemental awards, Title II AIDS Drug Assistance Program (ADAP) supplemental awards, and Title III and IV awards. In contrast to formula awards, which are based exclusively on estimates of living AIDS cases (ELCs), these grants attempt to take into account other factors affecting severity of need. The Health Resources and Services Administration's HIV/AIDS Bureau (HRSA/HAB) defines severity of need as "the degree to which providing primary medical care to people with HIV disease in any given area is more complicated and costly than in other areas based on a combination of the adverse health and socio-economic circumstances of the populations to be served" (HRSA, 2003).

In the 2000 reauthorization, Congress asked the Institute of Medicine (IOM) Committee to examine "existing and needed epidemiological data and other analytic tools for resource planning and allocation decisions, specifically for estimating severity of need of a community and the relationship to the allocations process" (Ryan White CARE Act. 42 U.S.C. § 300ff-11 [2003]). The Committee focused its analysis on the application of severity-of-need criteria in determining Title I supplemental awards, the largest of these discretionary grant awards, because of the specific requests for assistance by Congress and HRSA/HAB in this area. Although this chapter does not discuss other discretionary grant programs that use severe-need criteria in allocating resources, the Committee's findings and recommendations may also be relevant to those programs. In the remainder of this chapter, the Committee uses the term "resource needs" instead of "severity of need" to reflect Congress' interest in the relationship between *need* and *resource* allocation. The Committee uses the term "severity of need," however, when referencing the specific severity-of-need component of the Title I application.

Congress specified that "[Title I] supplemental awards are to be directed principally to those eligible areas with 'severe need,' or the greatest or expanding public health challenges in confronting the epidemic" (U.S. Congress, 2000). Reflecting this notion, Congress increased the weight assigned to severity of need in determining the supplemental award from 25 percent to 33 percent in the 2000 reauthorization (Ryan White CARE Act. 42. U.S.C. § 300ff-13 [2003]). In determining severity of need, Congress directed HRSA/HAB to consider factors such as: "(I) STDs, substance abuse, tuberculosis, severe mental illness, or other co-morbid factors; (II) new or growing populations of individuals with HIV; (III) homelessness; (IV) current prevalence of HIV; (V) increasing need for HIV services including the relative rates of increase in the number of cases of HIV disease; [and] (VI) unmet need for services" (Ryan White CARE Act. 42 U.S.C. §. 300ff-13 [2003]). Congress further directed HRSA/HAB to "employ standard, quantitative measures to the maximum extent possible in lieu of narrative self-reporting when awarding supplemental awards" (U.S. Congress, 2000).

In addressing its charge, the Committee organized its work into the following tasks:

1. Developing a conceptual framework for factors affecting resource needs;
2. Defining criteria for assessing measures of resource needs;
3. Evaluating the process and data currently used to award Title I supplemental funds;
4. Proposing a new way of identifying predictors of resource needs; and
5. Making recommendations to evaluate and implement this approach.

Although HRSA/HAB uses explicit criteria to evaluate resource needs and allocate Title I supplemental grants, no consistent indicators are used to evaluate *relative* need, and much of the evaluation process is subjective. The Committee also found that the process for awarding Title I supplemental grants focuses on the characteristics of individuals, such as the prevalence of comorbid conditions that often accompany HIV disease, and does not account for other important factors affecting resource needs, such as the cost of providing services and the availability of local resources. The Committee proposes a potential new approach to allocating Title I supplemental awards that is based on standardized, quantitative indicators of resource needs of different jurisdictions.

FACTORS AFFECTING RESOURCE NEEDS

A broad array of individual and social factors determines an area's resource needs. The Committee groups these factors into three categories: disease burden, the costs of providing care, and available resources. Resource needs can be viewed as a product of disease burden and cost of care minus available resources:

$$\text{Resource needs} = (\text{Disease burden} * \text{Costs of providing care}) - \text{Available resources}$$

Table 5-1 provides some examples of the types of measures that could be used to assess resource needs.

TABLE 5-1 Examples of Measures of Resource Needs

Factors Affecting Resource Needs	Example Measures[a]
Disease Burden	• Reported HIV cases • Reported AIDS cases • Incident reported HIV cases • Incident reported AIDS cases • Prevalent HIV infections (including undiagnosed) • Incident HIV infections (including undiagnosed) • Case mix
Costs	• Case mix • Wages of health care workers • Costs of medical supplies • Transportation costs
Resources	• Generosity of state Medicaid program • Number of primary care or HIV specialists per capita • Rates of insurance coverage • Per capita income • Poverty rate

[a]This is not intended to be a comprehensive list.

Disease Burden

Disease burden is commonly measured by the incidence or prevalence of a disease.[1] Incidence refers to the number of new cases of a condition during a specified period of time in a population at risk for developing the disease. Prevalence can be assessed in terms of either point prevalence or period prevalence. Point prevalence is defined as the proportion of persons in the population with the condition at a specific point in time (Gordis, 1996). Period prevalence is the proportion of people who have had the disease at any time during a certain period (e.g., a calendar year). Some people may have developed the disease during that time while others may have had the disease and died during that period (Gordis, 1996). Incident, or new, HIV infection is the ideal measure for understanding the dynamics, spread, and success of prevention programs. Prevalent known HIV infection is appropriate for estimating the clinical burden to apportion care resources. Current RWCA allocation formulas are based on estimated AIDS prevalence, based on data from states through their AIDS case-reporting systems.

It is important to note that the medical and financial significance of an AIDS diagnosis has changed as treatments have evolved. Thus, unlike the early period of the epidemic when the effects of therapy were small and transient, many people who currently have a diagnosis of AIDS have responded well to highly active antiretroviral therapy and are now at relatively low risk for opportunistic infections and are able to maintain an active and productive life. Estimates of HIV cases using a uniform methodology are not available (see Chapter 4).

Costs of Care

Costs of care may be driven by several factors, including the complexity of a person's medical condition. For instance, HIV-infected individuals who are at a later stage of disease generally require more resources for their care than HIV-infected people who are at earlier stages of disease (Bozzette et al., 2001).[2] The costs of care also depend on the cost of obtaining and providing services, such as the prevailing wages of health care

---

[1]Other measures of morbidity, mortality, or natality may be used to assess disease burden, but incidence and prevalence are the two most relevant for this report.

[2]While the rate of resource use is higher for HIV-infected individuals with more advanced disease, lifetime resource use is higher for individuals who receive state-of-the-art care from the earliest stages of their disease (Freedberg et al., 2001).

workers and the local costs of medical supplies. To receive comparable care, a patient in a costly metropolitan area may require greater financial resources than one residing in a less costly locality. Even with comparable patients and costs, some areas may have fewer resource needs because they are more efficient at providing care.

Available Resources

Available resources or fiscal capacity across regions or states also affect resource needs. Such resource disparities are important in many policy arenas. Formula allocations for Temporary Assistance to Needy Families (formerly Aid to Families with Dependent Children) and other federal programs have long been designed to assist less affluent states (NRC, 2003).

Defining "available resources" equitably is an extremely difficult task, however. The purchasing power of a dollar varies greatly across areas and many resources that affect the difficulty and cost of providing HIV care are not measured. Some programs use per capita income as a proxy to account for such variations. For example, Medicaid and several other formula allocation programs use a formula that adjusts allocations based on the ratio between the state per capita income and the national per capita income when determining what proportion of state program expenditures will be reimbursed by the federal government (NRC, 2003). A 1975 study of alternative formulas for the General Revenue Sharing (GRS) program recommended inclusion of a poverty factor in the intrastate allocation and allocations on a per capita basis for governmental jurisdictions for which reliable estimates of income and poverty were available (NRC, 2001).

In the arena of health services, advantages that accrue from higher per capita income are partly offset by higher labor costs and by higher costs of other resources required in patient care. Medicare addresses these issues through the use of adjusted average per capita cost (AAPCC) in determining capitation rates in different medical markets (CMS, 1999; MEDPAC, 1999). This method, which relies upon historical average reimbursements, is imperfect and controversial. The AAPCC is based on past Medicare reimbursements rather than differences in input prices. Thus, the AAPCC methodology appears to penalize cities and states that have historically made most efficient use of medical resources (Society of Actuaries, 1997). Despite these limitations, data regarding regional variation in medical costs and prices could provide a useful complement to existing data in determining RWCA formula allocations and supplemental awards.

Similarly, the coverage of private and public health insurance programs is a major factor affecting states' and Eligible Metropolitan Areas' (EMAs) resource needs. Medicaid programs in particular—by far the largest payer of care for people with HIV/AIDS—vary substantially in the benefits they cover and their eligibility criteria across states. For example, in some states, being medically needy is not an eligibility criterion for Medicaid; many states also have limitations on Medicaid drug coverage (Kaiser Family Foundation, 2000). The relative "generosity" of Medicaid programs can greatly influence regions' reliance on CARE Act funds, including its ADAP. All else equal, areas with a greater proportion of insured residents with HIV/AIDS should require fewer CARE Act funds than areas with a high proportion of uninsured patients with HIV/AIDS.

States further differ in the resources they devote to addressing the HIV/AIDS epidemic. For instance, some states have imposed one or more restrictions on ADAP, such as enrollment caps, limits on access to antiretroviral treatments, and expenditure caps (NASTAD et al., 2003). Furthermore, states vary a great deal in how much they contribute to ADAP programs. In some cases, lack of political will and emphasis on other priorities have contributed to these restrictions.

Title I supplemental awards, along with Title I and II formulas, do not take into account variations in the costs of providing care or other resources available to states and metropolitan areas. Including such information in allocation decisions could have a substantial impact on RWCA funding across states and EMAs. For example, an EMA in a state that has poor Medicaid coverage may choose to use more of its Title I funds on primary care services than an EMA in a state with more generous Medicaid coverage. The EMA in the state with poor Medicaid coverage will therefore have relatively fewer resources to devote to support services, since their RWCA funds must be used to cover basic primary medical care.

TITLE I SUPPLEMENTAL AWARD PROCESS

Congress divides Title I funds into two components, designating half for the formula-based awards and half for supplemental awards. After HRSA/HAB deducts funds for the Minority AIDS Initiative and the hold-harmless provision,[3] approximately 80 percent of the supplemental award amount remains available for distribution among EMAs.

---

[3]The hold-harmless provision is designed to prevent large reductions in funding from year to year.

The Review Process and Scoring Guide

Each application for a supplemental award can receive a maximum of 100 points (Box 5-1). Applications submitted for fiscal year (FY) 2002 could achieve up to the following number of points in each category:

BOX 5-1
Scoring of FY2002 Supplemental Application

Compliance with FY2000–2001 Title I requirements	26 points
Grant administration	5 points
Severe need	33 points
Impact of Title I funds	6 points
Planning council mandated roles/responsibilities	10 points
Update on assuring quality of services and evaluation activities	10 points
Progress in implementing the FY2001 plan	5 points
Plan for FY2002	5 points
MAXIMUM TOTAL	100 points

HRSA/HAB originally used an external review process to score Title I supplemental applications. However, beginning with the FY1999 review process, HRSA/HAB relied on Title I project officers as the primary reviewers, given their familiarity with grantees' programs. Because RWCA operates on a 5-year budget period, early reviews of applications for supplemental funding set the standard for the remaining budget period. HRSA still uses an external review process for the first year of the budget cycle.

At least two HRSA/HAB project officers review and score each application; the scores are then averaged. A guide helps reviewers assign scores to each component but also states clearly that such guidance is not definitive: "Reviewers should use their own judgment and expertise in determining a final score" (HRSA, 2001b). Hence, the subjective scores can deviate significantly from empirical indicators of need. HRSA/HAB also uses an algorithm that may vary from year to year, which may reduce disparities among supplemental allocations (HRSA, 2001c). The detailed algorithm for determining final supplemental awards is not made public.

It is important to note that even though severity of need accounts for one-third of the total points, it may not account for one-third of the *variation* in total points. That depends on both the relative variation in severity-of-need scores and the relative variation in other components of the application. If, for example, EMAs received identical scores for all items other than severity of need, 100 percent of the variation in scores—and thus in awards—would stem from severity of need. If, in contrast, all EMAs received similar severity-of-need scores, almost all the variation in scores and awards would stem from other components.

Severity-of-Need Component of the Application

Scoring of severity of need in the Title I application is based on three equally weighted components: (1) HIV/AIDS epidemiology; (2) comorbidity, poverty, and insurance status; and (3) assessment of populations with special needs.

HIV/AIDS Epidemiology

For this component, grantees supply data on AIDS incidence, AIDS prevalence, and HIV prevalence. Grantees also provide narrative detail on three issues:

- Trends and compositional changes in caseloads, based on a comparison of the estimated number of people living with HIV, the number of people living with AIDS, and the number of new AIDS cases reported within the last 2 years.
- The demographics of cases, based on populations in the EMA with disproportionately high HIV/AIDS prevalence compared with the general population.
- The level of unmet need among populations who are underrepresented in the CARE-funded system, based on utilization data for all covered services (HRSA, 2001a).[4]

Comorbidity, Poverty, and Insurance Status

The EMA must also provide information on the incidence of six comorbid conditions: tuberculosis, syphilis, gonorrhea, intravenous drug use, other substance use, and homelessness. The EMA also reports the

---

[4]In 2000, HRSA convened an unmet needs consultation with participants from HRSA, the Centers for Disease Control and Prevention (CDC), grantees, and researchers to assist HRSA in developing measures to estimate unmet need for HIV primary medical care. A number of issues emerged from that meeting including the need for common terms and definitions, methods and models for assessing unmet need, easy-to-use formulas to estimate the number of individuals not in care, and flexibility in meeting state and local needs and capabilities (HRSA, 2000; Kahn et al., 2003).

number and percentage of residents with incomes below 300 percent of the federal poverty line during the prior fiscal year, and the number and percentage of residents without public or private health insurance. Applicants must describe the overall effect of these components on their populations, and explain how they affect the cost of service and the complexity of providing care.

Populations with Special Needs

In the final severity-of-need component, applicants respond to 10 questions regarding six special populations. These populations are youth 13–24 years of age, injection drug users (IDUs), substance users other than IDUs, men of color who have sex with men, white/Anglo men who have sex with men, and women of childbearing age (13 years of age and older). Applicants can also report on other populations they deem to have special needs. Applicants are requested to provide information on HIV and AIDS prevalence, trends, and service needs for each special population (Box 5-2).

BOX 5-2
Information Requested for Special Populations

1. The estimated number of people in these populations in the EMA, regardless of HIV status.
2. The estimated number of people in each special population living with AIDS.
3. The estimated number of persons in these special populations with HIV infection, including AIDS.
4. The HIV prevalence rate for each special population.
5. A brief description of the special population, including its geographic distribution in the EMA, income level, language barriers, and other characteristics.
6. HIV infection and risk trends in the special population.
7. HIV/AIDS service needs of individuals in each special population who know their status and who are in primary care.
8. The extent to which members of this special population are not in HIV/AIDS care, and efforts by the planning council to identify and address their service needs.
9. HIV/AIDS service needs of individuals who know their status and who are not in primary care.
10. Information on the planning council's efforts to include this special population in its need assessment, used to determine its service priorities and allocate funds.

CRITERIA FOR ASSESSING MEASURES OF RESOURCE NEEDS

The Committee reviewed all 51 Title I applications submitted by grantees in FY2002. In reviewing the applications, the Committee considered whether the measures used by different jurisdictions were important, scientifically sound, and feasible for national use. Specifically, the Committee identified nine criteria to evaluate current measures that are similar to those used by previous IOM and National Research Council (NRC) committees (NRC, 1997; IOM, 2001a) (Box 5-3).

Measures should reflect important resource needs. A measure's importance encompasses its meaningfulness, the prevalence and seriousness of the needs being measured, the potential for changing the situation, and the overall impact of providing the resources under consideration.

BOX 5-3
Criteria for Selecting Measures of Resource Needs

Importance of the measure:

1. *Meaningfulness:* Is the measure meaningful to policy makers and grantees?
2. *Prevalence and seriousness of the problem:* How common is the problem being assessed? Is there a general deficit or significant variation in the need being measured?
3. *Potential for improvement:* How susceptible to improvement is the area being assessed?
4. *Potential impact:* Considering the prevalence, and seriousness of the problem, and the potential improvement, how much of an impact, in aggregate, would improvement have on resource needs?

Scientific soundness of the measure:

1. *Validity:* Does the measure capture what it purports to measure?
2. *Reliability:* Does the measure produce similar results when applied across the same populations and settings?
3. *Evidence:* Is there an evidence base to support this measure?

Feasibility of the measure:

1. *Data availability:* Are data collected in a timely manner with reasonable periodicity?
2. *Cost and burden of measurement:* Can the data be collected at a reasonable cost and with reasonable effort?

1. *Meaningfulness:* There should be consensus among clinicians, patients, or policy makers that the measure reflects an important area of need.

2. *Prevalence and seriousness of the problem:* Measures should focus on major problems that affect a sizable proportion of RWCA clients. Measures should focus on aspects of need that are unmet or for which there is significant variation across grantees.

3. *Potential for improvement:* Measures should reflect areas of need that can be improved most by additional resources.

4. *Potential impact:* Considering the prevalence and seriousness of the problem and the potential for improvement, measures of resources that could have the greatest impact on persons living with HIV infection are desirable.

Measures should be scientifically sound. Scientific soundness entails three major components: reliability, validity, and evidence base.

1. *Reliability:* Reliability can be enhanced by using standard data collection methods across EMAs, collecting data in a way that minimizes manipulation, and employing a common definition of the population of interest and the time period.

2. *Validity:* Measures should capture what they purport to measure. Measures should make sense logically (face validity), should correlate well with other measures of resource needs (construct validity), and should capture meaningful aspects of resource needs (content validity) (IOM, 2001a). If one is developing predictors of needs, then the measures should have predictive validity. That is, one should be able to show that they predict measured needs. As indicated elsewhere in the report, when comparable assessments across regions are important in determining allocations and absolute levels are not, valid measures can have a bias as long as the bias (e.g., a given percentage of underreporting) is consistent across allocation regions.

3. *Evidence base:* Measures should have strong empirical support. For instance, indicators of resource needs should be empirically linked to needs or costs.

Measures should be feasible. Feasibility includes the availability of data and the cost and burden of measurement.

1. *Availability of data:* Data should be available at the appropriate level. For example, for assessments at the EMA level, each EMA should have the same data. Data should also be available in a timely manner and collected with reasonable periodicity.

2. *Cost and burden of measurement:* Data should be collected at a reasonable cost and should not impose an excessive burden on grantees. Measures based on data that are already being collected for other purposes, or that are publicly available are more feasible than measures that require new data collection.

Ideally, each measure of resource needs would satisfy all these criteria; in reality, few, if any, do. Thus, these criteria should not be viewed as absolute, but rather as guidelines for assessing the relative strengths and weaknesses of different measures.

ANALYSIS OF TITLE I SUPPLEMENTAL APPLICATIONS

This section summarizes the various data sources and resource needs measures used by grantees in the severity-of-need sections of their FY2002 Title I supplemental applications. The Committee found considerable variability in the actual data sources and measures, and the quality of those data sources and measures, used by grantees to describe their severity of need.

HIV/AIDS Epidemiology

The first component of the severity-of-need section requires grantees to report data on AIDS incidence, AIDS prevalence, and HIV prevalence. The Committee found significant variability in the data sources and the quality of the data used by grantees to describe the prevalence of HIV and AIDS in their areas:

- 41 percent (21) used CDC's estimates of AIDS and/or HIV incidence and prevalence.[5]
- 25 percent (13) chose to use their own AIDS and/or HIV data and estimates (7 use state sources and 6 use local sources).
- 12 percent (6) used a combination of data from state and local health departments and CDC.
- 16 percent (3) applied their own adjustments to CDC's estimates.
- 16 percent (8) did not explicitly state the source of prevalence data.

[5]For states with code-based HIV reporting systems or name-based systems that have only been recently implemented, CDC provides EMAs with modeled estimates of HIV prevalence based on cases from the 25 states with the most experience with name-based reporting.

As discussed in Chapter 3, states have had AIDS case-reporting systems in place since the 1980s, and the overall completeness and quality of the data are very high. Thus, comparisons of AIDS incidence and AIDS prevalence (measured by newly reported AIDS cases or existing AIDS cases, respectively) across areas are possible. Estimates of HIV cases across EMAs using a consistent methodology are not currently available (see Chapter 4). The lack of complete coverage in states' case-reporting systems and methods for de-duplicating code-based states, and variability in system maturity and the quality of reported cases, hinder the ability to compare estimates of HIV case reports. Furthermore, data on HIV cases represent only partial HIV prevalence because they include only individuals who chose to be tested at confidential testing sites. No data exist on the incidence of HIV cases; the HIV case-reporting system does not capture all new infections, only newly diagnosed infections (IOM, 2001b). The limited maturity of HIV case-reporting systems in some states means that it is virtually impossible for EMAs to describe trends in HIV prevalence and the demographic characteristics of their cases, unless they have conducted local studies.

The methodologies and data EMAs use to describe unmet need also vary substantially. Researchers at the University of California, San Francisco (Kahn et al., 2003), conducted a systematic review of existing methods of estimating unmet need for HIV care, including those used by all 51 EMAs in their grant applications.[6] The researchers found that EMAs varied significantly in their definitions and measures of unmet need. Studies used different definitions for HIV care (for example, some included support services such as case management while others did not) and different samples (e.g., representative or convenience samples). The methods used by EMAs and others therefore varied widely in their usefulness in quantifying unmet need for HIV primary care. The most useful methods for estimating such unmet need were typically quantitative, although variability in the quality of the data sources and samples lessened the usefulness of some of these measures. Less useful methods for quantifying unmet need were generally qualitative studies that assessed population characteristics but not the size of the population, or focused on clinical outcomes.

[6]Kahn and colleagues (2003) reviewed 142 studies including all 51 RWCA Title I supplemental applications for FY2001 and 10 Title 1 FY2002 applications; 78 Title I and Title II needs assessments, comprehensive plans, and special studies by grantees; and 12 academic studies. Details on the review of methods to estimate unmet need are discussed in their report.

Comorbidities, Poverty, and Insurance Status

The Committee also reviewed the second component of the severity-of-need section of the Title I supplemental award application, which requires applicants to document comorbidity, poverty, and insurance status (Table 5-2).

Comorbidity Factors

Applicants provided estimates of comorbid conditions, but the validity, reporting period, and definition of these estimates varied significantly. All EMAs but one reported data on tuberculosis, syphilis, and gonorrhea. The most commonly used indicator was prevalence rate, although only 40 percent specified the time period for which they were reporting. EMAs used several categories to indicate the prevalence of syphilis, including primary and secondary disease rates (5 EMAs), congenital syphilis rates (2 EMAs), and syphilis incidence rate (1 EMA). Most EMAs (66 percent) tap their state health departments for these data, whose reliability is unknown.

All but one EMA reported on IDUs. Localities used six separate indicators of IDUs, with the estimated absolute number being the most common measure (86 percent). Other EMAs used more specific indicators, such as the estimated number of crack and cocaine abusers (2 EMAs), estimated number of IDUs with HIV (1 EMA), and the number of clients in methadone clinics (1 EMA). State health departments provided 32 percent of EMAs with these estimates, while state and county substance abuse agencies provided the other EMAs with these data (16 percent and 8 percent, respectively).

Forty-eight of 51 EMAs reported on "other substance abuse"—relying on 17 different indicators. A majority of EMAs estimated the number of alcohol abusers (47 percent), cocaine and crack cocaine abusers (45 percent), or substance abusers (38 percent). State health departments most often provided this information, although EMAs also relied on local health departments, state substance abuse agencies, and the federal Substance Abuse and Mental Health Services Administration (SAMHSA).

All but one EMA reported on homelessness, and they used six different indicators. EMAs most often cited the estimated number of homeless people (58 percent), the yearly number of homeless (26 percent), or the daily number of homeless (24 percent). A majority of EMAs cited community-based organizations as the source of these data. However, different localities appear to use different methods to count homeless people and such variability can affect the data. For example, estimates of homelessness based on shelter counts are likely to be significantly smaller than estimates based on population surveys that ask respondents whether they were homeless in the past month or year.

Although these six comorbid conditions (tuberculosis, syphilis, gonorrhea, injection drug use, other substance abuse, and homelessness) are of clear clinical and policy importance, their relationship to an area's need for resources for HIV care is not well documented. Without an evidence base and explicit model connecting indicators to resource needs, assessing the appropriateness of the current comorbid measures is extremely difficult.

Even if one could link comorbid conditions with resource needs, information on the prevalence of co-orbidities in the HIV-infected population is lacking. As a result, many EMAs provide information on the prevalence of comorbidities among the general population. Reliably estimating the number of HIV-positive people with comorbid conditions within an EMA would be difficult. For instance, homelessness is difficult to estimate for the general population as no universally recognized quantitative measures exist, much less for the HIV-infected population. Many applications do not provide documentation that would enable reviewers to evaluate the reliability of these data.

Another challenge is that different levels of government with varying priorities collect data (e.g., on substance abuse, STDs, corrections, and mental health) that grantees are required to or choose to report in their applications. EMAs' relationships with these data providers also vary widely: some EMA representatives reported good relationships with state correctional facilities and substance abuse agencies, for example, while others reported difficulty in obtaining data from them (Ryan White CARE Act 2002 Grantee Conference, August 22–23, 2003, Washington, DC: Meeting with Title I EMAs).

Poverty and Insurance Status

Fifty of the 51 EMAs reported information on poverty status. HRSA/HAB asks grantees to provide the number of people at or below 300 percent of the federal poverty level, and 68 percent of EMAs provided such an estimate. Other EMAs estimated the number at or below 100 percent of the poverty line (24 percent), while a few used other thresholds, such as 133 percent and 200 percent of the federal poverty line. EMAs primarily used data from the U.S. Census, although some relied on data from state health departments and other state agencies.

HRSA/HAB requires applicants to estimate the number of people without insurance, including those without Medicaid coverage, and all 51 EMAs did so, with 92 percent using the definition provided by HRSA/HAB. A few EMAs estimated the number of people living with HIV who

TABLE 5-2 Required Factors Used to Describe Severity of Need in FY2002 Title I Supplemental Applications

	Measures Used		Data Sources Used		
Indicators	# of EMAs Reporting the Measure	For Defined Time Period	SHD	LHD	CDC
COMORBIDITY INDICATORS					
TB (Total EMAs Reporting = 50)					
Prevalence rate	49	20	33	15	1
Incidence and prev rates	1	1		1	
Did not report	1				
Syphilis (Total EMAs Reporting = 50)					
Total prevalence rate	45	21	30	13	1
Primary & secondary rate	5	2	3	2	
Infectious syphilis	2	1	2		
Congenital rate	2	1	1	1	
Early latent rate	1	1	1		
Incidence rate	1	1		1	
Did not report	1				
Gonorrhea (Total EMAs Reporting = 50)					
Prevalence rate	49	20	33	14	1
Incidence rate	1	1		1	
Did not report	1				
Injection Drug Use (Total EMAs Reporting = 50)					
Estimated number of IDUs	43	4	16	3	1 (surveillance report)
IDUs, crack, and cocaine abusers	2				
Estimated number of uninfected IDUs	1				1
Estimated number of IDUs w/HIV	1		1		

Other State	Other Local	Other Federal or National Org	Academic Research	No Source
1 (state drug abuse agency)				
	1 (local DSS)			
7 (state drug abuse agency)	4 (county drug agency)	3 (SAMHSA) 1 (NHSDA) 1 (NIDA)	7	
	1 (CBO) 1 (local agency)			

Continued

TABLE 5-2 Continued

	Measures Used		Data Sources Used		
Indicators	# of EMAs Reporting the Measure	For Defined Time Period	SHD	LHD	CDC
Number of clients in methadone clinic	1			1	
Estimated number of heroin users	1	1	1		
Did not report	1				
Other Substance Abuse (Total EMAs Reporting = 48)					
Estimated number of alcohol abusers	22	5	8	6	
Estimated number of cocaine and crack cocaine abusers	21	5	7	5	
Estimated number of substance abusers (no clear definition)	18		7		1 (SHAS)
Estimated number using marijuana	9	2	2	1	
Use of illicit drugs	6	1	5		
Methamphetamine users	6	1		3	
Psychedelic/ hallucinogen users	4	1			
Did not report	3				
Estimated number needing treatment for SA problem	3		1	1	
Inhalant users	3	1			
Number of admissions for SA treatment	2		1	1	
Smoking/tobacco use	2				
Binge drinkers	2			1	
Estimated number using stimulants	2		1		
Meth, PCP, benzo,	1				

Other State	Other Local	Other Federal or National Org	Academic Research	No Source
4 (state drug abuse agency)	1 (county drug agency)	1 (SAMHSA) 1 (NHSDA)		1
4 (state drug abuse agency)	1 (county drug agency)	3 (NHSDA) 1 (SAMHSA)		
4 (state drug abuse agency)		4 (SAMHSA) 1 (NHSDA)	1	
2 (state drug abuse agency)	1 (county drug agency)	1 (SAMHSA) 1 (NHSDA)		1
		1 (NHSDA)		
2 (state drug abuse agency)		1 (NHSDA)		
3 (state drug abuse agency)		1 (NHSDA)		
1 (state drug abuse agency)				
2 (state drug abuse agency)		1 (NHSDA)		
		1 (NHSDA)		
		1 (NHSDA)		
		1 (NHSDA)		
		1 (SAMHSA)		1

Continued

TABLE 5-2 Continued

	Measures Used		Data Sources Used		
Indicators	# of EMAs Reporting the Measure	For Defined Time Period	SHD	LHD	CDC
barbituates, tranquilizers, sedatives					
Users of sedatives	1				
Problem drinkers and nonnarcotic users in need of treatment	1		1		
Percent population using alcohol, marijuana, hallucinogenics/cocaine and inhalants	1				
No definition included	1		1		
Homelessness (Total EMAs Reporting = 50)					
Estimated number of homeless	29			3	
Yearly number of homeless (cumulative)	13			3	
Daily number of homeless (point prevalence)	12			1	
Number homeless among PLWH/A	2		1		
Number of shelter beds provided (1 year)	1				
Low-income and working poor families and individuals for FY2000	1	1			
Not reported	1				
POVERTY AND INSURANCE STATUS INDICATORS					
Insurance Status (Total EMAs Reporting = 51)					
Estimated # of people without insurance, including without Medicaid	48		12	2	

Other State	Other Local	Other Federal or National Org	Academic Research	No Source
1 (state drug abuse agency)				
		1 (NHSDA)		
2 (Dept of Housing)	18 (CBO) 3 (city agency)	1 (HUD)	2	
1 (state DSS)	6 (CBO) 3 (local DSS)			
1 (state DSS)	6 (CBO) 2 (local DSS) 2 (city agency)			
	1 (local DSS)			
	1 (CBO)			
1 (state DSS)				
3	2 (community planning report)	9 (census) 3 (CPS) 2 (KFF) 1 (HRSA)	5	11

Continued

TABLE 5-2 Continued

	Measures Used		Data Sources Used		
Indicators	# of EMAs Reporting the Measure	For Defined Time Period	SHD	LHD	CDC
Estimated # of living HIV cases uninsured at time of HIV diagnosis	2		1		
Estimated # of living AIDS cases uninsured at time of AIDS diagnosis	1				
Poverty (Total EMAs Reporting = 50)					
Number people at/ below 300% FPL	34		4	2	
Number people at/ below 100% FPL	12		2		
Number adults at/ below 300%, 200%, 133%, and 100% of FPL	2		1		
Number people at/ below 200% FPL	1				
Number of children (<18) below poverty	3		2		
Not reported	1				

CDC = Centers for Disease Control and Prevention
CPS = Current Population Survey
SHD = State health department
DOL = Department of Labor
LHD = Local health department
HRSA = Health Services and Resources Administration
SAMHSA = Substance Abuse and Mental Health Services Administration
NIMH = National Institute for Mental Health

Other State	Other Local	Other Federal or National Org	Academic Research	No Source
		1 (KFF)		
3 (state agency)				
2 (DOL)	1 (community planning report)			
	1 (city agency)	12 (census)		
		1 (CHSI)		
		1 (CPS)		8
4		5 (census) 1 (KFF)		
		1 (census)		
		1 (census)		
			1	

CHSI = Community Health Status Indicators
NIDA = National Institute for Drug Abuse
DSS = Department of social services
CBO = Community-based organization
KFF = Kaiser Family Foundation
BRFS = Behavioral Risk Factor Survey
NHSDA = National Household Drug Abuse Survey
SHAS = Supplement to HIV/AIDS Surveillance

were uninsured at the time of HIV diagnosis (2 EMAs) or AIDS diagnosis (1 EMA). Many EMAs obtained their insurance data from the state health department (27 percent) or the U.S. Census (18 percent), although other EMAs used the Census Bureau's Current Population Survey (CPS),[7] the Kaiser Family Foundation's State Health Facts,[8] and other state agencies. Each source uses different definitions and measures of insurance status.

These data sources have several limitations. While the U.S. Census provides comprehensive data on poverty rates at the substate level, this information becomes less reliable as time from the decennial U.S. Census increases. The CPS provides more timely data than the decennial census, but does not provide data at the county level. One potential new source is the American Community Survey,[9] which if funded as planned will provide annual data on poverty rates for states and areas with a population of 250,000 or more (NRC, 2000).

Data on insurance rates are not uniformly available at the substate level. While many states and areas have conducted surveys of uninsurance rates, these tend not to be comparable from state to state because of differences in sample size and methods. For comparisons of uninsured rates at

[7]The CPS is a monthly survey of about 50,000 households conducted by the Bureau of the Census for the Bureau of Labor Statistics. The sample is representative of the civilian noninstitutional population. Estimates obtained from the CPS include employment, unemployment, earnings, hours of work, and other indicators. They are available by a variety of demographic characteristics including age, sex, race, marital status, and educational attainment. They are also available by occupation, industry, and class of worker. Supplemental questions to produce estimates on a variety of topics including school enrollment, income, previous work experience, health, employee benefits, and work schedules are also often added to the regular CPS questionnaire. See http://www.bls.census.gov/cps/cpsmain.htm for more information.

[8]The Kaiser Family Foundation has compiled an online resource containing state-level data on demographics, health, and health policy (including HIV/AIDS), including health coverage, access, financing, and state legislation. Data presented on State Health Facts Online are collected from a variety of public and private sources, including original Kaiser Family Foundation reports, data from public websites, and information purchased from private organizations. See http://www.statehealthfacts.kff.org/ for more information.

[9]The American Community Survey is planned as a large-scale, monthly sample survey of U.S. households similar to the census long-form version in content but is administered continuously (NRC, 2000). If implemented as planned (pending congressional funding), the annual sample size will include approximately 3 million addresses, and would provide the same sort of data as the census long form, updated every year. The survey will provide demographic, social, economic, and housing profiles annually for areas and subgroups with 65,000 or more people. For communities of less than 65,000, 3 to 5 years will be required to provide estimates similar in quality to those based on the census long form (http://www.census.gov/acs/www/, accessed July 8, 2003).

the state level, the Census Bureau and others often calculate averages over 2 to 3 years so that all the estimates have similar power (IOM, 2003).

Optional Factors

Several EMAs submitted additional information to describe severity of need (Table 5-3). These optional factors included chlamydia prevalence (26 EMAs), mental illness (18 EMAs), hepatitis (17 EMAs), incarceration and probation (4 EMAs), domestic violence (2 EMAs), other STDs (2 EMAs), coccidiomycosis (1 EMA), and teenage childbearing rates (1 EMA).

For mental illness, applicants used 13 different measures. General prevalence of mental illness was the most common indicator (55 percent of EMAs), followed by the number of residents receiving mental health services (17 percent) and the estimated number of severely mentally ill (11 percent). Variations across states and localities in collecting and reporting these data call into question their reliability and validity.

The majority of EMAs obtained optional data on comorbid and other conditions from the state health department, while a few relied on data from CDC and other federal agencies such as the Substance Abuse and Mental Health Services Administration and the National Institute of Mental Health. Again, the lack of standardization of measures and inconsistency in the quality of the data makes comparison across areas very difficult.

Populations with Special Needs

EMAs included assessments of the following populations with special needs (Table 5-4):

- Homeless (17 EMAs, or 33 percent of total EMAs)
- African Americans (10 EMAs, or 20 percent)
- Latinos (8 EMAs, or 17 percent)
- Recently or soon-to-be released from jail or prison (7 EMAs, or 14 percent)
- Rural individuals (6 EMAs, or 12 percent)
- Incarcerated (5 EMAs, or 10 percent)
- Mentally ill (5 EMAs, or 10 percent)
- Immigrants/undocumented (3 EMAs, or 6 percent)
- Haitians (2 EMAs, or 4 percent)
- Deaf people (2 EMAs, or 4 percent)
- Transgender people (2 EMAs, or 4 percent)

TABLE 5-3 Optional Factors Used to Describe Severity of Need in FY2002 Title I Supplemental Applications

	Measures Used		Data Sources Used		
Indicators	# of EMAs Reporting the Measure	For Defined Time Period	SHD	LHD	CDC
OPTIONAL COMORBIDITY INDICATORS					
Chlamydia (Total EMAs Reporting = 26)					
Prevalence rate	25	8	17	7	1
Rate among women	1			1	
Mental Illness (Total EMAs Reporting = 18)					
General prevalence of mental illness	10		4		1 (BRFS) 1(SHAS)
Number receiving mental health services	3	1	2	1	
Estimated total severely mentally ill	2		1	1	
Daily average in mental health hospitals	1		1		
Mentally ill chemically addicted	1				
Estimated # PLWH with severe mental illness	1		1		
Multiply diagnosed (SMI, SA, HIV)	1		1		
Mental illness based on psychiatric hospital data	1				
Estimated # with schizophrenia	1		1		
Estimated # with bi-polar	1		1		
Estimated # with major depression	1		1		

Other State	Other Local	Other Federal or National Org	Academic Research	No Source
	1 (county mental health agency)	1 (SAMHSA) 1 (NIMH) 1 (Surgeon General report)		
		1 (National Alliance for the Mentally Ill)		
	1 (pysch hospital)			

Continued

TABLE 5-3 Continued

	Measures Used		Data Sources Used		
Indicators	# of EMAs Reporting the Measure	For Defined Time Period	SHD	LHD	CDC
Estimated # with personality disorder	1		1		
Nonseverely mentally ill	1		1		
Hepatitis (Total EMAs Reporting = 17)					
Hep C prevalence rate	5	4	3	2	
Hep B and C	4	4	2	1	
Hep A, B, C separately	3		1	2	
Hep A and B	1	1	1		
Hep C incidence rate	1	1		1	
Hep C, chronic and acute	1	1		1	
Incarceration/Probation (Total EMAs Reporting = 4)					
Incarcerated	3				
Number on parole or probation	1				
Domestic Violence (Total EMAs Reporting = 2)					
Number of domestic violence victims	1				
Case rate per 100,000	1				
Other Venereal Diseases (Total EMAs Reporting = 2)					
Herpes, Tricomonas, N.S. Uteritis, Escabiosis, V. Bacteria	1	1	1		
Herpes and other ulcerative STDs	1		1		

Other State	Other Local	Other Federal or National Org	Academic Research	No Source
			1	
2 (Bureau of Justice)				1
				1
		1 (fed/city justice dept)		
			1 (nat'l study estimating % HIV+ women seeking care who are DV survivors)	

Continued

TABLE 5-3 Continued

	Measures Used		Data Sources Used		
Indicators	# of EMAs Reporting the Measure	For Defined Time Period	SHD	LHD	CDC
Coccidiomycosis (Total EMAs Reporting = 1)					
Prevalence rate	1			1	
Teen Births (Total EMAs Reporting = 1)					
Birth rate among 13–19 yo women (1)	1		1		

CDC = Centers for Disease Control and Prevention
CHSI = Community Health Status Indicators
CPS = Current Population Survey
NIDA = National Institute for Drug Abuse
SHD = State health department
DSS = Department of social services
DOL = Department of Labor
CBO = Community-based organization
LHD = Local health department
KFF = Kaiser Family Foundation
HRSA = Health Services and Resources Administration
BRFS = Behavioral Risk Factor Survey
SAMHSA = Substance Abuse and Mental Health Services Administrations
NHSDA = National Household Drug Abuse Survey
NIMH = National Institute for Mental Health
SHAS = Supplement to HIV/AIDS Surveillance

Other State	Other Local	Other Federal or National Org	Academic Research	No Source

TABLE 5-4 EMAs Reporting on Populations with Special Needs FY2002

EMA	Homeless	African Americans	Latinos	Recently/ Soon-To-Be Released from Jail or Prison
SUBPOPULATIONS DESCRIBED IN TABLE 6 OF THE SUPPLEMENTAL APPLICATION*				
Atlanta, GA	x			
Austin, TX				
Baltimore, MD	x			
Bergen-Passaic, NJ	x	x	x	x
Boston, MA				
Caguas, PR				
Chicago, IL	x		x	
Cleveland, OH		x		
Dallas, TX		x		
Denver, CO				
Detroit, MI				
Dutchess County, NY				
Ft. Lauderdale, FL	x			
Ft. Worth, TX				
Hartford, CN	x			x
Houston, TX				x
Hudson County, NJ		x	x	
Jacksonville, FL				
Kansas City, MO				
Las Vegas, NV				
Los Angeles, CA	x			
Miami, FL	x			
Middlesex-Somerset, NJ	x			
Minneapolis-St. Paul, MN		x	x	
Nassau-Suffolk, NY				
New Haven, CN				
New Orleans, LA	x			x
New York, NY	x			x
Newark, NJ	x			
Norfolk, VA				
Oakland, CA		x		
Orange County, CA		x	x	
Orlando, FL				
Philadelphia, PA				
Phoenix, AZ		x	x	
Ponce, PR	x			
Portland, OR				
Riverside-San Bern., CA				
Sacramento, CA				

Rural Individuals	Incarcerated	Mentally Ill	Immigrants & Undocumented	Other
	x			
				Surrounding counties
				Suburban residents
		x		
	x			Haitians
x				
		x		
x			x	Pediatric patients
		x		
				Transgender
			x	
		x		
x				
			x	
				45 and over
				Deaf; Native Americans
	x	x		
x	x			Relocated <2 yrs to C. Valley

Continued

TABLE 5-4 Continued

EMA	Homeless	African Americans	Latinos	Recently/ Soon-To-Be Released from Jail or Prison
San Antonio, TX				
San Diego, CA	x	x	x	x
San Francisco, CA	x	x	x	
San Jose, CA				
San Juan, PR				
Santa Rosa/Sonoma, CA				
Seattle, WA	x			
St. Louis, MO				
Tampa-St. Pete, FL				
Vineland-Millville, NJ				x
Washington, DC	x			
West Palm Beach, FL				
TOTAL	17	10	8	7

NOTE: X indicates that EMA selected this population as being disproportionately afffected by the HIV epidemic.
*(In addition to the required populations of: youth, IDUs, other substance users, men of color MSM, white MSM, and women of childbearing age)

Other special populations described by only one EMA include migrant workers, pediatric patients, people in surrounding counties, suburban residents, Native Americans, people 45 years and over, people who have relocated in the past 2 years, and people living in a particular part of a county.

Information on populations with special needs is difficult to compare, as the special population categories vary across EMAs, and as consistent data are not available on HIV cases across EMAs. In addition, no reliable estimates exist for the overall size of several of the special populations, such as homeless or transgender populations, much less for the proportion of those populations with HIV.

FINDINGS

Applicants for Title I supplemental awards are asked to supply a tremendous amount of information about the epidemiology of HIV infection and AIDS, the prevalence of various comorbid conditions, poverty and insurance status, and populations with special needs. The Committee found that many of the measures requested in the application did not meet scientific soundness standards of reliability, validity, or empirical

Rural Individuals	Incarcerated	Mentally Ill	Immigrants & Undocumented	Other
				Deaf; hemopheliacs
				Transgender
				PLWH in S/E King Cnty
x				
				Migrant workers
x	x			
				Haitians
6	5	5	3	

support. Many measures lacked standard definitions of the population of interest, time period, and measurement procedure. There was also enormous variation in the data sources used by grantees. Some measures also lacked validity. For example, the application asks grantees to provide HIV prevalence information for their area and for "special populations," but consistent estimates of HIV cases are not available at the EMA level, much less for special populations such as homeless or transgenders. Furthermore, many measures (e.g., comorbidities) lack a scientific evidence base linking them to resource needs. While such measures may have face validity, in that they are logical and are viewed as important by policy makers and grantees, scientific evidence should link them to direct measures of resource needs (such as costs of care, unmet needs, needs for additional services).

Overall, there is little consistency in the factors described in applications, and even when EMAs do describe comparable factors, there is tremendous variability in the types of indicators they use. Thus, it is virtually impossible to make objective comparative assessments of relative needs across areas. Furthermore, except for some information on insurance status and poverty rates, the applications do not describe variations in the costs of providing care in different areas or on the availability of other resources. HRSA/HAB provides a scoring guide for reviewers of applications, but it also emphasizes the importance of reviewer judgment. Perhaps as a result of the difficulty in assessing the variation in resource needs across regions, over and above those due to differences in the prevalence of AIDS, EMAs' Title I supplemental awards are highly correlated with their Title I formula (base) award. In FY2002, for example, the correlation in per-ELC supplemental and base awards was 0.87, indicating a close correspondence between the base and supplemental awards.

Although the use of idiosyncratic indicators of need makes comparisons across EMAs nearly impossible, discussions with Title I representatives suggest that some EMAs find the process of compiling a supplemental application useful for their own local planning efforts (Ryan White CARE Act 2002 Grantee Conference, August 22–23, 2003, Washington, DC: Meeting with Title I EMAs). Thus, EMAs may find value in retaining some aspects of this process for local planning and evaluation. The Committee also notes that the special needs of jurisdictions may not be completely captured by quantitative measures, and that one possibility is to have grantees include a brief (e.g., two pages) summary of their special needs with their application.

Finding 5-1 Resource needs are determined by a complex array of factors, including disease burden, the costs of providing care, and available resources. These factors, for example insurance coverage or costs of care, vary widely across regions. RWCA formula allocations rely primarily on one measure of disease burden (i.e., ELCs) in determining awards, although this measure does not well reflect underlying variations in resource needs. The Title I supplemental award is the largest RWCA grant program that attempts to take into account other factors affecting the complexity and costs of care.

Finding 5-2 The current Title I supplemental award process, which is determined by competitive application, relies on nonstandard and unvalidated measures of local need. Simple, commensurable measures are preferable to complex idiosyncratic measures in allocating resources and their use would improve the award process and resulting allocations.

Finding 5-3 The current Title I supplemental application process is burdensome for grantees. Given the high correlation between grantees' per-ELC supplemental and base awards, the effort required for grantees to complete the application seems unjustified.

One solution to these challenges would be to specify a set of direct or indirect measures of resource needs. An example of the former would be to interview patients and ask them about the kinds of services they need.

An example of the latter would be to develop predictors for areas that are likely to have extra resource needs, such as those with a high proportion of residents with incomes below the poverty level. These issues are discussed in the following sections.

AVAILABLE DATA SOURCES

There are numerous data that could be used to develop indicators of resource needs. CDC and HRSA are conducting a comprehensive review of available data sources as part of the development of guidelines for epidemiologic profiles (CDC, 2003a). The epidemiologic profile is intended to assist RWCA grantees and HIV prevention community planning groups in resource and program planning, evaluation, and allocation decisions (CDC, 2003a). This review will provide information about each data source, the relevant population of interest, its strengths and limitations, and its availability. The report will include information on data sources such as HIV/AIDS reporting and supplemental surveillance efforts, other disease-reporting systems (e.g., STDs, tuberculosis), census data, and vital records information.

The Agency for Healthcare Research and Quality (AHRQ) and HRSA have also compiled a number of potentially relevant variables from a collection of data sources as part of a joint Safety Net Monitoring Initiative in response to a 2000 IOM report, *America's Health Care Safety Net: Intact but Endangered*. One of the recommendations of the IOM report is that "concerted efforts be directed to improving the Nation's capacity and ability to monitor the changing structure, capacity and financial stability of the safety net to meet the health care needs of the uninsured and other vulnerable populations." (p. 10)

AHRQ and HRSA compiled two data books to assist with this effort: one for county and metropolitan areas and one for states. The first book presents data from 90 metropolitan areas in 30 states and the District of Columbia, including 354 counties and 171 cities. The data describe the health care safety net where 80 percent of Americans with family incomes below the federal poverty line live. The second book has similar information for all 1,818 counties in these 30 states (nonmetropolitan and metropolitan counties) (AHRQ, 2003). Data have been compiled on a number of variables that are potentially relevant in determining an area's need for resources. Examples of data collected include rates of uninsurance, Medicaid coverage, presence of a community health center, level of uncompensated care, physician supply per 100,000 population, as well as economic indices, population data, information on immigrant population, and sociodemographic factors.

CDC conducts a number of supplemental surveillance studies (Table

5-5) that could provide information on resource needs, as well as quality of care. CDC is currently in the process of developing a new Morbidity Monitoring System that will use interview and chart data and will allow CDC to collect HIV/AIDS data from a representative population sample. A meeting regarding the design of the new system is planned for early 2004. CDC has announced plans to discontinue the use of two of its supplemental data collection systems, the Adult Spectrum of HIV/AIDS Disease (ASD) and the Supplement to HIV/AIDS Surveillance Project (SHAS) beginning in mid-2004 in favor of this project (Personal communication, CDC, October 16, 2003).

HRSA has also recently undertaken a major effort to standardize the types of data collected from grantees. All grantees now report data to HRSA using the Ryan White CARE Act Data Report (CADR).[10] The CADR asks grantees to provide information on hundreds of data elements, such as client characteristics, service provision, and the costs of providing care. Unfortunately, the amount of data requested might preclude precise estimates of the most important elements, and the cost data are not compiled in a way that could be used to estimate the relative costs of providing a comparable element of care in different areas. Nevertheless, forms such as the CADR, if simplified and designed to provide specific types of information, such as estimates of resource needs and quality of care, could help standardize the plethora of data now submitted and evaluated for Title I supplemental awards. Redesign and coordination of these efforts across CDC and HRSA would enhance the usability of these data in assessing needs for both care and prevention resources and quality of care.

Finding 5-4 Many publicly available data sources, including data routinely collected by HRSA/HAB and CDC, could be used to assess resource needs using indicators that are comparable across areas. Direct measures probably would yield the most valid measures of need, but would be more expensive and perhaps less feasible than indirect measures.

PROPOSED APPROACH

The Committee recommends several steps for addressing some of the limitations of the current Title I supplemental award approach and the desire of Congress for HRSA/HAB to develop more quantitative indicators of need. The first step is to identify direct measures or predictors of resource needs that meet acceptable standards of scientific importance,

[10]http://www.careactdatasupport.hrsa.gov/CADRforms/form_rev.pdf.

soundness, and feasibility. The second step is to develop a more explicit definition of the factors that applicants should consider when defining their resource needs.

One strategy for identifying predictors of needs, sometimes referred to as social area analysis, attempts to relate the characteristics of geographically defined populations to variations in disease or service use (Shevky and Bell, 1955; Pittman et al., 1986; Kessler, 1998). In a social area analysis, one relates the characteristics of an area to the needs of individuals in that area (Shevsky and Bell, 1955; Pittman et al., 1986; Kessler, 1998). This technique is potentially useful when it is difficult or infeasible to routinely ascertain the variable of direct interest (e.g., individual needs) but when the characteristics of an area allow one to predict the distribution of the variable of interest. For example, the Alcohol, Drug Abuse & Mental Health Administration Reorganization Act (P.L. 102-321 [1992]) required states to provide estimates of the prevalence of serious mental illness in their applications for block grant funds (Kessler, 1998). Since such data are not routinely collected, it was necessary to develop a way of estimating prevalence. A technical expert committee developed prevalence estimates for sociodemographic subgroups that then could be applied to the population counts in each state to produce final state estimates. To do this, they used data from a mental health study to estimate prediction equations in which area characteristics were used to predict the prevalence of mental disorders.

To illustrate how this type of approach might be used to estimate resource needs in the context of RWCA allocations, the Committee developed an example of a model that related publicly available county characteristics to direct measures of need. The Committee selected several publicly available variables as example predictors of need. Although the Committee did not find any direct measures of resource needs, the HIV Cost and Services Utilization Study (HCSUS)—an interview study of a probability sample of noninstitutionalized HIV-infected U.S. residents—did collect data on reported needs and quality of care (Bozzette et al., 1998; Shapiro et al., 1999).[11] Using these data, the Committee identified significant predictors for reported needs and an indicator of care quality, whether a patient received treatment with highly active antiretroviral

[11]HCSUS (Bozzette et al., 1998; Shapiro et al., 1999) was an interview study of a national probability sample of noninstitutionalized persons with HIV infection. HCSUS interviewed a total of 2,864 patients. Several members of the Committee were members of the HCSUS consortium, so the Committee was able to access internal data allowing it to match 2,360 of the patients to their primary site of care in 82 counties. See Appendix D for more information.

TABLE 5-5 Selected Supplemental Surveillance Studies (CDC)

Project	Start Date	Description
Supplement to HIV/AIDS Surveillance Project (SHAS)	1989	The SHAS was begun in 1989 to obtain increased descriptive information on persons over 18 years of age with newly reported cases of HIV infection and AIDS. Information is collected from persons reported as having HIV infection or AIDS using a standardized questionnaire administered by trained interviewers. The questionnaire consists of modules involving demographic-socioeconomic information; drug use history, both injected and noninjected; sexual behavior history, including information about STDs, and use of health care services; reproductive history and children's health of women with HIV infection or AIDS, and information on disabilities treatment and adherence. This information supplements the data routinely collected through national HIV and AIDS surveillance and is used to improve our understanding of a variety of issues related to the epidemic of HIV infections for use by prevention programs.
Survey of HIV Disease and Care (SHDC)	2000	The SHDC is a population-based, medical record abstraction project which collects information from the medical records of HIV-infected persons. In the pilot phase of the project, the data elements collected have included: opportunistic illness diagnoses, prescription of prophylactic medications, and other prophylactic practices, such as influenza vaccination and TB skin testing. Prescription of antiretroviral therapies, laboratory markers of state of HIV disease, and comorbid conditions, such as homelessness, mental illness, and substance use. The outcome measures of the project are estimates of proportions of HIV-infected persons receiving a certain medication or with a certain clinical outcome, with confidence intervals. The SHDC uses a two-stage, cluster sampling methodology to allow the calculation of estimates of clinical endpoints generalizable to the population of HIV-infected persons in care; the cluster sampling also improves the efficiency of the study by limiting the number of medical facilities where medical record abstraction must be done.

	Funding Information	
Locations	Year	Total
Arizona	2000	$1,937,637
Atlanta, GA	2001	$2,110,588
Austin, TX	2002	$2,903,831
Chicago, IL		
Delaware		
Denver, CO		
Detroit, MI		
Hartford, CT		
Houston, TX		
Jacksonville, FL		
Jersey City, NJ		
Kansas		
Los Angeles County, CA		
Maryland		
Miami, FL		
Minnesota		
New Haven, CT		
New Mexico		
Philadelphia, PA		
Richland and Charleston Counties, SC		
Tampa, FL		
Washington		
Houston, TX	2000	$243,061
Louisiana	2001	$559,364
Maryland	2002	$235,532
Michigan		
New Jersey		
Ohio		
Philadelphia, PA		
Puerto Rico		
Virginia		
Washington		

Continued

TABLE 5-5 Continued

Project	Start Date	Description
Survey of HIV Disease and Care Plus (SHDC+)	2001	The purpose of this project is to estimate the proportion of HIV-related morbidity that results from the known behavioral determinants of access to care and adherence to medical treatment in association with clinical and laboratory indicators of HIV morbidity, selected sites participating in the SHDC interview patients included in the chart abstraction portion of the Survey. The interview project incorporates standard behavioral surveillance questions on HIV testing, risk, care-seeking, and other related behaviors. This project allows the evaluation of behavioral findings (including access to care, HIV and OI therapy adherence, client perception of value of therapies, disclosure of HIV infection, etc.) and clinical outcomes (virological and immunologic markers or occurrence of OIs, prescription of antiretroviral and OI therapies, etc.).
Adult/ Adolescent Spectrum of Disease (ASD)	1990	The ASD is a national surveillance project which collects demographic, clinical, laboratory, surveillance, health care utilization, and other related data on HIV-infected persons 13 years of age and over through a broad range of participating facilities in 10 U.S. cities. The geographic diversity of participating sites is further enhanced by the diversity of race, sex, sexual orientation, and socioeconomic status of the participants. Cases are drawn from hospital inpatient and outpatient facilities, infectious disease practitioners specializing in HIV infection, private practice medical groups, HIV treatment facilities, and health maintenance organizations. Since the inception of ASD in 1990, over 43,000 patients have been observed. Currently, ASD follows HIV/AIDS patients accessing care at participating sites to retrieve clinical, treatment, and laboratory data at 6 month intervals, beginning with the induction of the patient into ASD and ending with the patient's demise. The ASD project is currently the principal source of national surveillance data on HIV-related morbidity.

	Funding Information	
Locations	Year	Total
Michigan	2001	$328,367
New Jersey	2002	$240,000
Seattle, WA		
Atlanta, GA	2000	$2,005,836
Bayamon, PR	2001	$2,371,683
Dallas, TX	2002	$2,094,018
Denver, CO		
Detroit, MI		
Houston, TX		
Los Angeles County, CA		
New Orleans, LA		
New York, City, NY		
Seattle, WA		

Continued

TABLE 5-5 Continued

Project	Start Date	Description
HIV Testing Survey (HITS)	1996	Some public health and community groups remain concerned that implementing HIV case reporting may deter some at-risk persons from seeking HIV testing. The primary objective of the HITS is to identify the reasons that persons at risk for HIV infection may seek or defer HIV testing and HIV-related health care, and the role state HIV testing and reporting policies play in the decision, to assess whether HIV case reports underrepresent some populations and to improve HIV prevention planning. Additional objectives for HITS are to evaluate the influence of recent events, such as availability of drug therapies and new testing methodologies, on persons' decisions to seek HIV testing. HITS is an anonymous, cross-sectional survey of persons at risk for HIV. Project areas use a standardized protocol based on targeted venue-based sampling methods. Specific recruitment sites and methods will be developed locally, in order to provide a generalizable understanding of HIV testing patterns in at-risk racial/ethnic minority populations.

	Funding Information	
Locations	Year	Total
Arizona	2000	$199,999
California	2001	$1,252,205
Colorado	2002	$1,581,088
Florida		
Houston, TX		
Illinois		
Kansas		
Los Angeles, County, CA		
Louisiana		
Maryland		
Michigan		
Mississippi		
Missouri		
Nevada		
New Jersey		
New Mexico		
New York		
New York City, NY		
North Carolina		
Ohio		
Oregon		
Philadelphia, PA		
Portland, OR		
San Francisco, CA		
Seattle, WA		
Texas		
Vermont		
Washington		

Continued

TABLE 5-5 Continued

Project	Start Date	Description
Enhanced Perinatal Surveillance (EPS)	1990	EPS activities include two main activities in addition to those activities that are considered core pediatric surveillance. Participating areas are expected to match birth registries to HIV/AIDS registries in order to improve ascertainment of mother-infant pairs, and to collect supplemental information on both mothers and infants from a variety of medical records, including mother's prenatal care chart, labor and delivery chart, and the infant's birth chart and pediatric chart. In areas where HIV infection is not reportable by name a hospital-based approach to identify mother-infant pairs is pursued rather than the population-based approach which is feasible in HIV-reporting states only. Twenty-six areas were funded with 1999 supplemental funds to participate in EPS.
AIDS Progression Study (APS)	2001	The APS was designed to understand the characteristics of people who are infected with HIV who progress to or die from AIDS and to explain why progression to AIDS occurs. In addition, this time-limited study examines reasons for progression from AIDS to death among deceased AIDS cases. Abstracted from medical records during the 12-month period preceding AIDS diagnosis, the data include patient characteristics, HIV/AIDS-related history, testing history, AIDS defining conditions, HIV exposure, and laboratory data.

SOURCE: CDC, 2003b.

	Funding Information	
Locations	Year	Total
Alabama	2000	$1,866,553
California	2001	$1,874,431
Chicago, IL	2002	$1,814,324
Connecticut		
District of Columbia		
Houston, TX		
Los Angeles, CA		
Louisiana		
Maryland		
Massachusetts		
Michigan		
New Jersey		
New York		
New York City, NY		
North Carolina		
Ohio		
Pennsylvania		
Philadelphia, PA		
Puerto Rico		
South Carolina		
Tennessee		
Texas		
Virginia		
Boston, MA	2000	$199,999
Chicago, IL	2001	$319,593
Denver, CO		
Hartford, CT		
Los Angeles, CA		
San Francisco, CA		

therapy (HAART).[12] Details of the sample and analyses are represented in Appendix D. Below we summarize the approach and results.

As examples of indicators of need, the Committee used the number of needs reported by the patients and whether the patients had been treated with HAART drugs. In the HCSUS interview, each patient was asked the following questions:

1. Did you need income assistance such as SSI, SSDI, AFDC, or health care benefits from Medicaid or the Veterans Administration in the last 6 months?
2. Did you need to find a place to live in the last 6 months?
3. Did you need home health care in the last 6 months?
4. Did you need mental health or emotional care or counseling in the last 6 months?
5. Did you need drug or alcohol treatment in the last 6 months?

Using these data, the Committee calculated a variable called "number of needs," which is simply the number of these questions that the respondent answered affirmatively.

The Committee selected several county characteristics that it considered representative of the kinds of variables that are likely to be related to resource needs for HIV care.

Examples of indicators of medical resources are:

1. Total general practitioners in 1996 divided by the total population in 1990,
2. Total number of medical specialists in 1996 divided by the total population in 1990.

Examples of area sociodemographic characteristics are:

1. Percent of the population that was African American in 1990,
2. Percent of the population that is foreign born in 1990,
3. Percent of population that lives in urban areas in 1990,
4. Percent of population who live in poverty in 1990,
5. Percent of population who are college graduates in 1990.

---

[12]At the time of the HCSUS study, the recommended therapy for HIV disease was HAART. Recommendations for therapy change over time are updated in the treatment guidelines published by the Department of Health and Human Services (http://www.aidsinfo.nih.gov/) and others.

Using publicly available data (the U.S. Census and a compilation of information called the Area Resource File [ARF]), the Committee compiled data on several characteristics of each county.

The Committee then used the data to estimate models that assessed how well these area characteristics and regions predicted the number of reported needs and receipt of HAART. The models (Appendix D) indicate that the education in an area, the number of general practice physicians, and the number of specialists in an area are statistically significant predictors of the number of needs reported by individuals. Specifically, persons reported more needs if they lived in areas with fewer college educated persons, fewer general practitioners, and more medical specialists. The relationships with education and general practitioners seem reasonable. The relationship for medical specialists is counterintuitive, but it might be a reflection of an emphasis on more expensive care at the expense of more basic services. The strongest predictors of not receiving HAART therapy were living in a county with a high percent of African Americans, a high percentage of families below the poverty level, and an area with more general practitioners. Some of these effects imply striking differences. For example, the average percentage of persons with a college education in the counties studied was 16 percent, with a standard deviation of 5 percent. The coefficient in the model for percent of persons with a college education implies that if one went from a county with a percentage of college educated persons that is a standard deviation below the mean (11 percent) to a county that is a standard deviation above the mean (21 percent), the average need score, which has a range of 0 to 5 and a mean of 1.29 would increase by 0.33. This model illustrates an approach that could be used to select and calibrate variables that predict various types of resource needs.

This example has several limitations. For example, the HCSUS sample was not designed to support the analysis of county effects. The Committee selected variables that were readily available for modeling. Thus, the Committee mainly included variables representing the general availability of medical personnel in an area and its socioeconomic characteristics. Undoubtedly, other variables are more likely to be related to the needs of HIV persons. For example, the health provider shortage areas and medically underserved areas (designated by HRSA's Bureau of Primary Care) may have particularly high resource needs. The predictive value of such variables needs to be tested. However, it is important to recognize that many of the measures that grantees now report on their supplemental applications might not be related to resource needs. None of the applications the Committee reviewed provided empirical support for the association between resource needs and a specific "need factor."

An alternative approach would be to develop a set of direct indicators. There currently are no such indicators that are comparable across regions. It might be possible, however, to coordinate and/or consolidate current efforts conducted by HRSA/HAB and CDC. One would need to assess the tradeoff between scientific accuracy and cost. Surveying a scientifically valid random sample of HIV-infected persons would probably produce the most accurate assessment of needs and would allow one to develop measures directly related to the conceptualization of need proposed by HRSA. However, such an approach would be difficult and expensive to implement. The HCSUS study was able to identify and survey a probability sample of HIV-infected persons in treatment, but it was a complicated and expensive study. Presumably this would be less so for entities with legal surveillance authority. An indirect modeling approach could use available measures. The limitations of such a model are that it might be a poor predictor of interregional variations in needs and might be relatively insensitive to changes over time, if the predictor variables are not updated with sufficient frequency.

RECOMMENDATIONS

Recommendation 5-1 HRSA should modify the Title I supplemental application process. The severity-of-need component of the Title I supplemental award should be based on two components:

- Quantitatively defined need, based on a small number of measures that can be calculated by HRSA/HAB.
- Locally defined need described in a short narrative by the applicant.

Recommendation 5-2 A predominance of the weight for determining Title I awards should be given to the quantitative measure of resource needs that reflect variations in costs of care and fiscal capacity across EMAs.

Recommendation 5-3 HRSA/HAB should evaluate the feasibility and usefulness of using social area indicator models based on publicly available data that are collected in standardized ways across jurisdictions, to estimate EMA-level resource needs for the Title I supplemental award. This approach also might be useful in assessing resource needs for other RWCA discretionary grant programs.

Such an evaluation would entail several steps:

- First, HRSA/HAB should review with additional experts the potential data sources and develop recommendations for additional measures to be considered. HRSA/HAB should determine the availability of data to support these measures. The potential measures and corresponding data sources should be evaluated according to their importance, scientific soundness, and feasibility.

- Second, HRSA/HAB should determine an appropriate definition of resource needs that could be measured directly. Examples used in this report were needs and unmet needs reported by persons living with HIV infection and total costs of care. However, none of these measures captures the resource needs that are most appropriately provided by RWCA funds. Such a definition might take into account whether an individual had alternative sources of public or private health insurance, generosity of that insurance, and/or the cost of providing services in a given area. Thus, estimating need might involve determining both the needs of individuals living with HIV as well as the costs of meeting those needs in a particular area.
- Third, HRSA/HAB should develop a strategy for directly determining need in an adequate number of areas so the relationship between social area indicators and actual need can be estimated. The Committee knows of no such measures now available and so this step will involve consultation with survey experts and statisticians skilled in developing and estimating such models.
- Finally, HRSA/HAB should develop models and assess the association between social area indicators and direct measures of need. It likely will be not be feasible to collect enough data to do this at the EMA level, but models for county variability should be created and data from those models used to assess their ability to explain between-EMA variability.

It is important to evaluate whether a periodic direct assessment of needs or a model-based approach would be more feasible and useful. Resource needs change rapidly and many area-level predictors (e.g., census data) do not change frequently enough to capture such changes. Thus, it may be better to periodically review and update the quantitative indicators used to allocate Title I supplemental award funds.

Recommendation 5-4 The Secretary of Health and Human Services (HHS) should evaluate the cost and utility of redesigning and coordinating studies conducted by HRSA/HAB and CDC to assess the specific needs and circumstances of people living with HIV. These data can be used to estimate resource needs and as part of quality assessment activities. The Secretary of HHS should also assess the cost and utility of the indirect modeling approach described in Recommendation 5-3 for assessing regional variations in resource requirements.

REFERENCES

AHRQ (Agency for Healthcare Research and Quality). 2003. *Fact Sheet: Safety Net Monitoring Initiative.* [Online]. Available: http://www.ahrq.gov/data/safetynet/netfact.htm [accessed September 3, 2003].

Bozzette SA, Berry SH, Duan N, Frankel MR, Leibowitz AA, Lefkowitz D, Emmons CA, Senterfitt JW, Berk ML, Morton SC, Shapiro MF. 1998. The care of HIV-infected adults in the United States. HIV Cost and Services Utilization Study Consortium. *New England Journal of Medicine* 339(26):1897–904.

Bozzette SA, Joyce G, McCaffrey DF, Leibowitz AA, Morton SC, Berry SH, Rastegar A, Timberlake D, Shapiro MF, Goldman DP, and the HIV Cost and Services Utilization Study Consortium. 2001. Expenditures for the care of HIV-infected patients in the era of highly active antiretroviral therapy. *New England Journal of Medicine* 344(11):817–23.

CDC (Centers for Disease Control and Prevention). 2003a. Data for decision making: HIV epidemiologic profiles, HIV program evaluation. *Developing Epidemiologic Profiles for HIV Prevention and Ryan White CARE Act Community Planning—Grantee Training Meeting.* Atlanta, GA: CDC.

CDC. 2003b. Selected Programs Under Program Announcement 00005. (Email communication, Patricia Sweeney, CDC, May 2, 2003).

CMS (Centers for Medicare and Medicaid Services). 1999. Report to Congress: Proposed Method of Incorporating Health Status Risk Adjusters into Medicare+Choice Payments. [Online]. Available: http://cms.hhs.gov/researchers/reports/1999/RTC_RiskAdjusters.pdf.

Freedberg KA, Losina E, Weinstein MC, Paltiel AD, Cohen CJ, Seage GR, Craven DE, Zhang H, Kimmel AD, Goldie SJ. 2001. The cost effectiveness of combination antiretroviral therapy for HIV disease. *New England Journal of Medicine* 344(11):824–31.

Gordis L. 1996. *Epidemiology.* Philadelphia, PA: W.B. Saunders Company.

HRSA (Health Resources and Services Administration). 2000. Unmet Need Consultation Report. *Meeting Sponsored by the Health Resources and Services Administration HIV/AIDS Bureau.* Rockville, MD: HRSA.

HRSA. 2001a. FY 2002 Grant Application Guidance. *The Ryan White Comprehensive AIDS Resources Emergency (CARE) Act: Title I HIV Emergency Relief Grant Program.* Rockville, MD: HRSA.

HRSA. 2001b. *FY 2002 Title I Application Supplemental Application Scoring Guide.* Rockville, MD: HRSA.

HRSA. 2001c. A Primer on Title I and Title II Formula Allocation Calculations. Unpublished document.

HRSA. 2003. Appendix 1: Glossary of Terms. *Ryan White Comprehensive AIDS Resources Emergency (CARE) Act: Needs Assessment Guide (2003 Version).* Rockville, MD: HRSA.

IOM (Institute of Medicine). 2000. *America's Health Care Safety Net: Intact But Endangered.* Lewin ME, Altman S, Eds. Washington, DC: National Academy Press.

IOM. 2001a. *Envisioning the National Health Care Quality Report.* Hurtado MP, Swift EK, Corrigan JM, Eds. Washington, DC: National Academy Press.

IOM. 2001b. *No Time to Lose: Getting More from HIV Prevention.* Ruiz MS, Gable AR, Kaplan EH, Stoto MA, Fineberg HV, Trussell J, Eds. Washington, DC: National Academy Press.

IOM. 2003. *A Shared Destiny: Community Effects of Uninsurance.* Washington, DC: The National Academies Press.

Kahn JG, Janney J, Franks PE. 2003. Interim Report: Measuring Unmet Need for HIV Care Project. Submitted to Office of Science and Epidemiology, HIV/AIDS Bureau, HRSA, U.S. DHHS.

Kaiser Family Foundation. 2000. Financing HIV/AIDS Care: A Quilt with Many Holes. *Capital Hill Briefing Series on HIV/AIDS.* Kaiser Family Foundation.

Kessler RC. 1998. A methodology for estimating 12-month prevalence of serious mental illness. *Mental Health, United States 1998.* DHHS Pub. No. (SMA) 99-3285 ed. Washington, DC: Government Printing Office.

MEDPAC (Medicare Payment Advisory Commission). 1999. Appendix A: Determining Medicare+choice payment rates. *Report to the Congress: Medicare Payment Policy.* [Online]. Available: http://www.medpac.gov/publications/congressional_reports/Mar99%20AppA.pdf.

NASTAD, Kaiser Family Foundation, AIDS Treatment Data Network. 2003. Prepared by Davis D, Aldridge C, Kates J, Chou L. *National ADAP Monitoring Project Annual Report.* NASTAD, Kaiser Family Foundation, AIDS Treatment Data Network.

NRC (National Research Council). 1997. *Assessment of Performance Measures for Public Health, Substance Abuse, and Mental Health.* Perrin EB, Koshel JJ, Eds. Washington, DC: National Academy Press.

NRC. 2000. *Small-Area Income and Poverty Estimates: Priorities for 2000 and Beyond.* Citro CF, Kalton G, Eds. Washington, DC: National Academy Press.

NRC. 2001. *Choosing the Right Formula.* Jabine TB, Louis TA, Schirm AL, Eds. Washington, DC: National Academy Press.

NRC. 2003. *Statistical Issues in Allocating Funds by Formula.* Louis TA, Jabine TB, Gerstein MA, Eds. Washington, DC: The National Academies Press.

Pittman J, Andrews H, Struening E. 1986. The use of zip coded population data in social area studies of service utilization. *Evaluation and Program Planning* 9(4): 309–17.

Shapiro MF, Morton SC, McCaffrey DF, Senterfitt JW, Fleishman JA, Perlman JF, Athey LA, Keesey JW, Goldman DP, Berry SH, Bozzette SA. 1999. Variations in the care of HIV-infected adults in the United States: results from the HIV Cost and Services Utilization Study. *Journal of the American Medical Association* 281(24):2305–15.

Shevky E, Bell W. 1955. *Social Area Analysis.* Stanford: Stanford University Press.

Society of Actuaries. 1997. Medicare/Medicaid risk contracting—profitability. *RECORD* 22(2):1–20.

U.S. Congress. 2000. *Congressional Record.* 146(123):S10032.

6

Measuring Quality of Care

Morbidity and mortality from HIV disease declined dramatically in the mid-to-late 1990s due in large part to improvements in antiretroviral therapy and an increase in the proportion of individuals receiving therapy (Karon et al., 2001). The declines were unevenly distributed across HIV-infected populations, however, due to factors such as unequal access to care and variability in quality of care (Bozzette et al., 1998; Shapiro et al., 1999). A major focus of the Ryan White Comprehensive AIDS Resources Emergency (CARE) Act is not only to eliminate barriers to accessing care, but also to improve the quality of care that its clients receive.

Two major provisions of the 2000 CARE Act reauthorization emphasized aspects of quality of care. The first provision required that all Ryan White CARE Act (RWCA) grantees establish a quality-management program. Although Title III and IV grantees already had such programs in place, the new provision required Title I and II grantees to implement them.[1] The purpose of the quality-management programs is to ensure that service providers adhere to established HIV clinical practices and Department of Health and Human Services (DHHS) guidelines to the extent possible; to ensure that quality-improvement strategies include support services that help people receive appropriate HIV health care

[1]Some Title I and II grantees already had quality-management programs in place prior to the reauthorization.

(e.g., transportation assistance, case management); and to ensure that demographic, clinical, and health care utilization information is used to monitor trends in the spectrum of HIV-related illnesses and the local epidemic (U.S. Congress, 2000a).

The second provision in the reauthorization of RWCA directed the Institute of Medicine (IOM) to study two aspects of quality assessment:

1. "The availability and utility of health outcomes measures and data for HIV primary care and support services and the extent to which those measures and data could be used to measure the quality of such funded services" (Ryan White CARE Act. 42 U.S.C. § 300ff-11 [2003]).
2. "Other factors determined to be relevant to assessing an individual's or community's ability to gain and sustain access to quality HIV services" (Ryan White CARE Act. 42 U.S.C. § 300ff-11 [2003]).

The focus on quality in the most recent reauthorization reflects several national trends in quality improvement and accountability. First, the health sector has seen growing interest in measuring and improving quality (IOM 2000, 2001a).[2,3] In addition, numerous reports have identified a gap between care that should be provided based on available professional knowledge and technology and the care that patients actually receive (Advisory Commission on Consumer Protection and Quality in the Health Care Industry, 1988; IOM and NRC, 1999; IOM, 2000, 2001b). Significant disparities have also been identified in the quality of care for persons living with HIV disease (Cunningham et al., 1999; Shapiro et al., 1999; Stein et al., 2000). As a result, quality measurement and improvement efforts have become a central focus of the Health Resources and Services Administration HIV/AIDS Bureau (HRSA/HAB) and RWCA grantees.

Another major trend in quality improvement and accountability is the fact that federal policy and funding decisions are increasingly being based on performance indicators. The passage of the Government Performance Results Act (GPRA)[4] in 1993 and other legislation[5] emphasized accountability across federal government sectors and programs by requiring all federal programs to establish measurable performance goals

---

[2]Major groups with quality initiatives include the National Committee for Quality Assurance (NCQA), the Agency for Healthcare Research and Quality (AHRQ), the Foundation for Accountability (FACCT), the National Quality Forum, and the Leapfrog Group, among others.

[3]For a more comprehensive review of quality-of-care activities in health care, see IOM, 2000, 2001a,b.

[4]Government Performance Results Act., H.R. 826., 103d Cong., 1st Sess. 1993.

[5]Federal Management Improvement Act of 1996 (P.L. 104-208); Chief Financial Officers Act of 1990.

and to document actual results that can be linked to the budgetary process (Kates et al., 2001). As a result, HRSA/HAB and RWCA grantees must document the impact of CARE Act funds on improving access to care and treatment and in addressing unmet needs. Key GPRA performance measures for HRSA regarding RWCA include eliminating barriers to care, eliminating health disparities, assuring quality of care, and improving public health and health care access.

Progress on this broad agenda cannot be adequately measured by outcomes alone. Considering this context, the Committee interpreted this charge as a request to examine and make recommendations regarding the availability and usefulness of not only outcomes, but a broad continuum of measures for assessing and improving the quality of both primary care and support services funded through the CARE Act. Knowledge about what constitutes the best possible HIV/AIDS care is constantly changing, and the applicability of specific measures is limited by the evolving nature of the epidemic, including changes in the affected populations, the course and outcomes of infection, treatment standards, and policies and programs for financing and delivering care. Accordingly, while the Committee makes recommendations regarding measures that HRSA and grantees can use to monitor quality of care (see Recommendation 6-1), the Committee felt it could best contribute by providing a framework, criteria, and process for selecting measures that can evolve with the epidemic.

The Committee divided its work into several discrete tasks:

- Reviewing current HRSA/HAB quality-of-care activities;
- Developing a conceptual framework for indicators that reflects the availability and quality of the full range of services across populations and organizations;
- Developing criteria for selecting indicators for assessing and improving HIV/AIDS services funded through RWCA;
- Reviewing quality measures used by RWCA grantees and other major HIV providers, recommended by authoritative groups, and contained in the research literature;
- Identifying areas that require further development;
- Developing a process HRSA might use to select and regularly update measures; and
- Offering recommendations based on the analysis and findings presented here.

CURRENT HRSA/HAB QUALITY-OF-CARE ACTIVITIES

HRSA/HAB and RWCA grantees have undertaken a variety of efforts to address the quality of care, treatment, and training in RWCA programs.[6] HAB has sponsored several major quality-of-care initiatives and provides a variety of technical assistance tools and training opportunities for grantees designed to help them implement quality-management programs targeting clinical, administrative, and supportive services. HAB's quality initiatives focus on the service delivery system at various levels, including individual providers, Title I Eligible Metropolitan Areas (EMAs), and regions. Several of the initiatives have focused specifically on Title III/IV clinics and providers, although significant work is being done to implement quality-management programs through Title I and II. This section reviews the major quality initiatives of HRSA/HAB. A number of other quality efforts by HRSA/HAB, including special research projects and technical assistance guides, are presented in Table 6-1.

HIV Quality of Care Project (HIVQUAL)

Adapted from a model of quality improvement consultation developed by New York State, the HIVQUAL builds skills and capacity among Titles III and IV grantees to sustain quality improvement. The project is sponsored by HRSA/HAB and administered by the New York State Department of Health's AIDS Institute. The project aims to improve the quality of care delivered to persons with HIV by using data to measure performance, tracking clinical indicators based on clinical practice guidelines, and providing consultations regarding Continuous Quality Improvement. The HIVQUAL project collects information on a number of quality indicators, which are discussed later in this chapter. Grantees submit collected data to the HIVQUAL Project, where they are compiled into aggregate reports and comparative tables for participants and HRSA. A software program (HIVQUAL 3) is used to facilitate the measurement of quality indicators. Participation among grantees is encouraged, but not required (HRSA, 2003c).

Institute for Health Care Improvement HIV/AIDS Collaborative

The Institute for Healthcare Improvement (IHI) HIV/AIDS Collaborative was an effort to use rapid improvement strategies to accelerate the pace of quality improvement among CARE Act grantees. IHI focused on developing a systemwide model to ensure the delivery of evidence-based clinical care and provide strong support for self-management. The long-range goal of the IHI Collaborative was to maximize the length and qual-

---

[6]See McKinney and Marconi (2002) for a review of CARE Act–funded research on quality of care.

TABLE 6-1 Other HRSA/HAB Quality-of-Care Activities

HRSA/HAB Quality Initiative	Description
Outcomes Evaluation Tools	HRSA/HAB has developed several outcome evaluation guides that provide a framework for outcomes evaluation and sample measures (HRSA, 2003f): • The *Outcomes Evaluation Technical Assistance Guide: Primary Medical Care Outcomes* (2000) includes suggested outcomes indicators for primary medical care. • The *Outcomes Evaluation Technical Assistance Guide for Case Management Services* (2001) includes suggested outcomes indicators for case management and information on validated quality-of-life instruments. • *Outcomes Evaluation: Getting Started* (2001). • *HRSA Care Action: The Resource Gap. Measuring Success: Evaluation, Outcomes, and Quality of HIV Care.*
Special Projects of National Significance	HRSA/HAB has sponsored a number of Special Projects of National Significance (SPNS) that have examined access, quality of care, and outcomes (HRSA, 2003d). Some projects include: • *Assessing Existing Efforts to Increase Adherence to Medications* (1999). • *Evaluating the Impact of IT on Improving Delivery and Quality of Care for HIV Seropositive Individuals* (2002). • *Improving HIV Quality of Care Cooperative Agreement* (1999). For more information on SPNS projects see: http://hab.hrsa.gov/special/evaluation2g.htm.
HIV/AIDS Evaluation Monograph Series	The monograph series of publications was created by HRSA/HAB to assist RWCA grantees in designing and implementing evaluation studies (HRSA, 2003c). Example publications include: • *Using Data to Assess HIV/AIDS Service Needs: A Guide for Ryan White CARE Act Planning Groups*, Report #2. • *An Approach to Evaluating HAART Utilization & Outcomes in CARE Act–Funded Clinics*, Report #5. • *Delivering HIV Services to Vulnerable Populations: What Have We Learned*, Report #6.
HRSA Center for HIV Quality Care	The HRSA Center for Quality Care focuses on defining appropriate standards of care for clients of HRSA programs, determining the cost of that care, and conducting research on and comparing benefit packages and capitation rates in Medicaid managed care plans. The Center is also documenting community-based provider experience with managed care plans (HRSA, 2003a).

ity of life for patients with HIV/AIDS and satisfy patient and caregiver needs while maintaining or decreasing the total cost of care. Each participating health system identified a specific population of patients (either a subset of their patients or all of them) that could be monitored for the duration of the collaborative. Grantees then changed practices and systems to improve clinical management and office efficiency. Participants identified a set of quality-of-care indicators (discussed later in this chapter), while IHI provided guidance about how to implement and test changes in the care of their pilot population. Over 80 Title III and Title IV grantee organizations participated in the first collaborative, and Title I grantees are currently participating in a new collaborative (HRSA, 2003b; IHI, 2003).

Client Demonstration Project

The Client Demonstration Project collects client data on HIV-infected clients (tracked by unique identifiers) receiving services at CARE Act–funded providers at designated sites (EMAs or states). The client-level data permit analyses of various combinations of information on client demographics, medical status, and service utilization. The analysis of several characteristics, including CD4+ cell counts, CDC-defined disease stage, and tuberculosis status, is also possible. Though the project was originally designed to include clients who receive services from Title I and II providers, a substantial number of providers participating in the demonstration projects also receive funding from Title III and IV (HRSA, 2001, 2003a).

Primary Care Assessment Tool

The Primary Care Assessment Tool (PCAT) is a site-visit protocol developed for Title III–funded CARE Act programs. The tool, which includes a quality improvement component in the clinical section, is used to evaluate the clinical, fiscal, administrative, and support services of the grantees (HRSA, 2003e).

CARE Act Data Report

Each year all providers funded by CARE Act grantees are required to submit a CARE Act Data Report (CADR) to HRSA. Implemented in January 2002, CADR consolidated and replaced previous reporting instruments. The purpose of the CADR is to collect information on all clients who receive at least one CARE Act–eligible service during a calendar year, including information on the number and characteristics of clients served, types of services provided, and characteristics of provider agencies. CADR also requires medical service providers to provide information on the number of clients who have been screened or treated for comorbid conditions, diagnosed with an AIDS-defining condition, and prescribed combination antiretroviral therapy. An unduplicated count of patients is not currently possible in CADR, so clients may be reported more than one time. CAREWare is a free software program that assists grantees in producing the CADR. Data from CADR are used to assess program effectiveness and quality under the GPRA (HRSA, 2002).

Other HRSA Quality Initiatives

HRSA also supports a number of other quality-of-care activities, including outcome evaluation tools, several Special Projects of National Significance, and the HIV/AIDS Evaluation Monograph Series (Table 6-1).

FOUR-DIMENSIONAL CONCEPTUAL FRAMEWORK FOR HIV QUALITY ASSESSMENT

In this section, the Committee presents a conceptual framework for assessing the quality of HIV/AIDS care. In developing its framework, the Committee relied on previous work for definitions and theory of patient-level quality, and coupled this with a public health perspective in extending previous work to include quality of care for populations.

The Committee adopted the definition of health care quality first developed by the IOM in 1990. This report defined health care quality as "the degree to which health services for individuals and populations increase the likelihood of desired health outcomes and are consistent with current professional knowledge" (IOM, 1990). This definition highlights several important aspects of quality (IOM, 2001a). First, numerous persons, providers, and organizations provide care to patients and all must be of good quality. Second, the definition acknowledges that good quality health care should produce outcomes that patients desire and that patients' preference for treatment options may vary. Third, high-quality care does not necessarily lead to desirable outcomes. There are many factors beyond the control of providers or organizations, such as environmental or social factors, that can affect outcomes. The corollary is also true; desirable outcomes may occur despite poor quality of care. Finally, it speaks to the obligation of providers to inform themselves of most recent advances in their discipline (IOM, 2001a).

The Committee also relied heavily on the seminal work of Avedis Donabedian who conceptualized quality along three dimensions: structure ("the settings in which [health care] takes place and the instrumentalities of which it is the product"), process ("whether what is known as 'good' medical care has been applied") and outcomes ("in terms of recovery, restoration of function and of survival") (Donabedian, 1966). The Committee also based its framework on a model developed by Holzemer and Reilly (1995) that extends the work of Donabedian by focusing on the interactions and linkages between structure, process, and outcomes at the client, provider, and the care setting levels.

The Committee conceptualizes HIV quality assessment as having four key dimensions: the population of interest, the level assessed, the type of measures employed, and the spectrum of services to be evaluated (Figure 6-1).

I.	**Population of Interest** • Group I: Not diagnosed, not in care • Group II: Diagnosed, not in care • Group III: Diagnosed, in care
II.	**Level of Assessment** • Individual • Provider or clinic • Population or area (e.g., EMA, state)
III.	**Type of Measure** • Structure • Process • Outcome
IV.	**Spectrum of Services** • Counseling and testing • Referral to treatment • Social support services • Prevention of transmission • Prevention of AIDS • Prophylaxis • Treatment • Service integration and coordination

FIGURE 6-1 Dimensions of quality assessment.

Population of Interest

The HIV-infected population consists of three groups with respect to use of services: (I) those who are not yet diagnosed and thus are not in care, (II) those who are diagnosed but are not currently in care,[7] and (III) those who are diagnosed and are receiving care. These categories represent a dynamic continuum. Changes in HIV prevalence and the effectiveness of screening efforts affect the flow of persons from group I to groups II and III. Shifts between groups II and III can be rapid and frequent as individuals move in and out of care owing to changes in insurance coverage or as the need for hospital or other urgent care related to an HIV-related comorbid condition arises.

When assessing care quality, the CARE Act has traditionally focused on individuals who are diagnosed and currently in care. Grantees have long sought to improve continuity of care for persons who drop out of care or receive only episodic care, and there has recently been an increased emphasis on those who are diagnosed but not yet in care. To date, few CARE Act resources have been directed to those who are not yet diagnosed. However, providers, consumers, public health officials, and Congress are focusing more attention on ensuring access to high-quality services for *all* who are HIV-infected (U.S. Congress, 2000b).

Among those with HIV disease, many of those not receiving care were once in care and lost access or withdrew; it is generally agreed that a high proportion of these individuals would benefit from a return to regular care. A similar argument applies to those who know of their infection but have never sought or have been unable to gain access to care, as they may well have advanced disease amenable to chemotherapy. Those with early disease will benefit from monitoring and counseling regarding their general health before their disease progresses, and indications for antiretroviral therapy could be extended to this group in the future. In addition, society benefits from efforts to prevent transmission from all currently infected individuals. Thus, knowing the relative numbers of persons in groups I, II, and III gives direct information on the overall effectiveness of the health care system in providing access to needed care. Knowing the proportions of infected persons who are undiagnosed across areas allows inference regarding access to screening and case-finding services, and about the attractance associated with the perceived high quality of care in an area. Knowing the proportions of persons who are diagnosed but not in care across areas allows inference regarding the accessibility of existing care facilities and the ability of those facilities to maintain continuity of care for treated persons.

---

[7]The category of those who are "not in care" also includes those who are not in *regular care.*

Level of Assessment

The fundamental level for assessing quality of care is the individual patient. For example, if a clinician were assessing whether his or her patients were receiving high-quality care, it would be important to know whether patients for whom high active antiretroviral therapy (HAART) is indicated were offered such therapy. Such individual levels of quality also aggregate to the program level. For example, a measure of the quality of care provided by Title III clinics is the proportion of appropriate patients who are receiving HAART therapy. Provider organizations, including HRSA and its grantees, now commonly employ a variety of aggregated client-level measures of treatment quality in assessing clinics or practices, including monitoring, chemoprophylaxis, and antiretroviral therapy.[8] However, the scientific community has given little attention to assessing the quality of care across whole communities, metropolitan areas, or states, regardless of whether patients get care at any particular facility.[9]

The measures and data available to assess quality vary markedly according to both the target population and the level of the assessment. For example, in assessing the quality of and access to services at the clinic level, one might assess the average wait time for an initial appointment or the use of appropriate chemoprophylaxis. While analysts have much less experience in measuring quality at the population level, they might assess access and chemoprophylaxis by measuring the average time elapsed between HIV and AIDS diagnoses. In addition, as indicated above, one might measure the overall accessibility of care by measuring the proportion of HIV-infected people who are in care, those who are diagnosed but not in care, and those who are not diagnosed.

Type of Measure

The Committee adopted the widely accepted taxonomy that classifies measures into three domains (Donabedian, 1966). *Structural measures* assess the characteristics and resources of an organization, such as staffing, supplies, equipment, and training. The influence of physical surroundings, availability of services, and staffing mix on the quality and costs of care is poorly understood. However, an abundance of literature has demonstrated a link between the experience of individual and institu-

---

[8]While the data for these indicators of the quality of medical care are collected at the patient level, they are generally aggregated to make assessments at the provider, clinic, and program level.

[9]HRSA, however, has recently initiated some work focused on developing quality measures at the EMA level.

tional providers (in terms of the volume and complexity of HIV services they offer) and improved clinical and economic outcomes (Kitahata et al., 1996; Turner et al., 1998; Aiken et al., 2002; Landon et al., 2002, 2003).

Process measures focus on the actions taken in the course of providing medical care, such as conducting diagnostic tests, offering appropriate therapies, promoting self-care. Process measures are important because they "cause" outcomes to the extent that medical interventions have an effect and because the acts of providing care are convenient targets for quality improvement. Although information for process measures is usually obtained from medical records, analysts can also obtain important information by asking patients about their experiences (Cleary and Edgman-Levitan, 1997; Cleary, 1999; Wilson et al., 2002). Quality assessment often aims primarily at improving processes as the key to improving outcomes because they are easier to track and modify than outcomes.

Outcome measures assess the changes in a patient's health status. Intermediate outcome measures may assess patients' viral load or CD4+ cell count, while longer-term outcome measures might examine morbidity, mortality, and health-related quality of life. These three major elements are interrelated and theoretically causally linked; that is, the structure of care affects the probability of good processes of care, which can in turn affect outcomes such as health status, quality of life, and patient satisfaction.

Despite compelling arguments for analyzing outcomes as ultimate indicators of quality, there are practical and theoretical impediments to doing so, at least for the individual patient and the small (in a statistical sense) aggregations of patients often used to assess providers. First, individual patient outcomes are often not closely linked to quality of care offered or provided. A broad range of factors, many of which providers do not control, determines clients' health outcomes. Accounting for these influences is extremely difficult (Brook et al., 1996). Strong links between care and outcomes are more likely when considering a large patient group that is well defined by medical condition or demographics, when interventions target outcomes, and when well-accepted physiological, biochemical, and psychological mechanisms link medical interventions with outcomes. When assessing the quality of specific clinics or programs, it is therefore important to ensure that the outcome measures are primarily affected by the program being assessed rather than some characteristic of the subpopulation being served, and that there is evidence for the quality of the actions and programs at that clinic. For this reason, process measures are often used in lieu of outcome measures at the program or clinic level, while monitoring outcomes is a simpler and more compelling way of assessing the impact of all care provided in an area.

Spectrum of Services

Congress clearly intended to develop measures that could be used to assess the quality of both primary care and support services, and the Committee concurs that both are essential components of high-quality care (Ryan White CARE Act. 42 U.S.C. § 300ff-11). Research also shows that support services such as case management are important in reducing barriers to care (Katz et al., 2000, 2001). However, quality measurement has focused almost exclusively on clinical care.

As an individual moves along the continuum of diagnosis and care, the services that compose quality of care also change. For those not yet diagnosed, strong efforts to find, screen, and counsel them are essential; while those who are diagnosed but not in care need finding, referral, support services, and strategies for preventing transmission. Those in care, meanwhile, need not only a wide range of clinical services, including monitoring, prophylaxis, and treatment, but also social support services and efforts to prevent transmission (Figure 6-2).

Spectrum of Services	**Population with HIV/AIDS**		
	Group I Not diagnosed, not in care	**Group II** Diagnosed, not in care	**Group III** Diagnosed, in care
Counseling and testing	✓	✓	
Referral to treatment		✓	
Social support services		✓	✓
Prevention of transmission		✓	✓
Prevention of AIDS			✓
Prophylaxis			✓
Monitoring			✓
Treatment			✓
Service integration and coordination		✓	✓

FIGURE 6-2 Spectrum of services across the HIV/AIDS population.
KEY: ✓ = service appropriate to group.
NOTE: This figure includes examples of services, rather than a comprehensive listing.

PRINCIPLES FOR SELECTING QUALITY-OF-CARE MEASURES

Chapter 5 discussed three overarching criteria—importance, scientific soundness, and feasibility—that could be used to evaluate measures of resource needs (Chapter 5, Box 5-2). These same criteria can be applied to evaluation of quality-of-care measures.

Importance

1. *Meaningfulness:* There should be consensus among clinicians, patients, or policy makers that the measure reflects an important aspect of quality of care.

2. *Prevalence and seriousness of the problem:* Measures should focus on common problems or care procedures that affect a sizable proportion of RWCA clients. Measures should focus on aspects of quality of care that are a general problem, or for which there is significant variation across grantees.

3. *Potential for improvement:* Measures should reflect aspects of care that can be improved most by RWCA grantees or through administrative changes.

4. *Potential impact:* Considering the prevalence and seriousness of the problem and the potential for improvement, measures should reflect the prevalence and seriousness of the problem and the potential for improvement. Measures should be selected that reflect aspects of care that can have the greatest impact on persons living with HIV infection.

Scientific Soundness

1. *Reliability:* Measures should be reproducible and yield consistent results when repeated in the same populations and settings. Reliability is enhanced by using standard data collection methods across clinics or populations, collecting data in a way that minimizes manipulation, and employing a common definition of the population of interest and the time period.

2. *Validity:* Measures should capture what they purport to measure. Measures should make sense logically or clinically (face validity), should correlate well with other measures of the same aspects of quality of care (construct validity), and should capture meaningful aspects of quality of care (content validity) (IOM, 2001a).

3. *Evidence base:* Measures should have a strong evidence base to support their use. For instance, structure and process measures should be clearly linked to outcomes. A number of established systems for scoring

the strength of evidence have been used to evaluate potential quality measures (Gross et al., 2000).

Feasibility

1. *Availability of data:* Data should be available at the appropriate level. For example, if the measure is to be used to assess the quality of medical clinics, each clinic should have the data; likewise, if the assessment will occur at the EMA level, each EMA should have the same data. Data should also be available in a timely manner and collected with reasonable periodicity.

2. *Cost or burden of measurement:* Data should be collected at reasonable cost and should not impose an excessive burden on grantees. Measures based on data that are already being collected for other purposes, or that are publicly available, are more feasible than measures that require new data collection. Similarly, the use of a small set of indicators rather than lengthy questionnaires would reduce the burden on patients and providers. Feasible measures should also be robust to different documentation practices.

There is an implied hierarchy in applying these criteria. Measures should first be considered for their importance, then scientific soundness and feasibility. Measures that are scientifically sound and feasible but do not reflect an area of importance should not be included. HRSA and grantees should select measures that are the most important in terms of the potential impact on the clients served by RWCA. Measures that are important and scientifically sound but not feasible should not be automatically discarded but considered for the future.

The feasibility criterion is particularly important in assessing quality of care under RWCA. The Committee is well aware of the data-collecting and -reporting burden experienced by grantees. RWCA grantees often receive funds from numerous other public and private sources, each of which has their own data-reporting requirements, format, and timeframes (Ryan White CARE Act 2002 Grantee Conference, August 22–23, 2003, Washington, DC: Meeting with Title I EMAs). Even within the RWCA, collecting and reporting required data is a substantial burden. For example, the CADR, which all grantees are required to complete annually, asks literally hundreds of questions, many of which are difficult to answer. HRSA could both reduce the burden of data collection on RWCA grantees and obtain more useful information on quality of care by focusing on a limited set of measures.

EXISTING QUALITY-OF-CARE MEASURES FOR HIV/AIDS

The Committee reviewed the quality measures commonly used by key organizations and often-cited studies. The Committee summarizes measures used by following nine sources: HIVQUAL, Institute for Healthcare Improvement Collaborative on HIV/AIDS (Title III), Evaluation of Quality Improvement for HIV Care (EQHIV), HIV Cost and Services Utilization Study (HCSUS), Infectious Disease Society of America (IDSA), FACCT, California Health Care Foundation Quality Assessment tool (developed by RAND), HIV Quality Enhancement Research Initiative (HIV-QUERI), and University Health System Consortium (UHC) (Table 6-2).

While there is some consistency in the measures used across these sources, there is also a great deal of variation in how the measures are defined and implemented. This review also indicates that many sources use numerous process measures and, to a lesser extent, outcomes measures. Process measures, almost all of which were closely related to well-accepted clinical guidelines,[10] were over 10 times more frequent than outcome measures. Comparable attention has not been devoted to measures of structure, such as the availability of clinicians with the appropriate expertise and experience, despite studies linking increased provider expertise, capacity, and number of HIV-specific services to longer patient survival and prevention of opportunistic conditions (Kitahata et al., 1996; Bennett et al., 1989; Ball and Turner, 1991; Turner et al., 1998). The Committee identified relatively few measures of support services, and no systematic efforts to assess patient experiences with care. Finally, the Committee found that all measures focused on the provider level. No population-level process or outcome measures of quality were in routine use, although they serve as important indicators of the overall impact of the epidemic and prevention/treatment/support programs in an area.[11] A brief summary of the provider-level quality-of-care measures used by different sources is included below. A detailed review of measures used by these sources is included in Appendix E.

Summary of Provider-Level Quality-of-Care Measures

Measures are organized according Donnabedian's structure, process, and outcome framework.

---

[10]See DHHS guidelines (http://www.aidsinfo.nih.gov/guidelines/) and International AIDS Society-USA guidelines (Yeni et al., 2002; http://www.iasusa.org/).

[11]HRSA/HAB is working with the Institute for Healthcare Improvement and grantees to develop population-based measures for Title I EMAs.

Structural Measures

The Committee found no structural measures of quality recommended or used by these sources, although certain process measures, such as visits with HIV specialists, imply the availability of appropriate healthcare services.

Process Measures

Aggregations of patient-level process-of-care measures dominated this group. The measures of process quality used by the programs divide into five categories: prevention, screening and monitoring, antiretroviral treatment, prophylactic treatment for opportunistic infections, and social and support services.

Prevention

Three sources had quality measures focused on prevention activities. One monitored counseling and testing of pregnant women, one measured counseling regarding high-risk behaviors, and another measured tobacco use assessment.

Screening and Monitoring

Eight sources measured viral load monitoring. Seven sources measured cervical cancer screening and CD4+ cell counts; six monitored tuberculosis screening; six monitored hepatitis B and/or C screening; five monitored toxoplasmosis and syphilis screening; three tracked screening for cytomegalovirus disease; two sources each monitored complete blood count, whether individuals were in care (outpatient visits), and lipid screening. One source tracked each of the following: hepatitis A, oral health/dental exam, and visits with an HIV specialist (Figure 6-3).

Antiretroviral Treatment

All nine sources had measures of antiretroviral therapy. Eight sources had measures of provision of indicated antiretroviral therapy (ART). Four sources had measures of adherence counseling and/or monitoring. One source measured appropriate management of patients on ART, and another monitored changes in treatment regimens (Figure 6-4).

TABLE 6-2 Selected Sources of Commonly Used Quality Measures

Source	Sponsor
HIV Quality of Care Program (HIVQUAL) http://hab.hrsa.gov/special/hivqual.htm	HRSA/HAB and the New York State Department of Health AIDS Institute
Institute for Health Care Improvement (IHI) Collaborative for Improving Care for People with HIV/AIDS http://hab.hrsa.gov/special/breakthrough.htm	HRSA/HAB
Evaluation of Quality Improvement for HIV Care (EQHIV)[a]	AHRQ
HIV Cost and Services Utilization Study (HCSUS) http://www.rand.org/health/hcsus/	A consortium of private and government sponsors; work conducted by The RAND Corporation

Description
Adapted from a model of quality-improvement consultation first developed by New York State, HIVQUAL (sponsored by HAB and administered by the New York State Department of Health AIDS Institute) builds capacity and capability among Title III and IV grantees to sustain quality improvement. The project aims to improve the quality of care delivered to persons with HIV through the use of aggregate data to measure performance, the measurement of clinical indicators that are based on clinical practice guidelines, and provision of continuous quality-improvement consultations and coaching. The HIVQUAL project measures a number of quality indicators (discussed later in this chapter). The data collected by grantees are submitted to the HIVQUAL Project, where they are compiled into aggregate reports and comparative tables for participants and HRSA. A software program (HIVQUAL 3) developed through this project helps facilitate the measurement of quality indicators. Participation among grantees is encouraged but not required (HRSA, 2003c)
The IHI HIV/AIDS Collaborative was a collaborative effort to accelerate the pace of quality improvement among CARE Act grantees. IHI focused on developing a systemwide model of care to ensure the delivery of evidence-based clinical care, and strong support for self-management. Through the Collaborative, participating grantee organizations identified a set of quality-of-care indicators. IHI provided guidance about how to implement and test changes in the care of pilot populations. More than 80 Title III and Title IV grantee organizations participated in the first Collaborative, and Title I grantees are currently participating in a new Collaborative (HRSA, 2003b; IHI, 2003).
Starting in 1999, HRSA required Title III grantees to undergo continuous quality improvement (CQI) training using the IHI breakthrough series approach. The goal of this project is to assess the quality of care provided by participating clinics, changes in such care subsequent to quality training, and the organizational characteristics and policies related to such changes. EQHIV is a controlled observational study examining the outcomes of the CQI training. The study will compare three groups of Title III clinics: (1) clinical HIV programs receiving new Title III funds as of July 1999 that receive CQI training; (2) clinical HIV programs already receiving Title III funding that will receive CQI training; and (3) clinical HIV programs already receiving Title III funding that will not receive CQI training.
HCSUS was the first major research effort to collect information on a nationally representative sample of people in care for HIV infection. The study provides information on the health care services persons with HIV disease are receiving, and on the costs of those services, to inform policy making and resource allocation. The study was conducted May 1994 through October 2000. HCSUS consisted of a core study and seven supplemental studies. The core study used data on over 3,700 HIV-positive persons in care in hospitals, clinics, and private practices in 28 urban areas and 24 clusters of rural counties in the United States. The core study examined cost, use, andquality of care; access to care; unmet needs for care; quality of life; social support; knowledge of HIV; clinical outcomes mental health; and the relationship of

Continued

TABLE 6-2 Continued

Source	Sponsor
Gross et al. (2000) http://www.idsociety.org/HIV/CEN/PGindex_HIV.htm	IDSA
FACCT Quality-of-Care Indicators for HIV/AIDS http://www.facct.org/facct/doclibFiles/documentFile_302.pdf	FACCT
California Health Care Foundation QA Tool (developed by RAND) http://www.rand.org/publications/MR/MR1281/	California Health Care Foundation
HIV-QUERI http://www.va.gov/chrr/active_trials/queri_factsheetHIV.pdf	Veterans Health Administration
University Health System Consortium (UHC) (UHC, 2002)	UHC, an allianceof the clinical enterprises of 87 academic health centers

[a]Personal communication, P. Cleary, Harvard University, 2003.

Description
these variables to provider type and patient characteristics. Seven supplemental studies used data from the core study to examine HIV in rural areas, early disease stages, mental health, older persons with HIV, drug use, oral health, and antiretroviral therapy (HRSA, 2003c).
These measures are extracted from the 1999 U.S. Public Health Service/IDSA guidelines on the prevention of opportunistic infections in persons infected with HIV. In an accompanying article, Gross et al. (2000) identify performance measures to assess compliance with the guidelines on preventing opportunistic infections and to assist in their implementation.
Wu and colleagues produced a discussion paper in 1998 for the FACCT that examines issues related to quality-of-care assessment for people with HIV/AIDS. Specifically, Wu et al. discuss potential indicators "that could be used to examine the performance of providers and organizations in managed care organizations, to compare organizations, and to inform quality improvement activities" (Wu et al., 1998). The paper includes a discussion of practical issues in collecting indicator data, sampling issues, and a review of a number of potential indicators. Wu and colleagues published an article adapted from the report in 2000 (Wu et al., 2000).
The RAND Corporation produced the report *Quality of Care for Oncological Conditions and HIV: A Review of the Literature and Quality Indicators*, for the California Health Care Foundation in 2000 (Asch et al., 2000). RAND developed quality indicators for HIV disease using six practice guidelines, five reviews, and an extensive MEDLINE search of medical literature from 1993 to 1996.
HIV-QUERI seeks to develop a "comprehensive and continuously improving HIV disease management system that integrates administrators, physicians, nurses, pharmacists and patients in a coordinated fashion" within the Veterans Health Administration (VHA). Building on guidelines for standards of HIV care from entities such as the International AIDS Society and the IDSA, as well as the DHHS, CDC, VHA, FACCT, and the NCQA, HIV-QUERI has collected and adapted these guidelines to the VHA to generate indicators of best practice. (VA, 2003).
This study was conducted to help participants improve clinical processes based on comparative information from actual practice in the era of combination antiretroviral therapy (as opposed to pre-CART, to which most of the published studies on adherence to recommended guidelines in HIV patient care refer). Institutional enrollment in the project was voluntary and self-selected. Selected members of the National Association of Public Hospitals and Health Systems are also eligible to participate in UHC benchmarking studies. Forty organizations participated. Project participation included the selection of a minimum of 40 patients and submission of a patient log, completion of a cross-sectional survey on clinic organizational structure and processes, and a retrospective patient-level medical record abstraction tool.

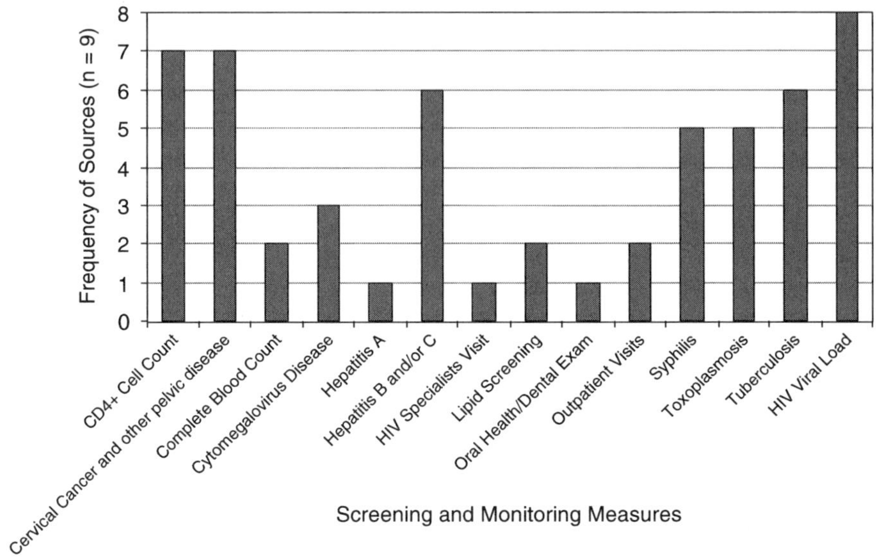

FIGURE 6-3 Frequency of screening and monitoring quality measures among select sources.

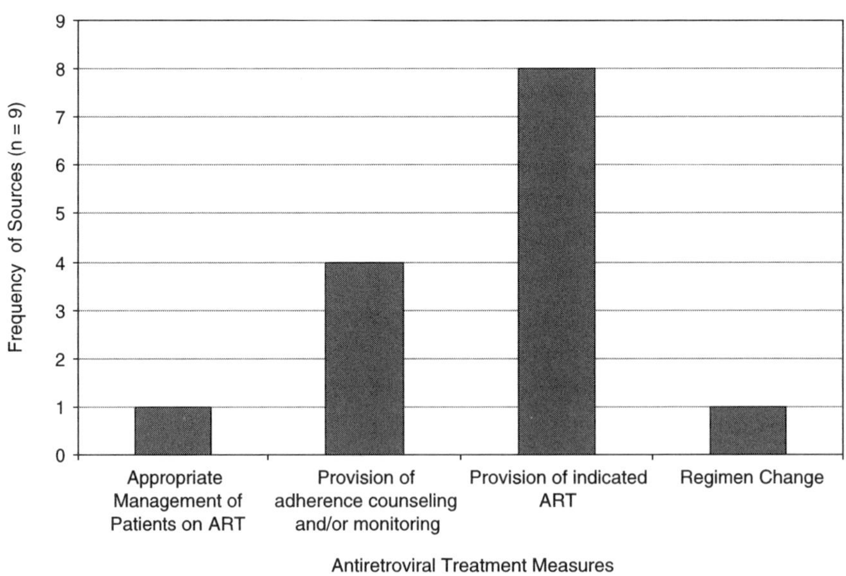

FIGURE 6-4 Frequency of antiretroviral treatment quality measures among select sources.

Prophylactic Treatment for Opportunistic Infections

Prophylaxis for opportunistic infections, such as *Pneumocystis carinii* pneumonia (PCP) (n = 8) and *Mycobacterium avium* vomplex (MAC) (n = 6), are the next most commonly used indicators, generally for patients who have a low or very low CD4+ cell count, respectively. Five sources collected data on patients' receipt of influenza and pneumococcal ("pneumonia") vaccines. Two sources measured patients' receipt of the hepatitis B vaccination series and prophylaxis for tuberculosis and toxoplasmosis (Figure 6-5).

Social and Support Services

Only three sources reviewed by the Committee monitored indicators of social and support services. IHI had optional indicators for self-management/goal setting and support services. HIVQUAL had indicators for mental health assessment and substance abuse treatment. The HCSUS study asked patients to assess their access to critical support services by indicating whether, in the previous six months, they had needed any of five types of services: income assistance, housing assistance, home health

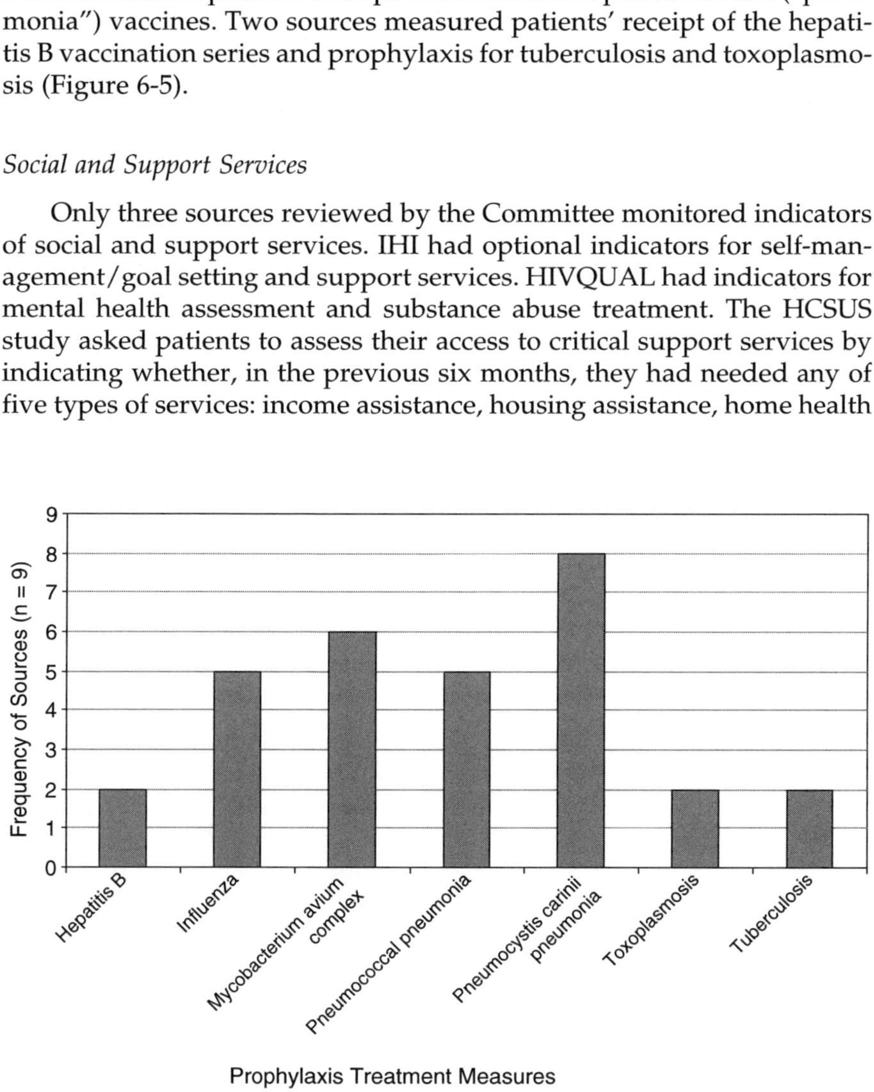

FIGURE 6-5 Frequency of prophylactic treatment quality measures among select sources.

care, mental health care, and substance abuse treatment. Any subject who answered yes to any of these questions was asked if those needs were met.

Health Outcomes

Outcome measures used are classified into three major groups: CD4+ cell counts, viral load counts, and emergency room visits and hospitalizations. Two sources measured CD4+ cell counts and viral load levels, and one source each measured patients' emergency room visits and hospitalizations.

Population-Level Quality-of-Care Measures

Most quality assessment is designed to improve service quality and patient care, and thus focuses on the provider level, which by definition covers only people receiving treatment at a defined set of facilities or enrolled in a specific HMO. However, population-based measures are important in assessing the overall impact of RWCA in a region. Although several potential measures have been developed, research in this area has been limited.

One recent study utilized a *Pneumocystis carinii* pneumonia (PCP) index, defined by zip code as the number of PCP-related hospitalizations for residents divided by the number of residents living with AIDS), to identify geographic areas within New York City where residents were at increased risk for PCP (Arno et al., 2002). The PCP index is an example of a population-based measure that can be used to identify areas in need of public health interventions and improvements in HIV service delivery. This measure has the added advantage of being easy to generate and requiring only a few data sources (surveillance and service utilization data).

In a separate analysis, the Committee examined another potential population-level measure—the 12-month case fatality rate—which measures the proportion of people who die within 12 months after they are diagnosed with HIV infection. Figures 6-6 and 6-7 show a general decline in the 12-month case fatality rate after the introduction of HAART in the mid-1990s before the measure levels off. One notable aspect of these graphs is that they show two- and threefold variations in fatality rates among EMAs, and several EMAs show rising rates.

Another potential population-based quality measure is the proportion of patients in an area who have an AIDS diagnosis within 12 months of their HIV diagnosis. This measure can be calculated using data from the HIV and AIDS reporting system. Currently, these data are only avail-

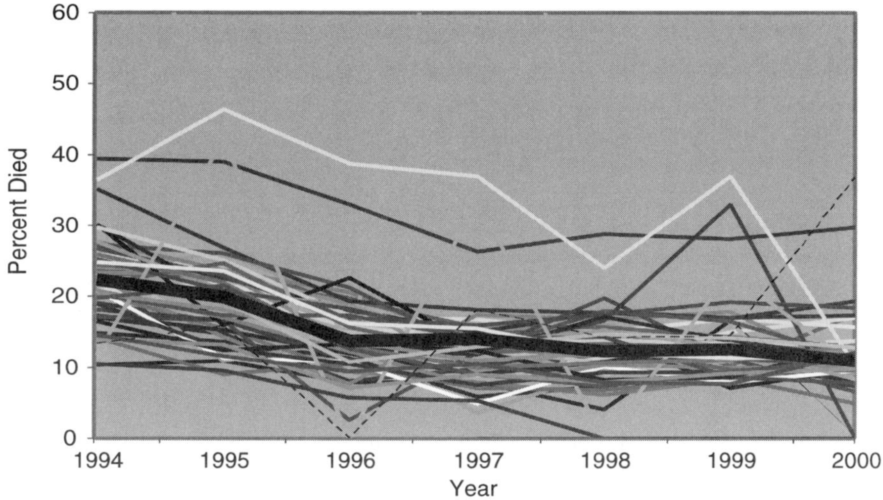

FIGURE 6-6 Percent of people who died within 12 months of AIDS diagnosis, by state/territory, 1994–2000.

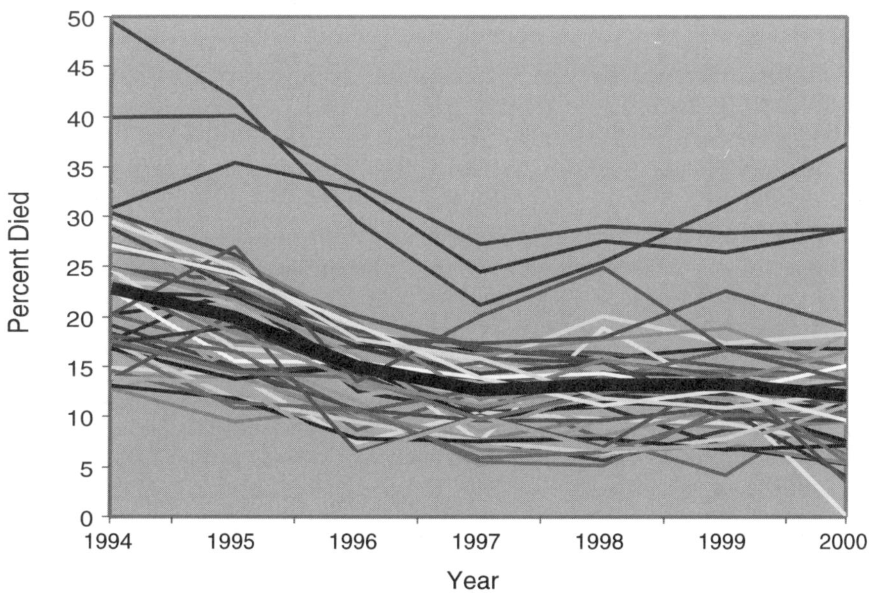

FIGURE 6-7 Percent of people who died within 12 months of AIDS diagnosis, by EMA, 1994–2000.

able for states with name-based HIV reporting in place as CDC does not accept code-based data.

A recent report by the CDC highlights other potential measures that could be applied at the population level (CDC, 2003a). Using data from four supplemental surveillance studies[12] conducted in selected geographic areas, CDC reports on a number of measures including: HIV-infected persons ever prescribed ART; HIV-infected persons currently prescribed ART; HIV-infected persons ever diagnosed with PCP; HIV-infected persons currently prescribed prophylaxis for PCP; and HIV-infected persons receiving a tuberculin skin test. Such measures would be difficult to obtain routinely from all relevant jurisdictions because they require estimates of the number of persons in a defined area who are infected and in care. However, a combination of intensive, targeted surveys, the current population surveys, the Area Resource File, and regional and local data could be used to estimate these populations.

While population measures are critical in monitoring the overall health of the population in a region, population-based outcomes and other measures may be influenced by a number of factors. Kates and colleagues (2001) refer to this as the "problem of attribution," that is the difficulty of ascribing client-level or local-level outcomes to a state or federal program. They note several challenges to the effective measurement of health programs: "Variation in health systems infrastructure, market dynamics, epidemiology, and demographics makes it difficult to connect federal level activities to effects at the local level. In addition, because clients of federal programs may receive services at multiple locations, each with multiple funding sources, it is difficult to align a federal program activity (or grant dollar) with a client level outcome such as reduction in morbidity and mortality. Indeed, individual client characteristics and varying levels of disease severity may require sophisticated case mix adjustment to make comparisons meaningful" (Kates et al., 2001, p. 147).

---

[12]Data in the report are from (1) the Adult/Adolescent Spectrum of HIV Disease (ASD) project, a longitudinal medical record review study conducted in >100 selected facilities in 11 major U.S. cities; (2) the Survey of HIV Disease and Care (SHDC), a cross-sectional, population-based medical record review project conducted in 3 areas; (3) the Supplement to HIV/AIDS Surveillance (SHAS) project, an interview project of persons with HIV/AIDS conducted by 12 state/local health departments; and (4) the Missed Opportunities for Tuberculosis Prevention study, a medical record review of a population-based sample of persons newly diagnosed with HIV or AIDS in three major U.S. cities (CDC, 2003a). CDC has announced plans to discontinue two of these projects, ASD and SHAS, beginning in mid-2004. CDC is currently in the process of developing a new Morbidity Monitoring System that will use interview and chart data and will allow collection of HIV/AIDS data from a representative population sample (CDC, 2003c).

FINDINGS

HRSA and RWCA-funded clinics and programs are doing an admirable job of defining, assessing, and attempting to improve the quality of care received by HIV-infected individuals. RWCA-funded clinics have established quality management and improvement programs, and states and EMAs either have or are establishing such programs. HRSA has sponsored numerous research and demonstration projects and a national quality-improvement collaborative to enable RWCA clients to receive the best-possible care. In many ways, RWCA-funded programs have a more advanced approach to measuring and improving quality of care than most general medical facilities. Yet, HRSA, RWCA grantees, and providers could still do much more to measure and improve quality of care. Current efforts are not guided by a common conceptual framework and measures are often not standardized. This is understandable given the recent development of quality-management programs, particularly under Titles I and II. From a programmatic point of view, the primary limitation is that the measures are not defined and measured in a comparable manner across jurisdictions. Thus, it would be very hard for HRSA to assess the relative quality of care across clinics, EMAs, or states, using the data currently available. A more organized and coherent approach would be beneficial.

Based on its review of selected quality-of-care measure sets in the previous section, the Committee recommends a standardized set of structure, process, and outcome quality measures for assessing and facilitating quality improvement at the clinic level and at the EMA/state levels (see Recommendation 6-1). For the well-developed process measures of clinical care, measures were selected if at least four of the nine groups included them. Other measures were identified using the expert judgment of the Committee.

A critical step in improving the current situation of uncoordinated data collection would be reaching a consensus on how different indicators should be defined and implemented and then putting into place a mechanism for ensuring the quality of the ensuing data. Although there are many ways of doing this, the NCQA and the National Quality Forum have developed procedures and policies that could be emulated or modified. For example, NCQA has technical advisory groups that provide advice on the importance, scientific soundness, and feasibility of possible measures, and it maintains a standing Committee on Performance Measurement that evaluates recommendations from technical experts and staff. The Committee on Performance Measurement includes representatives from the Office of Personnel Management, a state Medical Association, corporate health care purchasers, health care systems, business coalitions, professional organizations, the American Association of Health Plans, patient advocacy groups, insurance companies, a state department of human services, researchers, Centers for Medicare & Medicaid Services (CMS), CDC, the Veterans Administration, and the AHRQ. A comparable set of procedures could be established by HRSA.

Finding 6-1 The RWCA legislation's emphasis on development of outcome measures is appropriate because tracking outcomes is a crucial element for accountability, and helpful in quality improvement. However, outcome measures alone are not sufficient because outcomes may be influenced by many factors not under the control of grantees, and because structure and process measures can uniquely identify areas for specific improvement.

Finding 6-2 Quality measures for HIV/AIDS that are in wide use are based on broadly accepted clinical guidelines and are appropriate. However, these measures are not standardized, which has hindered efficient evaluation of RWCA programs. Moreover, these measures are generally restricted to evaluating providers via examination of aggregated patient-level clinical data. Measures examining a more complete spectrum of services including, for example, those assessing support services, are important but are not yet in wide enough use to allow for consensus to emerge about specific measures for HIV care. Examples of potential measures of supportive services include the provision of case management, benefits advocacy, or substance abuse and mental health services.

Finding 6-3 Measures of access to needed medical and nonmedical services are also lacking. Such measures have been developed for other diseases (e.g., cancer and heart disease) and could be adapted to HIV/AIDS. Examples of potential access measures include those that focus on continuity of care (e.g., identification of primary care provider), access to needed specialty care, and access to needed nonmedical care.

Finding 6-4 Population-based measures are essential in monitoring HIV care in an EMA, region, or state and identifying areas for improvement. Current efforts to assess overall quality of care in EMAs and states are rudimentary and no population-based measures are in wide use. These measures should not be interpreted as direct measures of the quality of care being provided by specific clinics, but rather as reflecting the cumulative effects of many influences on case quality and outcomes. Additional work is needed to further develop these measures.

RECOMMENDATIONS

The Committee's recommendations are an effort to support and extend the excellent work of HRSA and RWCA grantees in quality assessment and improvement.

Recommendation 6-1 Quality measures: HRSA should adopt quality measures that are comprehensive with respect to populations (diagnosed in care; diagnosed but not in care; not diagnosed, not in care), level of assessment (provider and population levels), types of measures (structure, process, and outcome), and spectrum of services (clinical and supportive services). At a minimum, HRSA and grantees should strongly consider inclusion of the following standard set of measures to assess the quality of care provided by RWCA-funded providers and EMA and state-level programs. Standard definitions and detailed criteria for these measures need to be developed by HRSA in collaboration with grantees, affected communities, and other stakeholders after a rigorous examination of the importance, scientific soundness, and feasibility of potential measures.

I. CLINIC LEVEL MEASURES

A. Structure

1. Proportion of providers with appropriate expertise and experience in treating patients with HIV*
2. Availability of case management services

B. Process

Screening for:

3. Cervical cancer*
4. Hepatitis B
   a. And administration of hepatitis B vaccine if negative
5. Hepatitis C*
6. Syphilis*
7. Toxoplasmosis
8. Tuberculosis*

Performance of the following clinical monitoring tests:

9. CD4+ cell count and HIV viral load (process)*

Antiretroviral Treatment:

10. Provision of indicated antiretroviral treatment*
11. Provision of adherence counseling and monitoring

Vaccinations and Prophylaxis for Opportunistic Infections:

12. Influenza vaccination
13. Pneumoccocal pneumonia vaccination
14. Hepatitis B vaccination if patient not immune
15. If indicated, *Mycobacterium avium* complex (MAC)
16. If indicated, *Pneumocystis carinii* pneumonia* (PCP)

C. Outcomes 17. Monitoring of CD4+ cell count and viral load values*
18. Proportion of patients with a history of an AIDS-defining opportunistic condition*
19. Proportion of patients who have >2 missed scheduled clinic appointments per year
20. Hospitalizations and emergency room visits without hospital admission*
21. Proportion of patients with unmet need for support services (e.g., assistance with obtaining housing).^

II. AREA (E.G., EMA OR STATE) LEVEL MEASURES

Outcome measures related to access and care:
22. Proportion of HIV-infected persons in an area who are not diagnosed^
23. Proportion of diagnosed persons in area who are receiving regular care^
24. Proportion of people with HIV who died within 12 months of an HIV diagnosis*
25. Proportion of people with HIV who progressed to AIDS within 12 months of initial HIV diagnosis*

Key: * indicates high priority; ^ indicates high priority, but may require further development. Other measures are important, but of lower priority.

Recommendation 6-2 Infrastructure development: The Secretary of Health and Human Services (HHS) should provide additional resources to HRSA and CDC to develop infrastructure for monitoring quality at the patient, clinic, and population levels. This infrastructure development strategy has three major components:

a. HRSA should enhance support for information technology and personnel to enable clinics to collect, aggregate, and report a focused set of clinical and patient-reported data.

b. HRSA should collaborate with CDC and other agencies to develop innovative population-based measures that can be captured using existing data sources or other community-based information-gathering activities, such as surveys of unmet needs.

c. Congress should enhance flexibility in the administrative caps at the grantee level to promote infrastructure development.

Recommendation 6-3 Collaborative quality activities: The Secretary of HHS should convene a working group, not restricted to, but including the NCQA, state insurance commissioners, state Medicaid officials, and representatives from HRSA, CDC, the CMS, providers of community, outpatient, and inpatient care, and members of the relevant research communities, to consider strategies for promoting greater collaboration between public health departments and public- and private-sector providers in order establish tools and methods to assess systems of care and quality, building on the successful collaborative models developed by the CDC for immunization (e.g., Clinic Assessment Software Application and Assessment Feedback Incentives Exchange).

REFERENCES

Advisory Commission on Consumer Protection and Quality in the Health Care Industry. 1998. *Quality First: Better Health Care for All Americans.* Washington, DC: U.S. Government Printing Office.

Aiken L, Clarke S, Sloane D, Sochalski J, Silber J. 2002. Hospital nurse staffing and patient mortality, burse burnout, and job dissatisfaction. *Journal of the American Medical Association* 288(16):1987–93.

Arno PS, Gourevitch MN, Drucker E, Fang J, Goldberg C, Memmott M, Bonuck K, Deb N, Schoenbaum E. 2002. Analysis of a population-based *Pneumocystis carinii* pneumonia index as an outcome measure of access and quality of care for the treatment of HIV disease. *American Journal of Public Health* 92(3):395–8.

Asch SM, Kerr EA, Hamilton EG, Reifel JL, McGlynn EA, Eds. 2000. *Quality of Care for Oncologic Conditions and HIV: A Review of the Literature and Quality Indicators.* Santa Monica, CA: Rand Health.

Ball JK, Turner BJ. 1991. *AIDS in U.S. Hospitals in 1986-1987: A National Perspective.* Rockville, MD: Agency for Health Care Policy and Research.

Bennett CL, Garfinkle JB, Greenfield S, Draper D, Rogers W, Mathews C, Kanouse DE. 1989. The relation between hospital experience and in-hospital mortality for patients with AIDS-related PCP. *Journal of the American Medical Association* 261:2975–9.

Bozzette SA, Berry SH, Duan N, Frankel MR, Leibowitz AA, Lefkowitz D, Emmons CA, Senterfitt JW, Berk ML, Morton SC, Shapiro MF. 1998. The care of HIV-infected adults in the United States. HIV Cost and Services Utilization Study Consortium. *New England Journal of Medicine* 339(26):1897–904.

Bozzette SA, Phillips B, Asch S, Gifford AL, Lenert L, Menke T, Ortiz E, Owens D, Deyton L. 2000. Quality Enhancement Research Initiative for Human Immunodeficiency Virus/Acquired Immunodeficiency Syndrome: Framework and Plan. *Medical Care* 38(6 Suppl 1):160–9.

Brook RH, McGlynn EA, Cleary PD. 1996. Quality of health care. Part 2: Measuring quality of care. *New England Journal of Medicine* 335(13):966–70.

CDC (Centers for Disease Control and Prevention). 2003a. *Selected measures of access to and utilization of treatment and prophylaxis for HIV-infected persons.* HIV/AIDS Surveillance Supplemental Report. 9(3).

CDC. 2003b. IOM Request: Data on Early Progression and Early Deaths. (Email commuication P. Sweeney, CDC, March 20, 2003).

CDC. 2003c. Morbidity Monitoring System. (Email communication, Patricia Sweeney, October 16, 2003).

Cleary PD. 1999. The increasing importance of patient surveys. *British Medical Journal* 319:720–1.

Cleary PD, Edgman-Levitan S. 1997. Health care quality: Incorporating consumer perspectives. *Journal of the American Medical Association* 278(19):1608–12.

Cunningham W, Andersen R, Katz M, Stein M, Turner B, Crystal S, Zierler S, Kuromiya K, Morton S, St Clair P, Bozzette S, Shapiro M. 1999. The impact of competing subsistence needs and barriers on access to medical care for persons with human immunodeficiency virus receiving care in the United States. *Medical Care* 37(12):1270–81.

Donabedian A. 1966. Evaluating the quality of medical care. *The Milbank Memorial Fund Quarterly* 44(3 Supp):166–206.

Gross PA, Asch S, Kitahata M, Freedberg KA, Barr D, Melnick DA, Bozzette S. 2000. Performance measures for guidelines on preventing opportunistic infections in patients infected with human immunodeficiency virus. *Clinical Infectious Diseases* 30(Suppl 1):S85–S93.

Holzemer W, Reilly CA. 1995. Variables, variability, and variations research: Implications for medical informatics. *Journal of the American Medical Informatics Association* 2(3):183–9.

HRSA (Health Resources and Services Administration). 2001. *The Ryan White CARE Act*. [Online]. Available: http://hab.hrsa.gov/data2/cdemosum.htm [accessed July 31, 2003].

HRSA. 2002. Instruction for completing the Ryan White CARE Act data report (CARE Act Data Report): Cross—Title Data Report. January, 2002. [Online]. Available: http://www.careactdatasupport.hrsa.gov/CADRforms/instruct.pdf [accessed July 31, 2003].

HRSA. 2003a. Report and Studies: Client Demonstration Projects. [Online]. Available: http://hab.hrsa.gov/data2/cdemosum.htm [accessed July 31, 2003].

HRSA. 2003b. Special Initiatives: HIV/AIDS Breakthrough Series Collaborative. [Online]. Available: http://hab.hrsa.gov/special/breakthrough.htm [accessed June 30, 2003].

HRSA. 2003c. Special Initiatives: HIV/QUAL Continuous Quality Program. [Online]. Available: http://hab.hrsa/gov/special/hivqual.htm [accessed June 30, 2003].

HRSA. 2003d. Special Initiatives: Initiatives/Collaboratives (by topic). [Online]. Available: http://www.hab.hrsa.gov/special/evaluation2g.htm [accessed July 31, 2003].

HRSA. 2003e. Tools for Grantees: Primary Care Assessment Tool (PCAT). [Online]. Available: http://hab.hrsa.gov/tools/pcat.htm [accessed July 31, 2003].

HRSA. 2003f. Outcomes Evaluation Technical Assistance Guide: Primary Medical Care Outcomes, Titles I and II of the Ryan White CARE Act. [Online]. Available: ftp://ftp.hrsa.gov/hab/guide.pdf [accessed July 31, 2003].

IHI (Institute for Healthcare Improvement). 2003. Improving Care for People Infected with HIV. [Online]. Available: http://www.ihi.org/collaboratives/breakthroughseries/HIV/charter.asp [accessed July 31, 2003].

IOM (Institute of Medicine). 1990. *Medicare: A Strategy for Quality Assurance. Vol. 2*. Lohr K, Ed. Washington, DC: National Academy Press.

IOM. 2000. *To Err Is Human: Building a Safer Health System*. Washington, DC: National Academy Press.

IOM. 2001a. *Envisioning the National Health Care Quality Report*. Hurtado MP, Swift EK, Corrigan JM, Eds. Washington, DC: National Academy Press.

IOM. 2001b. *Crossing the Quality Chasm: A New Health System for the 21st Century*. Washington, DC: National Academy Press.

IOM and NRC (Institute of Medicine and National Research Council). 1999. *Ensuring Quality Cancer Care*. Hewitt M, Simone JV, Eds. Washington, DC: National Academy Press.

Karon JM, Fleming PL, Steketee RW, De Cock KM. 2001. HIV in the United States at the turn of the century: An epidemic in transition. *American Journal of Public Health* 91(7):1060–8.

Kates K, Marconi K, Mannie TE. 2001. Developing a performance management system for a federal public health program: The Ryan White CARE ACT Titles 1 and 2. *Evaluation and Programs Planning* 24:145–55.

Katz M, Cunningham W, Mor V, Andersen R, Kellogg T, Zierler S, Crystal S, Stein M, Cylar K, Bozzette S, Shapiro M. 2000. Prevalence and predictors of unmet need for supportive services among HIV-infected persons: impact of case management. *Medical Care* 38(1):58–69.

Katz M, Cunningham W, Fleishman J, Andersen R, Kellogg T, Bozzette S, Shapiro M. 2001. Effect of case management on unmet needs and utilization of medical care and medications among HIV-infected persons. *Annals of Internal Medicine* 135(8 Pt 1):557–65.

Kitahata MM, Koepsell TD, Deyo RA, Maxwell CL, Dodge WT, Wagner EH. 1996. Physicians' experience with the acquired immunodeficiency syndrome as a factor in patients' survival. *New England Journal of Medicine* 334(11):701–6.

Landon BE, Wilson IB, Wenger NS, Cohn SE, Fichtenbaum CJ, Bozzette SA, Shapiro MF, Cleary PD. 2002. Specialty training and specialization among physicians who treat HIV/AIDS in the United States. *Journal of General Internal Medicine* 17(1):12–22.

Landon BE, Wilson IB, Cohn SE, Fichtenbaum CJ, Wong MD, Wenger NS, Bozzette SA, Shapiro MF, Cleary PD. 2003. Physician specialization and antiretroviral therapy for HIV: Adoption and use in a national probability sample of persons infected with HIV. *Journal of General Internal Medicine* 18(4):233–241.

McKinney M, Marconi K. 2002. Delivering HIV services to vulnerable populations: A review of CARE act-funded services. *Public Health Reports* 117:99–113.

Shapiro MF, Morton SC, McCaffrey DF, Senterfitt JW, Fleishman JA, Perlman JF, Athey LA, Keesey JW, Goldman DP, Berry SH, Bozzette SA. 1999. Variations in the care of HIV-infected adults in the United States: Results from the HIV Cost and Services Utilization Study. *Journal of the American Medical Association* 281(24):2305–15.

Stein MD, Crystal S, Cunningham WE, Ananthanarayanan A, Andersen RM, Turner BJ, Zierler S, Morton S, Katz MH, Bozzette SA, Shapiro MF, Schuster MA. 2000. Delays in seeking HIV care due to competing caregiver responsibilities. *American Journal of Public Health* 90(7):1138–40.

Turner B, Markson L, Cocroft J, Cosler L, Hauck WW. 1998. Clinic HIV-focused features and prevention of *Pneumocystis carinii* pneumonia. *Journal of General Internal Medicine* 13(1):16–23.

UHC (University Health System Consortium). 2002. HIV Ambulatory Care Clinical Benchmarking Executive Summary. 12.

U.S. Congress. 2000a. *Congressional Record* 146(123):S10032.

U.S. Congress, House of Representatives. Committee on Commerce. 2000b. *Report on Ryan White CARE Act Amendments of 2000 (106-788).* 106th Cong., 2d Sess. July 25, 2000.

VA (Veterans Health Administration). 2003. HIV Quality Enhancement Research Initiative (HIV-QUERI). [Online]. Available: http://www.va.gov/chrr/active_trials/queri_factsheetHIV.pdf [accessed July 31, 2003].

Wilson IB, Ding L, Hays RD, Shapiro MF, Bozzette SA, Cleary PD. 2002. HIV patients' experiences with inpatient and outpatient care: Results of a national survey. *Medical Care* 40(12):1149–60.

Wu A, Gifford A. 1998. Quality of Care Indicators for HIV/AIDS: A Discussion Paper for the Foundation for Accountability. [Online]. Available: http://www.facct.org/facct/doclibFiles/documentFile_302.pdf [accessed July 31, 2003].

Wu AW, Gifford A, Asch S, Cohn SE, Bozzette SA, Yurk R. 2000. Quality-of-care indicators for HIV/AIDS. *Disease Management and Health Outcomes* 7(6):315–30.

Yeni P, Hammer SM, Carpenter CC, Cooper DA, Fischl MA, Gatell JM, Gazzard BG, Hirsch MS, Jacobsen DM, Katzenstein DA, Montaner JS, Richman DD, Saag MS, Schechter M, Schooley RT, Thompson MA, Vella S, Volberding PA. 2002. Antiretroviral treatment for adult HIV infection in 2002: Updated recommendations of the International AIDS Society-USA Panel. *Journal of the American Medical Association* 288(2):222–35.

7

Findings and Recommendations

The Ryan White Comprehensive AIDS Resources Emergency (CARE) Act (RWCA) was first enacted in 1990 to provide funding to cities, states, and other public and private entities for care and support services to medically underserved, uninsured, and underinsured individuals with HIV disease. The CARE Act was refined and expanded during two subsequent reauthorizations in 1996 and 2000. The RWCA is the third-largest payer for HIV care behind Medicaid and Medicare, with a budget of $2 billion in fiscal year 2003 (HRSA, 2003). The RWCA is a program that has provided lifesaving care to millions of persons who otherwise would not have access to adequate services, and that has helped develop an infrastructure for providing high-quality care that would not exist in the absence of the Act. Furthermore, the Health Resources and Services Administration (HRSA), the agency that administers the RWCA, has been assertive and innovative in promoting quality-management and -improvement programs throughout the country.

Although the CARE Act program has been extremely successful, the complexity of the program and the changing HIV epidemic raise challenges with respect to the equitable allocation of resources and the maintenance of highest quality care. During the 2000 reauthorization of the Act, Congress asked the Institute of Medicine (IOM) to address three questions relating to (1) the inclusion of reported HIV cases, instead of only reported AIDS cases, in the RWCA Title I and II allocation formulas; (2) the data and methods that could be used to estimate severity of need and related resource needs; and (3) available health outcome and other data that could be used to assess the quality of RWCA-funded services.

These questions were motivated in part by several important aspects of the HIV epidemic and the health care system. Despite national guidelines recommending early access to medical care and treatment (Yeni et al., 2002; DHHS, 2003), an estimated 42 to 59 percent of the estimated 850,000-950,000 people living with HIV/AIDS in the United States are not in regular care (Fleming et al. 2002). Approximately one-quarter of all people with HIV do not know their HIV status (Fleming et al., 2002), and many others face financial and other barriers to accessing care (Kaiser Family Foundation, 2000). The cost of HIV care, which ranges between $10,000 and $12,000 annually per person for antiretroviral medications alone (Kahn et al., 2001), presents a formidable barrier to people with HIV/AIDS, many of whom are poor, unemployed, uninsured, or underinsured (Bozzette et al., 1998; Kaiser Family Foundation, 2000). Data suggest that although the quality of HIV/AIDS care has improved over time, both access to care and its quality vary by insurance status, race/ethnicity, and sex (Bozzette et al., 1998; Shapiro et al., 1999). Furthermore, many of the programs that provide care to individuals with HIV vary substantially in their eligibility and benefits across states, resulting in uneven access to care (Kaiser Family Foundation, 2000).

Because of these factors, Congress, HRSA, and grantees have raised questions about whether the original strategies for allocating resources to those in greatest need are consistent with the current distribution of the disease across states and Eligible Metropolitan Areas (EMAs) and associated resource needs. An overarching concern was that current RWCA allocation strategies might not be as equitable as they could be because of perceived changes in the HIV epidemic. There was also a desire to facilitate efforts by HRSA to monitor and improve the quality of care supported by RWCA. Over the past decade, knowledge about how to assess and improve health care quality has dramatically improved. These developments, coupled with growing knowledge about disparities between what is possible and what is routinely achieved in many areas of care, led Congress to suggest that the Committee review current knowledge about ways of monitoring the quality of HIV care in the RWCA.

The Committee focused on strategies and measures for federal resource allocation, evaluation of grantee applications, and assessments of the quality of care. The Committee's specific recommendations are described in Chapters 4, 5, and 6 and are summarized in Box 7-1. In brief, the key messages from this report are:

(1) While the Committee supports Congressional intent to incorporate data into the RWCA allocation formulas that reflect the evolving

needs of the epidemic, the Committee finds that states' HIV reporting systems are neither ready nor adequate for purposes of RWCA resource allocation. One state and one city have not implemented HIV case reporting, states' HIV reporting systems are in different stages of maturity across the United States, and the Centers for Disease Control and Prevention (CDC) does not accept HIV cases from code-based reporting states into the national database. HRSA should continue to use estimated living AIDS cases for at least the next 4 years to allow for improvement in HIV reporting data, and development of alternative strategies to case reporting, such as survey- or model-based estimation.

The Committee suggests two ways to improve HIV case reporting for RWCA resource allocation purposes. First, CDC should accept HIV data from all states, including code-based reporting states, into the national HIV/AIDS reporting database. CDC and code-based reporting states will need to develop algorithms to unduplicate these cases. Second, states and CDC should more fully utilize data from other sources, particularly laboratories, and potentially pharmacies, to enhance the relative completeness and timeliness of reporting across states and EMAs.

Concerted effort should also be devoted to improving the comparability of HIV case reporting as quickly as possible. The Committee also highlighted several structural features of the current Title I and II allocation formulas that may not support the goal of equitable allocation and that could obviate any potential advantage of including HIV data in the formulas.

(2) The current process for distributing Title I supplemental awards to EMAs relies on nonstandard and unvalidated measures of local need, making objective assessments of relative needs across areas virtually impossible. The Title I supplemental award should be modified so that assessment of resource needs is based mostly on a small number of objective quantitative indicators that can be calculated by HRSA. The Committee recommends evaluating a social area indicators model and direct indicators as potential new methods of estimating resource needs.

(3) HRSA's and RWCA grantees' efforts to measure the quality of RWCA services are commendable. These quality-measurement activities should be expanded, however, to be more comprehensive with respect to types of measures, level of assessment, target populations, and spectrum of services.

The questions Congress posed to the IOM were quite specific. Addressing these narrow questions, however, required consideration of several overarching issues that the Committee thinks Congress and HRSA should explore in future reauthorization discussions.

First, current RWCA Title I and II formula allocations do not appear to match the intent of the legislation to serve as a payer of last resort for uninsured and underinsured individuals with HIV/AIDS, because the formulas are based on all estimated living AIDS cases, with no adjustment for lack of or variations in insurance coverage across states and EMAs. Supplemental awards do consider variations in insurance coverage, but the data may be reported in inconsistent ways and the treatment of insurance is not explicit. Similarly, neither the formulas nor the supplemental award account for variations in the costs of providing care or among states and EMAs, or their fiscal capacity to provide care.

Second, there is a pressing need to expand the focus of RWCA to include the entire population of HIV-infected persons, both in identifying those who are infected but not diagnosed or in care, and measuring the overall quality of care provided to individuals with HIV/AIDS. Need for care services begins at the time of infection; outreach is needed to facilitate early entry into care for those who are diagnosed with HIV and to encourage others to be tested. Better linkages are also needed between HIV testing and treatment programs.

The ability of HRSA to assess variations in resource needs and quality of care is hampered by limitations in the available data. The ability to develop standardized, high-quality measures at the clinic and population level, in turn, is hindered by the limited resources of many grantees for collecting and reporting data. Future development of strategies for using data should consider the burden of data collection and reporting and help states and EMAs develop the technical skills and infrastructure necessary to provide standardized, timely information.

Despite the many challenges facing the Ryan White CARE Act, it is, in many ways, an extraordinarily successful health care policy. It has allowed communities throughout the country to develop an infrastructure for providing care that would not otherwise be available for many individuals with HIV disease. Since its inception, Congress, HRSA, RWCA grantees, and other public and private partners have worked together to continuously refine and improve the allocation of resources and provision of high-quality services. The Committee hopes that the implementation of the proffered recommendations will continue that tradition and in some small way contribute to better care for persons with HIV infection.

BOX 7-1
Findings and Recommendations

The Committee targets these and subsequent recommendations to several different entities including Congress, the Secretary of Health and Human Services (HHS), HRSA and CDC, and independent bodies. The Committee directs several recommendations (4.5, 5.2, 6.2c) to Congress that are related to the intent of the Ryan White CARE Act program. Many of the recommendations (4.2a, 4.2c, 4.4, 5.4, 6.2, 6.3) are targeted to the Secretary of HHS, who has broad oversight responsibilities for the implementation of the CARE Act. The Committee also targeted recommendations to the Secretary of HHS when the recommendations involved coordination among multiple agencies. Several recommendations involving specific technical issues are targeted to HRSA (4.1, 5.1, 5.3, 6.1, 6.2a, 6.2b) and CDC (4.2a, 4.2b, 4.2c, 4.3, 6.2b). In a few instances, the Committee makes recommendations that assessments be undertaken, or reviewed, by an independent body (4.3, 4.4). An independent body was specified when the recommendations required a broad assessment of the science base or when the Committee thought that an independent entity could protect the federal entities from any appearance of vested or conflict of interest, since those agencies would be applying the resulting methods. In some situations, an independent body was specified when it was thought that such an arrangement would minimize any inappropriate pressure on an agency from groups with vested interests in the outcomes of deliberations. Such pressure could inappropriately influence scientific assessments and/or result in strained relationships between agencies and their grantees or constituents. Additional resources may be required to implement some of the Committee's recommendations.

CHAPTER 4: HIV REPORTING DATA AND TITLE I AND II FORMULAS FINDINGS AND RECOMMENDATIONS

Finding 4-1 While the Committee supports Congressional intent to incorporate data into the RWCA allocation formulas that reflect the evolving needs of the epidemic, the Committee finds that states' HIV reporting systems are neither ready nor adequate for purposes of RWCA resource allocation. One state and one city have yet to implement HIV case reporting, states' HIV reporting systems are in different stages of maturity across the United States, and the national HIV database does not include HIV cases from code-based reporting states.

Finding 4-2 Different rates of completeness and timeliness of HIV reports across states and EMAs have the potential to create significant biases in RWCA formula allocations. To date, studies have not answered key questions about the comparability of HIV case-reporting data for use in resource allocation formulas. Additional studies are needed to examine the comparability of data from the HIV case-reporting system across states and EMAs.

Continued

BOX 7-1 Continued

Finding 4-3 The Committee could not confirm the hypothesis that the maturity of the HIV epidemic varies significantly across regions. If the ratio of reported AIDS cases to HIV cases differs across states or EMAs, including data on HIV cases in the RWCA formulas could affect the relative measure of disease burden and the allocations. Data examined by the Committee suggest that the rate of new HIV infections is somewhat greater in the southeastern region of the United States. Due to the lack of HIV case data in all areas, however, assumptions regarding interregional variability in epidemic maturity need further assessment.

Finding 4-4 When examining combined Title I and II funds, the Committee found that those awards depart from a nationwide standard of equivalent spending per unit of HIV burden. Although such departures may be appropriate, the justification for such departures was not clear. Such departures persist regardless of the measure of disease burden used, but they are most pronounced when using a combined measure of estimated HIV prevalence and AIDS prevalence.

Finding 4-5 With the exception of San Francisco, Title I formula allocations per estimated living AIDS case (ELC) are quite uniform across EMAs. Because of hold-harmless provisions, the San Francisco EMA receives significantly greater resources per ELC than do other EMAs. Removal of this provision would reduce San Francisco's allocation to within the reported range for other EMAs. However, removing the hold-harmless protection would have a small influence on other EMAs, which would observe a 2.6 percent increase in their allocation if San Francisco's allocation were reduced. As noted by others (GAO, 2000), hold-harmless provisions have a small overall effect on allocations to EMAs, yet a large effect on a single EMA.

Finding 4-6 Several structural features of the Title I and Title II funding formulas—most notably the counting of EMA cases in both Titles I and II state formula allocations, but also such measures as hold harmless provisions and set-asides for Emerging Communities—have a large influence on resulting allocations. Such structural features may dampen the effect of variation introduced by the addition of HIV cases, and could obviate the potential benefits of adding HIV cases to the CARE Act allocation formulas.

Finding 4-7 RWCA Title I and II formula allocations are determined by the estimated number of living AIDS cases. Thus, they do not take into account factors defining those for whom such funds were intended, such as lack of insurance and special needs. That is, there are no provisions to estimate the number of persons in need of a "payer of last resort."

Finding 4-8 The completeness of the data from existing HIV case-reporting systems can be improved by making changes, specifically counting all HIV cases that are reported to the national system rather than only those reported from states with name-based reporting, and more fully utilizing data from laboratories and other sources such as pharmacies to enhance the completeness of HIV reporting.

Finding 4-9 Techniques exist to estimate the prevalence of HIV infection independently of the HIV case-reporting systems. Sample-based surveys and modeling approaches permit estimates of the total HIV-infected population, regardless of diagnostic status.

Finding 4-10 A surveillance mechanism that provides information about the total population of persons with HIV infection, be they diagnosed or undiagnosed, is highly desirable. Knowing the size and distribution of the undiagnosed HIV-infected population is an important marker of success in providing care to all people with HIV.

Recommendation 4-1 For at least the next 4 years, HRSA should continue to use ELCs in the RWCA Title I and II formulas. During that period, concerted effort should be devoted to improving the consistency, quality, and comparability of HIV case reporting. Specific attention should be paid to two, complementary approaches in this regard: (1) the attainment of coverage, maturity, and comparability standards and the development of de-duplication strategies that permit full use of all reported HIV cases; and (2) implementation of alternative strategies for estimating HIV cases, such as survey or model-based estimation.

Recommendation 4-2 The following steps should be taken by states as quickly as possible to improve the consistency, quality, and comparability of HIV case reporting for RWCA allocation purposes.

a. The CDC should accept reported HIV cases from all states. Until this occurs, large numbers of HIV cases will not be included in the national HIV reporting system, and there will be no reliable centralized way to use reported HIV cases to apportion CARE Act funds. CDC should work with all states to develop and evaluate methods for unduplicating HIV cases regardless of whether such cases are code- or name-based. The Secretary of HHS should provide CDC with the funding to provide the technical assistance to states necessary to support the integration of code with name-based data into the national HIV reporting database. Because of the importance of obtaining consistent data from all jurisdictions, the CDC should include HIV reporting data from code-based states and estimate the degree of overcounting due to duplication while procedures and infrastructure for definitive unduplication are developed.

b. CDC should collaborate with all states to periodically assess and compare the completeness and timeliness of their HIV reporting systems.

c. The Secretary of HHS should provide additional funds to CDC to assist states in improving the completeness and timeliness and overall comparability of their HIV reporting systems. Enhancing electronic laboratory

Continued

BOX 7-1 Continued

reporting in all states is critical in achieving this goal. Pharmacy-based surveillance, with a focus on the AIDS Drug Assistance Program (ADAP), is another potential source of information for enhancing completeness.

Recommendation 4-3 CDC should obtain estimates of total HIV prevalence (including the undiagnosed population) and evaluate methods other than case reporting for use as an alternative or supplement in estimating HIV cases for RWCA Title I and II formula allocations, with advice and review by an independent body. This assessment should address the accuracy and costs of different strategies and should be repeated periodically.

Recommendation 4-4 Prior to future reauthorizations of the CARE Act, the Secretary of HHS should initiate studies to improve the evidence base for understanding how well HIV case reporting and other methods for estimating HIV cases reflect the relative burden of disease and the relative resources necessary to respond to those needs in different areas. The Secretary should engage an independent body to estimate the dollar allocations that would result for Title I and II grantees from alternative input data and alternative RWCA allocation formulas. Specifically:

a. "What-if" assessments should be reported every 5 years on the range of each EMA's and state's RWCA formula allocation, depending on whether ELCs or total HIV cases are used as the measure of disease burden.

b. Analyses should be conducted to estimate the dollar allocations that would result from modifying different structural elements of the formula, such as:
   - Hold-harmless provisions,
   - The eligibility requirements for becoming an EMA,
   - The percentage set-aside in the Title II base award for non-EMA states (currently 20 percent),
   - The minimum base Title II award (now $500,000 for states and $50,000 for territories),
   - The eligibility criteria for becoming a Tier 1 and Tier 2 emerging community.

c. Evaluate the extent of interregional variability in HIV epidemic maturity and its effect on relative resource needs.

These activities should be repeated periodically.

Recommendation 4-5 In keeping with the CARE Act's intent as a payer of last resort, Congress should reevaluate the RWCA formulas to determine whether they allocate resources in proportion to the estimated number of individuals with HIV/AIDS who are uninsured or underinsured in states and EMAs. Readily available data on the insurance coverage of the general population may mirror insurance coverage of people with HIV/AIDS, but additional estimation will likely be required.

CHAPTER 5: ESTIMATING RESOURCE NEEDS FINDINGS AND RECOMMENDATIONS

Finding 5-1 Resource needs are determined by a complex array of factors, including disease burden, the costs of providing care, and available resources. These factors, for example insurance coverage or costs of care, vary widely across regions. RWCA formula allocations rely primarily on one measure of disease burden (i.e., ELCs) in determining awards, although this measure does not well reflect underlying variations in resource needs. Title I supplemental award is the largest RWCA grant program that attempts to take into account other factors affecting the complexity and costs of care.

Finding 5-2 The current Title I supplemental award process, which is determined by competitive application, relies on nonstandard and unvalidated measures of local need. Simple, commensurable measures are preferable to complex idiosyncratic measures in allocating resources and their use would improve the award process and resulting allocations.

Finding 5-3 The current Title I supplemental application process is burdensome for grantees. Given the high correlation between grantees' per-ELC supplemental and base awards, the effort required for grantees to complete the application seems unjustified.

Finding 5-4 Many publicly available data sources, including data routinely collected by HRSA/HIV/AIDS Bureau (HAB) and CDC, could be used to assess resource needs using indicators that are comparable across areas. Direct measures probably would yield the most valid measures of need, but would be more expensive and perhaps less feasible than indirect measures.

Recommendation 5-1 HRSA should modify the Title I supplemental application process. The severity-of-need component of the Title I supplemental award should be based on two components:

- Quantitatively defined need, based on a small number of measures that can be calculated by HRSA/HAB.
- Locally defined need described in a short narrative by the applicant.

Recommendation 5-2 A predominance of the weight for determining Title I awards should be given to the quantitative measure of resource needs that reflect variations in costs of care and fiscal capacity across EMAs.

Recommendation 5-3 HRSA/HAB should evaluate the feasibility and usefulness of using social area indicator models based on publicly available data that are collected in standardized ways across jurisdictions, to estimate EMA-level resource needs for the Title I supplemental award. This approach also might be useful in assessing resource needs for other RWCA discretionary grant programs.

Continued

BOX 7-1 Continued

Recommendation 5-4 The Secretary of HHS should evaluate the cost and utility of redesigning and coordinating studies conducted by HRSA/HAB and CDC to assess the specific needs and circumstances of people living with HIV. These data can be used to estimate resource needs and as part of quality-assessment activities. The Secretary should also assess the cost and utility of the indirect modeling approach described in Recommendation 5-3 for assessing regional variations in resource requirements.

CHAPTER 6: MEASURING QUALITY OF CARE FINDINGS AND RECOMMENDATIONS

Finding 6-1 The RWCA legislation's emphasis on development of outcome measures is appropriate because tracking outcomes is a crucial element for accountability and helpful in quality improvement. However, outcome measures alone are not sufficient because outcomes may be influenced by many factors not under the control of grantees, and because structure and process measures can uniquely identify areas for specific improvement.

Finding 6-2 Quality measures for HIV/AIDS that are in wide use are based on broadly accepted clinical guidelines and are appropriate. However, these measures are not standardized, which has hindered efficient evaluation of RWCA programs. Moreover, these measures are generally restricted to evaluating providers via examination of aggregated patient-level clinical data. Measures examining a more complete spectrum of services including, for example, those assessing support services, are important but are not yet in wide enough use to allow for consensus to emerge about specific measures for HIV care. Examples of potential measures of supportive services include the provision of case management, benefits advocacy, or substance abuse and mental health services.

Finding 6-3 Measures of access to needed medical and nonmedical services are also lacking. Such measures have been developed for other diseases (e.g., cancer and heart disease) and could be adapted to HIV/AIDS. Examples of potential access measures include those that focus on continuity of care (e.g., identification of primary care provider), access to needed specialty care, and access to needed nonmedical care.

Finding 6-4 Population-based measures are essential in monitoring HIV care in an EMA, region, or state and identifying areas for improvement. Current efforts to assess overall quality of care in EMAs and states are rudimentary and no population-based measures are in wide use. These measures should not be interpreted as direct measures of the quality of care being provided by specific clinics, but rather as reflecting the cumulative effects of many influences on case quality and outcomes. Additional work is needed to further develop these measures.

Recommendation 6-1 Quality measures: HRSA should adopt quality measures that are comprehensive with respect to populations (diagnosed in care; diagnosed but not in care; not diagnosed, not in care), level of assessment (provider and population levels), types of measures (structure, process, and outcome), and spectrum of services (clinical and supportive services). At a minimum, HRSA and grantees should strongly consider inclusion of the following standard set of measures to assess the quality of care provided by RWCA-funded providers and EMA and state-level programs. Standard definitions and detailed criteria for these measures need to be developed by HRSA in collaboration with grantees, affected communities, and other stakeholders after a rigorous examination of the importance, scientific soundness, and feasibility of potential measures.

I. CLINIC LEVEL MEASURES

A. Structure

1. Proportion of providers with appropriate expertise and experience in treating patients with HIV*
2. Availability of case management services

B. Process

Screening for:

3. Cervical cancer*
4. Hepatitis B
   a. And administration of hepatitis B vaccine if negative
5. Hepatitis C*
6. Syphilis*
7. Toxoplasmosis
8. Tuberculosis*

Performance of the following clinical monitoring tests:

9. CD4+ cell count and HIV viral load (process)*

Antiretroviral treatment:

10. Provision of indicated antiretroviral treatment*
11. Provision of adherence counseling and monitoring

Vaccinations and prophylaxis for opportunistic infections:

12. Influenza vaccination
13. Pneumoccocal pneumonia vaccination
14. Hepatitis B vaccination if patient not immune
15. If indicated, *Mycobacterium avium* complex (MAC)
16. If indicated, *Pneumocystis carinii* pneumonia* (PCP)

C. Outcomes

17. Monitoring of CD4+ cell count and viral load values*
18. Proportion of patients with a history of an AIDS-defining opportunistic condition*
19. Proportion of patients who have >2 missed scheduled clinic appointments per year
20. Hospitalizations and emergency room visits without hospital admission*
21. Proportion of patients with unmet need for support services (e.g., assistance with obtaining housing).^

Continued

BOX 7-1 Continued

II. AREA (E.G., EMA OR STATE) LEVEL MEASURES

Outcome measures related to access and care:

22. Proportion of HIV-infected persons in an area who are not diagnosed^
23. Proportion of diagnosed persons in area who are receiving regular care^
24. Proportion of people with HIV who died within 12 months of an HIV diagnosis*
25. Proportion of people with HIV who progressed to AIDS within 12 months of initial HIV diagnosis*

Key: * indicates high priority; ^ indicates high priority, but may require further development. Other measures are important, but of lower priority.

Recommendation 6-2: Infrastructure development: The Secretary of Health and Human Services (HHS) should provide additional resources to HRSA and CDC to develop infrastructure for monitoring quality at the patient, clinic, and population levels. This infrastructure development strategy has three major components:

a. HRSA should enhance support for information technology and personnel to enable clinics to collect, aggregate, and report a focused set of clinical and patient-reported data.

b. HRSA should collaborate with CDC and other agencies to develop innovative population-based measures that can be captured using existing data sources or other community-based information-gathering activities, such as surveys of unmet needs.

c. Congress should enhance flexibility in the administrative caps at the grantee level to promote infrastructure development.

Recommendation 6-3 Collaborative quality activities: The Secretary of HHS should convene a working group, not restricted to, but including the National Committee on Quality Assurance (NCQA), state insurance commissioners, state Medicaid officials, and representatives from HRSA, CDC, the Centers for Medicare & Medicaid Services (CMS), providers of community, outpatient, and inpatient care, and members of the relevant research communities, to consider strategies for promoting greater collaboration between public health departments and public- and private-sector providers in order establish tools and methods to assess systems of care and quality, building on the successful collaborative models developed by the CDC for immunization (e.g., Clinic Assessment Software Application and Assessment Feedback Incentives Exchange).

REFERENCES

Bozzette S, Berry SH, Duan N, Frankel MR, Leibowitz AA, Lefkowitz D, Emmons CA, Senterfitt JW, Berk ML, Morton SC, Shapiro MF. 1998. The care of HIV-infected adults in the United States. HIV Cost and Services Utilization Study Consortium. *New England Journal of Medicine* 339(26):1897–904.

DHHS (Department of Health and Human Services). AIDSInfo: Overview of Guidelines. [Online]. Available: www.aidsinfo.nih.gov/guidelines [accessed July 31, 2003].

Fleming P, Byers R, Sweeney P, Daniels D, Karon J, Janssen R. 2002. HIV Prevalence in the United States, 2000. *Presented at the 9th Conference on Retroviruses and Opportunistic Infections, Seattle, WA* Abstract 11.

GAO (General Accounting Office). 2000. *Ryan White CARE Act: Opportunities to Enhance Funding Equity* GAO/T-HEHS-00-150. Washington, DC: GAO.

HRSA (Health Resources and Services Administration). 2003. CARE Act Overview and Funding History. [Online]. Available: ftp://ftp.hrsa.gov/hab/fundinghistory.pdf [accessed October 1, 2003].

Kahn JG, Haile B, Kates J, Chang S. 2001. Health and federal budgetary effects of increasing access to antiretroviral medications for HIV by expanding Medicaid. *American Journal of Public Health* 91(9):1464–73.

Kaiser Family Foundation. 2000. Financing HIV/AIDS Care: A Quilt with Many Holes. *Capital Hill Briefing Series on HIV/AIDS.*

Shapiro MF, Morton SC, McCaffrey DF, Senterfitt JW, Fleishman JA, Perlman JF, Athey LA, Keesey JW, Goldman DP, Berry SH, Bozzette SA. 1999. Variations in the care of HIV-infected adults in the United States: Results from the HIV Cost and Services Utilization Study. *Journal of the American Medical Association* 281(24):2305–15.

Yeni P, Hammer SM, Carpenter CC, Cooper DA, Fischl MA, Gatell JM, Gazzard BG, Hirsch MS, Jacobsen DM, Katzenstein DA, Montaner JS, Richman DD, Saag MS, Schechter M, Schooley RT, Thompson MA, Vella S, Volberding PA. 2002. Antiretroviral treatment for adult HIV infection in 2002: Updated Recommendations of the International AIDS Society-USA Panel. *Journal of the American Medical Association* 288(2):222–35.

Appendixes

A

Acronyms

AAPCC	Adjusted Average Per Capita Cost
ADAMHA	Alcohol, Drug Abuse & Mental Health Administration
ADAP	AIDS Drug Assistance Program
AETC	AIDS Education and Training Centers
AFIX	Assessment Feedback Incentives Exchange
AHRQ	Agency for Healthcare Research and Quality
AIDS	Acquired Immune Deficiency Syndrome
APS	AIDS Progression Study
ARF	Area resource file
ART	Antiretroviral treatment
ASD	Adult/Adolescent Spectrum of Disease Project
CADR	CARE Act Data Report
CARE	Comprehensive AIDS Resources Emergency
CASA	Clinical Assessment Software Application
CDC	Centers for Disease Control and Prevention
CPS	Current Population Survey
CSTE	Council of State and Territorial Epidemiologists
DHHS	Department of Health and Human Services
ELC	Estimated living (AIDS) case
EMA	Eligible Metropolitan Area
EQHIV	Evaluation of Quality Improvement for HIV Care
FACCT	Foundation for Accountability
FY	Fiscal year
GAO	General Accounting Office

GPRA	Government Performance Results Act
GRS	General revenue sharing
HAART	Highly active antiretroviral therapy
HARS	HIV/AIDS Reporting System
HCSUS	HIV Costs and Service Utilization Study
HEDIS	Health Plan Employer Data and Information Set
HIPPA	Health Insurance Portability and Accountability Act
HIS	Health Interview Survey
HIV	Human immunodeficiency virus
HIVQUAL	HIV Quality of Care Program
HPSA	Health Provider Shortage Area
HRSA	Health Resources and Services Administration
HRSA/HAB	Health Resources and Services Administration's HIV/AIDS Bureau
IDEP	Interstate de-duplication evaluation project
IDSA	Infectious Diseases Society of America
IDU	Injection drug user
IHI	Institute for Healthcare Improvement
IOM	Institute of Medicine
MAI	Minority AIDS Initiative
MSA	Metropolitan Statistical Area
MUA	Medically Underserved Area
NAS	National Academy of Sciences
NASTAD	National Alliance of State and Territorial AIDS Directors
NCQA	National Committee for Quality Assurance
NHANES	National Health and Nutrition Examination Survey
NNDSS	National Notifiable Disease Surveillance System
PCAT	Primary Care Assessment Tool
PHS	Public Health Service
QUERI	Quality Enhancement Research Initiative
RWCA	Ryan White Comprehensive AIDS Resources Emergency Act
SAMHSA	Substance Abuse and Mental Health Services Administration
SHAS	Supplement to HIV/AIDS Surveillance Project
SHDC	Survey of HIV Disease in Care
SPNS	Special Projects of National Significance
STAHRS	Serologic Testing Algorithm for Recent HIV Seroconversion
STD	Sexually transmitted disease
UHC	University Health System Consortium
UHDDS	Uniform Hospital Discharge Data Set

B

Financial Resources of States for HIV/AIDS Reporting

Several of the factors determining system accuracy, such as the ability to follow up on a backlog of cases, depend on the capacity to conduct surveillance. As one indicator of capacity, the Committee examined federal and state funding for HIV/AIDS case reporting. The Committee heard testimony from a small number of states, from the Centers for Disease Control and Prevention (CDC) staff, and from select Eligible Metropolitan Areas (EMAs) regarding surveillance capacity and funding. The Committee also reviewed information provided by state AIDS programs and from the CDC regarding state and federal contributions to HIV/AIDS surveillance for fiscal years 1999–2002.

With the exception of very large county or city health departments, state surveillance programs provide the HIV/AIDS surveillance data for Ryan White CARE Act (RWCA) planning and evaluation. While HIV reporting has been implemented in all states and cities, except Georgia and Philadelphia (as of October 2003), most states did not see a concurrent increase in financial resources to assist with the implementation of HIV reporting. Although the RWCA Amendments of 2000 authorized limited additional funds to assist states with the implementation of HIV reporting systems (Ryan White CARE Act. Sec. 300ff-13), that funding has yet to be appropriated. Even though HIV and AIDS data are perceived to be readily available for RWCA purposes at no additional cost, states must often provide specialized reports for RWCA planning that include different or more-detailed data than are provided in standard epidemiologic reports.[1] Such efforts can be costly.

[1]Subcommittee site visit to the CDC, April 4, 2002.

When considering the question of surveillance capacity, there are at least two levels of system cost: one associated with the implementation of HIV reporting, and the other associated with RWCA planning efforts at state and local levels. Cost issues are relevant to the question of capacity, particularly given the pervasive fiscal austerity of states and localities.

DATA EXAMINED

Financial resources clearly affect reporting capacity. In the absence of models to estimate surveillance costs, the Committee attempted to understand more about surveillance capacity by studying the distribution of federal and state funding for surveillance programs. The Committee reviewed two sources of funding for state HIV/AIDS surveillance programs for the years 1999 through 2002: (1) self-reported state general revenue contributions for HIV and AIDS surveillance, and (2) federal core surveillance funding to states through cooperative agreements with the CDC.[2]

The National Alliance of State and Territorial AIDS Directors (NASTAD) administered a request for information to state AIDS directors regarding states' general revenue contributions to their HIV/AIDS surveillance programs during fiscal years 1999–2002. Forty-one states responded to that request for information.[3] States were also asked to identify expected changes in general revenue (remain constant, decrease, increase). The CDC provided data to the Committee on federal funding to states for core surveillance and for other surveillance activities for corresponding fiscal years 1999 through 2002 (CDC, 2003).

The Committee reviewed data for 1999 through 2002 for three reasons: (1) approximately one-third of states implemented HIV reporting during this time period (see Table 3-1 in chapter 3), (2) state fiscal austerity was emerging during this time period, and (3) these data were readily available from most states.

---

[2]CDC provides "core funding" to states for their HIV/AIDS reporting systems. CDC provides additional funds to states, based on a competitive grant application process, for supplemental surveillance activities.

[3]States were asked not to include state general revenue contributions to the six cities/counties in their jurisdiction that receive direct funding from CDC for HIV/AIDS reporting (Chicago, Houston, New York, Los Angeles, Philadelphia, and San Francisco). A separate request for information was made to those areas. States were also asked to exclude in-kind contributions (e.g., staff on loan from another division) and funding for general communicable disease or sexually transmitted disease surveillance.

RESULTS

The Committee examined data provided by the CDC and NASTAD on federal and state contributions for HIV surveillance. The Committee converted the total spending to spending per capita, using data from the 2000 Census (U.S. Census Bureau, 2000). During 1999–2002, the majority of funds for AIDS and HIV surveillance programs came from the federal government, and in 32 states, funding was entirely from the federal government. Average federal and state funding was flat from 1999–2002. Relative state contributions were flat during the period with less than 10 percent of the total average $0.09–$0.10 spent per capita. Moreover, 33 of the 41 states that responded reported $0 of state general revenue funding for HIV/AIDS surveillance programs for fiscal years 1999, 2000, and 2002. Thirty-two states reported $0 state contributions in fiscal year 2001.

State-by-state comparisons of federal and state HIV/AIDS surveillance funding for 1999–2002 in dollar terms is found in Table B-1. State contributions to HIV/AIDS surveillance funding are only provided for the 41 states that responded to NASTAD's request for information. Federal contributions are provided for all 50 states and the District of Columbia.

The funding picture for state HIV/AIDS surveillance programs did not change appreciably during FY1999–2002 for the 41 states that responded to the request for information.[4]

Table B-2 shows state general revenue contributions for HIV/AIDS surveillance as a percentage of total surveillance budgets. The aggregate reliance on federal resources for HIV/AIDS surveillance does not change greatly from year to year.

Table B-3 presents data from the 11 states that implemented HIV reporting during the analysis period. These data show that for the majority of these states, there was little change in the amount of state or federal funding for surveillance during the period when they were implementing HIV reporting. Only California substantially increased funding in the years just prior to implementation of HIV reporting. Pennsylvania began general revenue contributions prior to implementing HIV reporting, but Kansas discontinued general revenue contributions the year following implementation of HIV reporting. Federal funding increased for Vermont, Hawaii, Alaska, and Kansas during this period, but was essentially flat for other states.

---

[4]Financial data were adjusted for inflation using the *All Items* Consumer Price Index. U.S. City average, nonseasonally adjusted, All Urban Consumers. (U.S. Department of Labor, Bureau of Labor Statistics). [Online] http://data.bls.gov. Series ID: CUUS0000SA0.

TABLE B-1 State and Federal Contributions for HIV/AIDS Surveillance for FY1999–2002, in Dollars (N=51)

	FY1999		FY2000	
State	State General Revenue (in $)	Federal Revenue (in $)	State General Revenue (in $)	Federal Revenue (in $)
Alabama	Not Available*	572,603	Not Available	786,712
Alaska	0	115,000	0	115,000
Arizona	125,000	340,573	125,000	398,133
Arkansas	0	238,727	0	207,653
California[a]	5,116,200	3,914,875	7,746,000	4,058,017
Colorado	0	537,822	0	467,772
Connecticut	Not Available	346,444	Not Available	298,319
Delaware	0	112,664	0	113,005
District of Columbia	Not Available	388,336	Not Available	485,865
Florida	634,227	1,806,242	634,227	1,760,761
Georgia	0	196,816	0	297,909
Hawaii	0	31,505	0	135,989
Idaho	0	75,000	0	75,000
Illinois	Not Available	1,010,508[b]	Not Available	1,409,531[b]
Indiana	0	274,633	0	280,708
Iowa	0	29,476	0	129,151
Kansas	42,900	90,200	42,900	127,301
Kentucky	0	109,852	0	117,000
Louisiana	7,500	772,966	7,500	774,042
Maine	0	112,947	0	72,319
Maryland	Not Available	956,359	Not Available	956,359
Massachusetts	0	226,901	0	483,925
Michigan	0	851,426	0	881,745
Minnesota	0	189,568	0	232,345
Mississippi	0	243,071	0	220,000
Missouri	0	550,203	0	577,455
Montana	0	68,105	0	67,124
Nebraska	0	83,635	0	120,000
Nevada	Not Available	310,600	Not Available	327,494
New Hampshire	Not Available	83,200	Not Available	77,985
New Jersey	616,000	2,202,177	553,000	2,089,025
New Mexico	Not Available	163,320	Not Available	213,479
New York	1,607,028	4,525,303[c]	1,809,183	4,394,123[c]
North Carolina	0	406,125	0	1,292[d]
North Dakota	0	59,675	0	59,251
Ohio	0	176,228	0	399,052
Oklahoma	0	286,509	0	286,509
Oregon	Not Available	330,108	Not Available	320,108
Pennsylvania	0	1,079,110[e]	0	1,092,184[e]
Rhode Island	Not Available	213,218	Not Available	214,304
South Carolina	0	446,217	0	486,314

FY2001		FY2002	
State General Revenue (in $)	Federal Revenue (in $)	State General Revenue (in $)	Federal Revenue (in $)
Not Available	551,606	Not Available	557,276
0	120,750	0	120,750
125,000	423,863	125,000	380,226
0	218,036	0	218,036
7,746,000	3,927,473	7,746,000	4,042,160
0	522,250	0	318,972
Not Available	433,988	Not Available	454,338
0	126,864	0	126,904
Not Available	487,435	Not Available	510,158
634,227	1,896,204	634,227	183,146
0	69,973	0	384,666
0	173,417	0	173,418
0	78,750	0	64,184
Not Available	750,838[b]	Not Available	988,642[b]
0	362,653	0	325,508
0	169,198	0	143,412
42,900	135,344	0	130,144
0	122,850	0	122,850
7,500	812,010	7,500	322,866
0	103,530	0	106,688
Not Available	988,653	Not Available	874,028
0	488,190	0	409,864
0	925,832	0	924,110
0	144,096	0	247,094
0	132,424	0	132,720
0	601,078	0	601,078
0	63,100	0	67,772
0	126,000	0	126,000
Not Available	343,869	Not Available	343,870
Not Available	87,681	Not Available	76,838
692,000	2,260,092	400,000	2,224,150
Not Available	179,071	Not Available	153,312
1,726,081	4,097,758[c]	1,590,230	4,484,826[c]
0	228,949	0	374,534
0	61,067	0	62,214
0	481,189	0	516,746
0	300,834	0	300,834
Not Available	326,113	Not Available	336,114
100,000	1,128,759[e]	100,000	966,010[e]
Not Available	226,169	Not Available	226,170
0	501,745	0	371,358

Continued

TABLE B-1 Continued

	FY1999		FY2000	
State	State General Revenue (in $)	Federal Revenue (in $)	State General Revenue (in $)	Federal Revenue (in $)
South Dakota	0	52,048	0	54,404
Tennessee	0	526,858	0	505,200
Texas	263,006	1,627,176[f]	263,006	1,401,897[f]
Utah	0	115,481	0	141,092
Vermont	0	64,294	0	75,056
Virginia	0	339,806	0	423,268
Washington	0	748,702	0	760,952
West Virginia	0	182,351	0	204,419
Wisconsin	0	342,445	0	342,445
Wyoming	0	52,690	0	52,689

[a]Includes funding for Los Angeles and San Francisco.
[b]Includes funding for Chicago.
[c]Includes funding for New York City.
[d]$1,292 was allocated to North Carolina in 2000 due to unexpended and carryover funding from the previous year.
[e]Includes funding for Philadelphia.
[f]Includes funding for Houston.
*Not available means there was no response to NASTAD's request for information.
NOTE: Data from states is self-reported and has not been independently verified.
SOURCE: NASTAD, 2003.

TABLE B-2 State Funding for HIV/AIDS Surveillance as a Percent of Total State HIV/AIDS Surveillance Budget, FY1999–2002 (N = 41)

Fiscal Year	Mean (%)
1999	4.48
2000	4.36
2001	4.65
2002	3.51

FY2001		FY2002	
State General Revenue (in $)	Federal Revenue (in $)	State General Revenue (in $)	Federal Revenue (in $)
0	47,024	0	44,454
0	581,102	0	616,100
268,872	1,308,762[f]	268,872	1,086,330[f]
0	168,719	0	179,268
0	128,832	0	82,526
0	444,332	0	393,084
0	802,181	0	770,510
0	199,627	0	225,750
0	383,851	0	341,914
0	51,555	0	57,954

TABLE B-3 State and Core Federal Funding for Surveillance by States Implementing HIV Surveillance per 1,000 Adult Population, FY1999–2002, by State (N = 11)

	State Funding (in $)				Federal Funding (in $)			
State	1999	2000	2001	2002	1999	2000	2001	2002
Alaska	0*	0	0	0	20*	20	190	190
California	150	230	230	230*	120	120	120	120*
Delaware	0	0	0*	0	160	140	160*	160
Hawaii	0	0	0*	0	30	110	140*	140
Kansas	20	20	20	0	30*	50	50	50
Kentucky	0	0*	0	0	30	30*	30	10
Maine	0*	0	0	0	90*	60	80	80
Montana	0	0*	0	0	80	70*	70	80
New York	80	100*	90	80	80	80*	90	80
Pennsylvania	0	0	10	10*	40	40	40	40*
Vermont	0	0*	0	0	110	120*	210	140

*Year of HIV surveillance implementation

As one of several potential indicators of capacity, these data imply that more financial resources might be required to accommodate the current and additional information needs or demands of the HIV/AIDS surveillance programs vis-à-vis use of information for RWCA planning, allocation, or evaluation. States are facing significant financial crises, and while several states are newly implementing HIV reporting, most programs do not anticipate additional state general revenue contributions. According to the 41 states that responded to the NASTAD request for information, 65 percent (27) reported that they expect their state's contributions for HIV/AIDS surveillance to remain constant; 7.3 percent (3) reported that they expect a decrease; while 2.4 percent (1) reported they expect an increase. State dependence upon federal funding for HIV surveillance activity, and for the provision of HIV/AIDS data for RWCA planning, evaluation, and allocation is apparent.

The use of financial data to understand capacity has limitations. For example, some resources used for other surveillance may partially support HIV/AIDS surveillance. Furthermore, the Committee did not have the ability to calculate the incremental costs of implementing specific HIV surveillance and reporting activities. Nevertheless, it appears that states are being required to engage in additional surveillance and reporting activities without a commensurate increase in state or federal resources. Additional assessments of the incremental costs of such activities would be helpful in determining overall funding needed to support HIV/AIDS surveillance activities.

REFERENCES

CDC (Centers for Disease Control and Prevention). 2003. FY02 Surveillance by State Final. (Email communication, Patricia Sweeney, CDC, May 2, 2003).

NASTAD. 2003. Request for Information: State/Local Funding for HIV/AIDS Surveillance.

U.S. Census Bureau. 2000. Population, Housing Units, Area and Density (geographies ranked by total population). [Online]. Available: http://factfinder.census.gov/ [accessed June 25, 2003].

U.S. Department of Labor. Bureau of Labor Statistics. [Online]. Available: http://data.bls.gov. Series ID: CUUS0000SA0.

C

Analyses of the Sensitivity of the Formula Allocations to Underlying Changes in Input Data

This appendix provides detailed analyses of the sensitivity of allocation formulas to changes in the underlying data. The Committee originally intended to conduct extensive "what-if" policy simulations. That is, it intended to compare different factors in the funding formulas to examine the impact of including HIV cases on resource allocations across regions, and to compare the inclusion of HIV cases to other features, such as hold-harmless provisions, set-asides, minimum funding thresholds, and the potential addition of new Eligible Metropolitan Areas (EMAs) based on a more inclusive definition of HIV disease burden. The Committee could not examine the impact of including HIV data in the formula because data on HIV cases were not available from all states, including several key states with a high disease burden. Since data from those states could have a large influence on results, any analyses based on partial data could be very misleading. Nevertheless, the analyses and policy assessment in this appendix highlight the implications of current policies. These findings should allow policy makers to explore the implications of proposed changes in funding allocations (see Chapter 3 and 4).

Given that constraint, the Committee chose instead to explore how assessments of the "fairness" of those awards might be influenced by including additional data regarding HIV prevalence. In particular, the Committee examined what the current allocation is, per unit of HIV disease burden, using two reasonable but distinct measures of that burden: the estimated number of living AIDS cases (ELCs) (the measure now used for Ryan White CARE Act [RWCA] resource allocation) and combined estimates of HIV prevalence and AIDS prevalence provided by the Centers for Disease Control and Prevention (CDC).[1] For states with mature name-based HIV reporting systems, estimates of HIV prevalence were based on data from their individual case-reporting systems. For code-based states or states without mature name-based reporting systems, CDC used modeling to produce the HIV prevalence estimates. California and Massachusetts declined to release CDC's estimates of HIV prevalence, and thus no data were available for these two states. Given that California and Massachusetts did not permit CDC to share CDC's modeled estimates of HIV prevalence in these states, we imputed the number of HIV cases for these states by assuming that the proportion of HIV to AIDS cases matched the reported proportion in New York. This is an important limitation. The Committee also employed multiple linear regression analysis to identify predictors of RWCA Title I and Title II funding.

In its analyses, the Committee examined "dollar allocations per case" across jurisdictions as a point of departure. The Committee acknowledges that there are many reasons why an equitable system would depart from this standard, including unequal costs of care, unequal need, differences in the efficiency with which jurisdictions apply funds, differences in the quality and comprehensiveness of the existing resource base from one jurisdiction to another, and differences in economies of scale.

In some instances, deviations from the "equal dollars per case" standard will highlight disparities to be corrected; in other instances, they will confirm the view that the system is applying appropriate flexibility to its standards to reflect legitimate differences in need from one jurisdiction to another. Viewed in this light, the Committee's goal is not to hold up equal dollar allocation as an absolute standard, but rather to make explicit the consequences of allocation formulas that are the product of complex political negotiation, epidemiological evidence, and competing conceptions of fairness.

Despite these limitations, analyses of current allocations are pertinent to stakeholders who wish to anticipate the distributive impact of changes to current formulas. If the current allocation appears unfavorable to states and EMAs that include a high proportion of reported HIV cases to ELCs, the move to a more inclusive definition of HIV burden may have large

[1]The Committee also examined current allocations using estimated AIDS prevalence alone. The differences in allocations using estimated AIDS prevalence and ELCs were not informative, suggesting that any methodological differences between the calculation of ELCs and the calculation of AIDS prevalence is not important for the purposes of identifying allocation variations.

distributional effects. If, in contrast, the ranking of states and EMA per-case RWCA spending is similar for different measures of HIV burden, epidemiological factors may be less important than other features of RWCA funding allocations in shaping real or perceived funding disparities. The Committee began by examining total RWCA allocations in fiscal year (FY) 2001 for the 50 states, DC, and Puerto Rico, and the nonterritory EMAs. FY2001 was especially pertinent because it was the most recent year in which the Committee could match available surveillance data with RWCA funding allocations. In that year, Title I awards totaled \$565,229,972 (HRSA, 2002a). Title II awards were significantly larger, totaling \$873,424,373 (HRSA, 2002b). Combined Title I and Title II awards therefore totaled \$1,438,654,345. These awards were determined based on the number of ELCs from the previous calendar year. In the year 2000, there were 280,759 ELCs, with 204,298 residing within EMAs (HRSA 2002a,b). If Title I and Title II funds were provided to funding units in strict proportion to the number of ELCs, the nationwide allocations per ELC would have been:

- Title I: \$2,767 per ELC (\$565,299,972 divided by 204,298)
- Title II: \$3,111 per ELC (\$873,424,373 divided by 280,759)
- Titles I and II: \$5,124 per ELC (\$1,438,654,345 divided by 280,759)

These summary statistics provide one benchmark of equity with which to compare actual awards per ELC.

Figure C-1 illustrates how the FY2001 Title I award per ELC varied across EMAs. With the exception of San Francisco, Title I awards per ELC spanned a narrow range across metropolitan areas (mean \$2,754; standard deviation: \$174). This uniform allocation reflects the strong role of ELCs in Title I funding. Thus, applying the standard of equal expenditures per ELC, the Title I formula allocations are highly equitable. This uniform pattern of per-ELC Title I expenditure is more open to question through other conceptions of equity, for example if one believes that formula allocations should vary in accordance with per-capita income, with the socioeconomic status of persons living with AIDS, or with other characteristics that systematically vary across EMAs.

The large allocation to San Francisco reflects the influence of the hold-harmless provision. Removal of this provision would reduce San Francisco's allocation to within the reported range for other EMAs. Under current allocation rules, however, removing the hold-harmless protection would have a small effect on other EMAs, which would observe a 2.6 percent increase in their allocation if San Francisco's allocation were reduced. As noted by GAO (2000), the hold-harmless provision has a small overall effect on allocations to EMAs, yet a large effect on a single EMA.

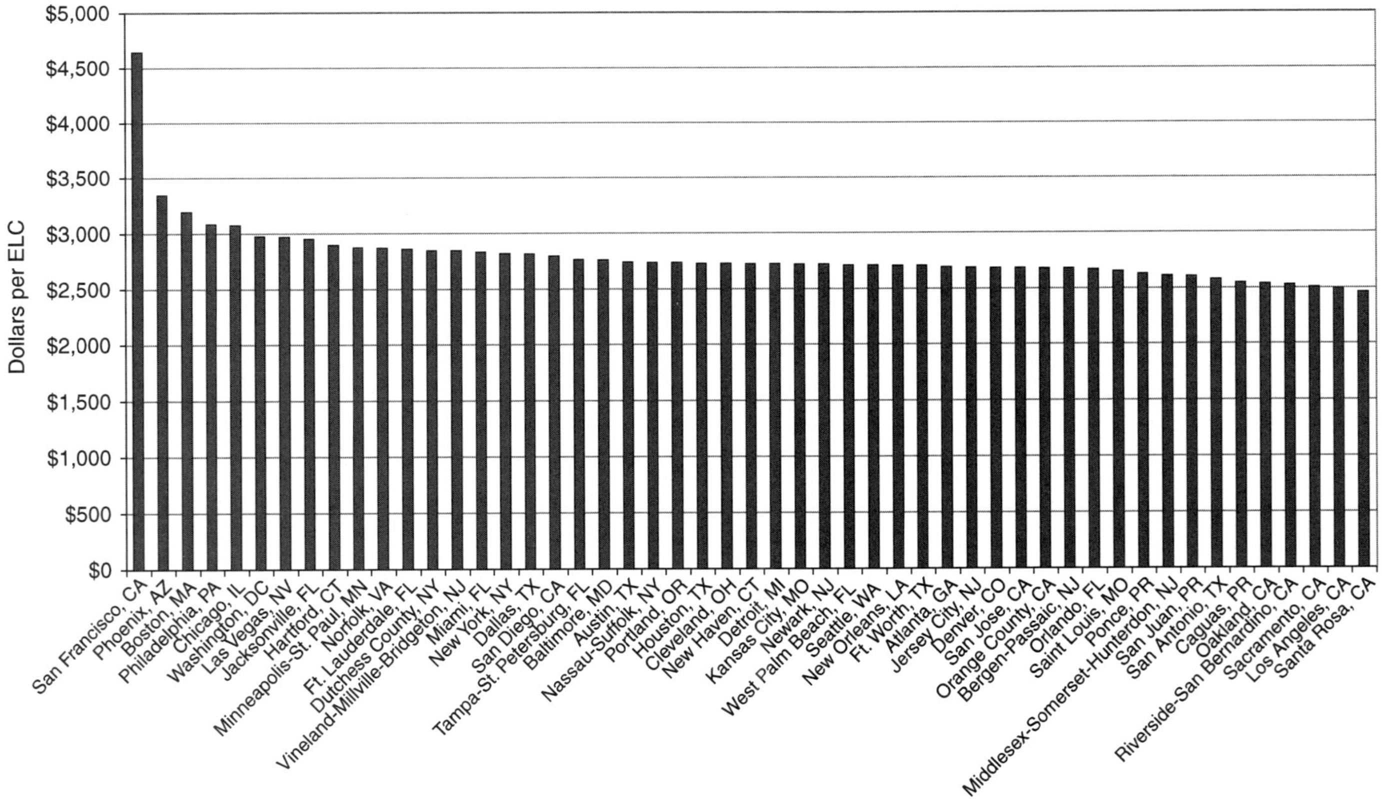

FIGURE C-1 FY2001 Title 1 allocations to EMAs per ELC.

USING HIV DATA IN FORMULAS

The Committee then examined other measures of HIV/AIDS burden. Not surprisingly, the number of ELCs was quite similar to estimated AIDS prevalence. Thus, moving from ELCs to AIDS prevalence appears to have a small impact on funding allocations. However, ELCs accounted for only about half of the total combined estimated HIV and AIDS prevalence. Combined estimated prevalence for the 50 states, DC, and Puerto Rico was 651,238 cases, with 449,898 of these cases associated with a specific EMA.

If Title I and Title II funds were provided in strict proportion to the total estimated HIV and AIDS prevalence, the nationwide allocations per case would be:

- Title I: $1,256 ($565,229,972 divided by 449,898),
- Title II: $1,341 ($873,424,373 divided by 651,238),
- Titles I and II: $2,209 ($1,438,654,345 divided by 651,238) (Figure C-2)

Again the EMA Title I award allocation is roughly proportional to the total number of HIV and AIDS cases (mean $1,198; standard deviation: $175), although using a combined HIV and AIDS measure accentuates the impact of the hold-harmless differential. This may be attributable to the relative maturity of the epidemic (and the resulting disproportion in the number of AIDS cases to HIV cases) in San Francisco compared with other areas (see discussion in Chapter 4).

Although this analysis does not directly address alternative allocation rules, EMAs listed on the right-hand side of Figure C-2 are most likely to benefit from an allocation formula that includes HIV cases, because these EMAs include the highest proportion of HIV cases to ELCs. It is important to note that if there is any random fluctuation or measurement error in reported HIV cases, one would expect to observe the variability found in Figure C-2. Because funding allocations are determined by ELCs, localities that understate true HIV prevalence would appear toward the left of the diagram, and those which overstate true HIV prevalence would appear closer to the right. Also note that because all figures for HIV and AIDS cases in California and Massachusetts are hard-wired, there is some uncertainty about the reliability of the results on the left side of Figure C-2. This does not change the relative allocations in other places.

Changing the unit of measurement to include HIV cases also appears to produce greater variance in funding allocation per unit of HIV burden. This suggests that states and localities vary in the ratio of HIV to AIDS cases. It is unclear whether such variation reflects variation in the matu-

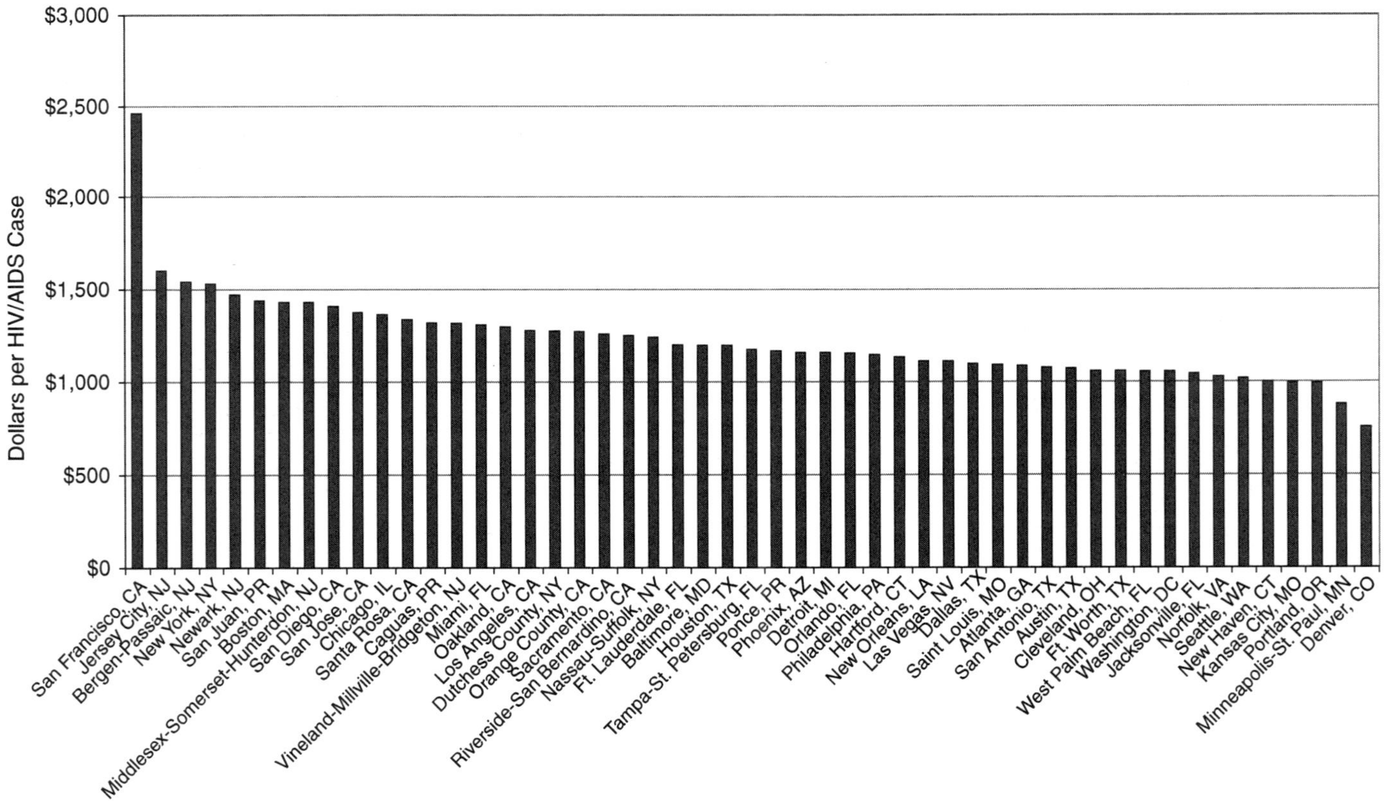

FIGURE C-2 FY2001 Title I allocations per HIV/AIDS case.

rity of the HIV/AIDS epidemic, HIV treatment practices that delay the onset of AIDS, or the quality and aggressiveness of HIV surveillance case finding.

Figures C-3 through C-6 illustrate the influence of the Title II formula on state-to-state allocation per unit of HIV disease burden. Non-EMA states receive somewhat greater per-ELC Title II funding than do EMA states ($3,985/ELC for non-EMA states, and $3,003/ELC for EMA states) (Figures C-3 and C-4). This difference is attributable to the 20 percent set-aside built into the Title II structure to favor non-EMA states (see Chapter 2). Title II awards per ELC are similar within each of the two groups: EMA and non-EMA states. Because every state receives at least $500,000 in Title II funding, some small non-EMA states receive high Title II awards per ELC. Kansas and New Hampshire have slightly lower allocations per ELC than other states, though the reasons for such variability are unclear.

The Title II funding advantage to non-EMA states diminishes when one shifts the unit of HIV burden to all HIV and AIDS cases (Figures C-5 and C-6). Average awards for non-EMA states ($1,339 per case) are virtually identical to the awards for EMA states ($1,342). This suggests that non-EMA states account for a greater proportion of HIV cases than they do of ELCs.

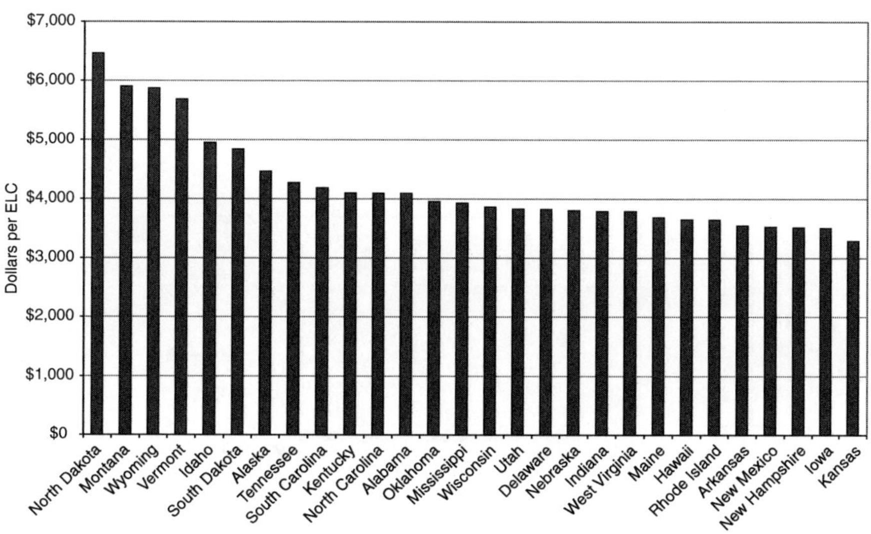

FIGURE C-3 FY2001 Title II allocations per ELC in states without an EMA.

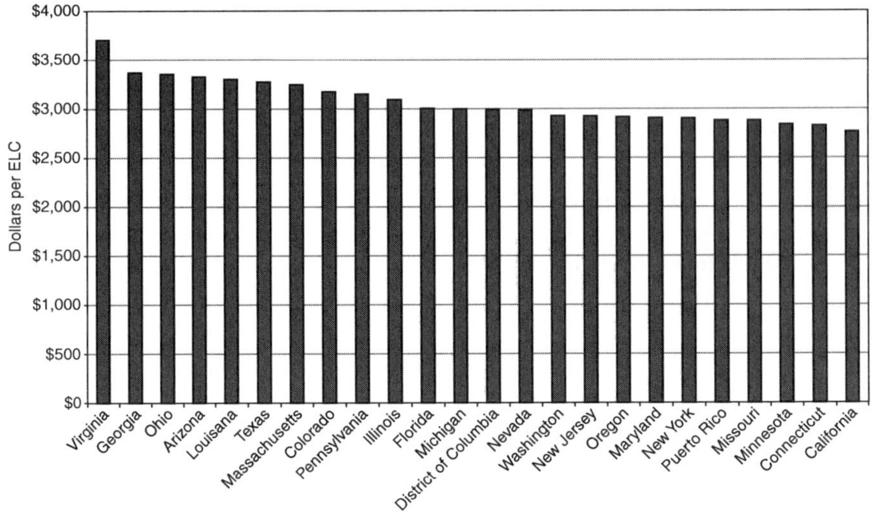

FIGURE C-4 FY2001 Title II allocations per ELC in states with an EMA.

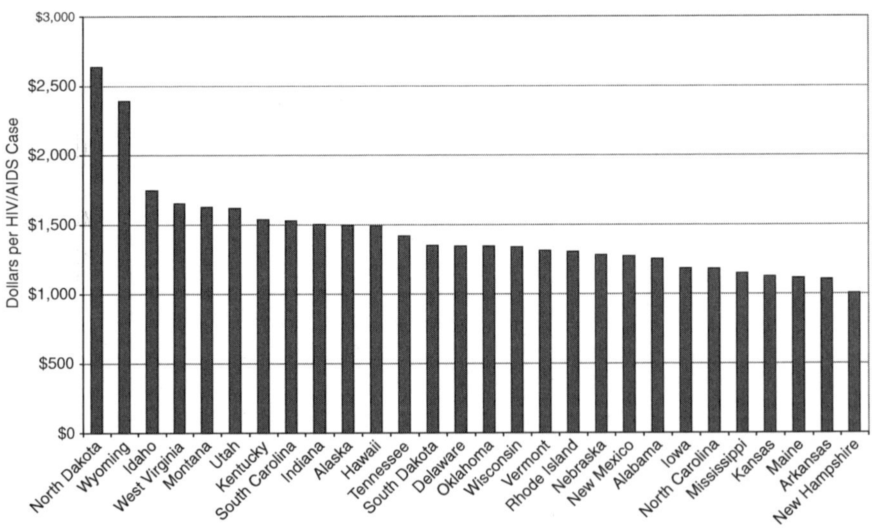

FIGURE C-5 FY2001 Title II allocations per HIV/AIDS case in states without an EMA.

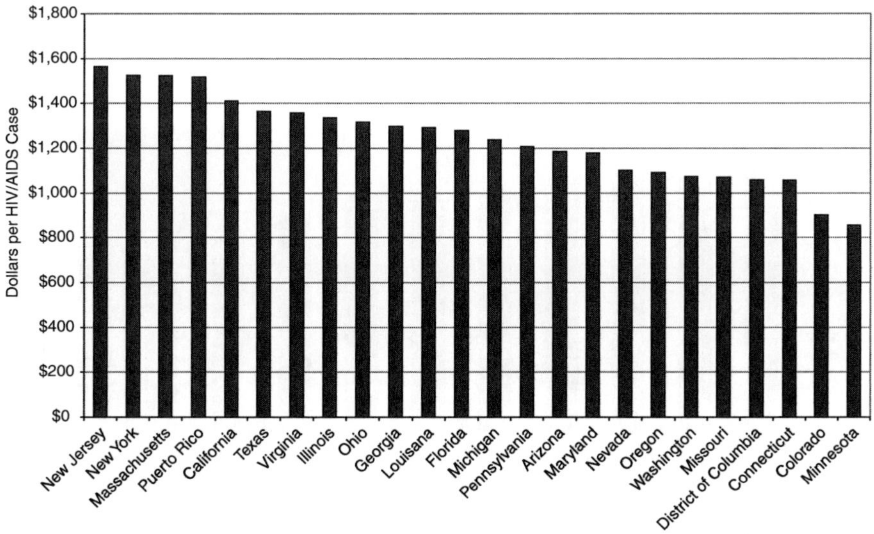

FIGURE C-6 FY 2001 Title II allocations per HIV/AIDS case in states with an EMA.

The Committee limited its analysis to the subgroup of states with more than 1,000 ELCs to avoid "outlier" states that account for a small proportion of overall ELCs and RWCA Title I and II allocations. Within this subgroup, Title I and II combined awards average $5,124 per ELC (and range between $3,290 and $8,285) (Figure C-7). On a per HIV/AIDS case basis, the average is $2,209 (ranging between $1,003 and $2,931) (Figure C-8).

Regional differences were evident in both figures, whether or not one uses reported HIV cases. In FY2001, southeastern states represented the four lowest allocations per HIV/AIDS case.

The other critical disparity arises between EMA and non-EMA states. In FY2001, 11 out of the 12 states receiving the fewest dollars on a per-ELC basis lacked an EMA. States whose ELCs were highly concentrated within EMAs received more funding than did other states whose EMAs accounted for a smaller proportion of state ELCs.

MULTIPLE REGRESSION ANALYSIS

The Committee performed several cross-sectional state regressions to examine characteristics associated with FY2001 RWCA funding. These

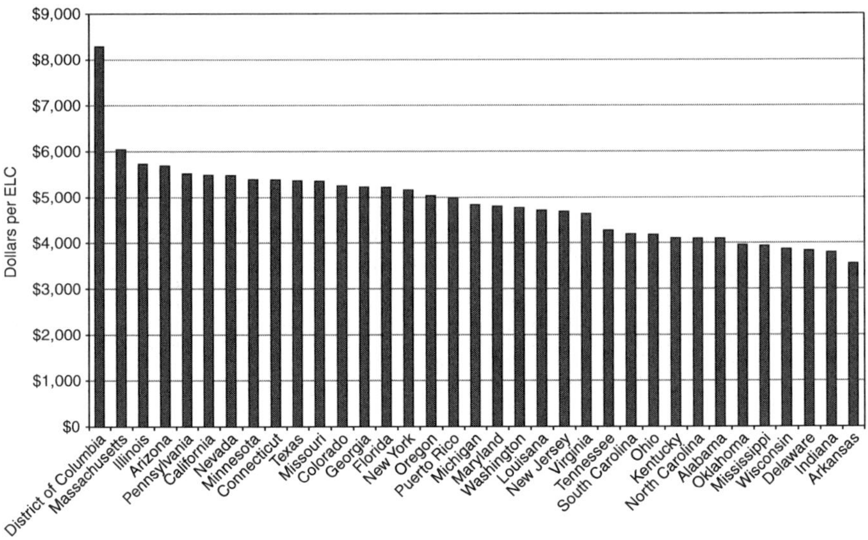

FIGURE C-7 FY2001 Total Title I and II allocations per ELC in states with more than 1,000 ELCs.

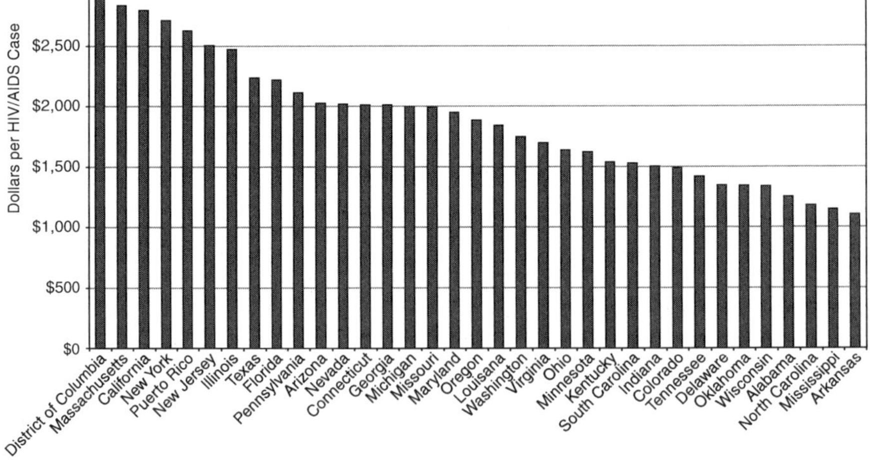

FIGURE C-8 FY2001 Total Title I and II allocations per HIV/AIDS in states with more than 1,000 ELCs.

analyses also allowed greater scrutiny of the qualitative patterns apparent in earlier figures. The resulting coefficients can then be evaluated in light of stakeholders' broader judgments regarding RWCA funding allocation. Multiple regression analysis indicates the influence of a specific explanatory variable on formula allocation, presuming that other explanatory variables remained unchanged. Regression analysis is useful to distinguish the likely impact of one variable, holding other correlated variables constant. In conducting simulations and considering policy implications of these results, readers are cautioned that localities and jurisdictions differ across many variables included in these models.

The analysis considered both Title I and Title II in examining RWCA resources available to states. Although Title II provides the primary funding to assist states, Title I funding is also pertinent, since these funds may augment or substitute for those provided by states. We examined funding per ELC and per HIV/AIDS case. In all four columns, regressions are weighted by state population size.

Given the small sample size of RWCA funding jurisdictions, we chose a deliberately sparse regression specification. Many advocates and policy makers contacted by the Committee noted the possibility that southern states receive lower funding allocations per unit of HIV burden. We therefore included an indicator variable set to one for southeastern states, and set to zero for others. The role of EMAs is widely discussed in comparing state RWCA funding allocations. We therefore included a dummy variable to indicate whether a state included an EMA. To capture potential differences related to race or ethnicity, we also included the percentage of African American or Hispanic residents in each state. To examine whether RWCA funding allocations favor low-income or high-income states, we included the logarithm of state median income in our preferred specification.

The coefficients in each column can be interpreted as a dollar change per unit of disease burden in RWCA funding associated with each unit change in the independent variable. Standard errors are shown in parentheses. For example, each percentage-point change in the fraction of the population that is Hispanic is associated with a –10.2 dollar change in Title II allocation per ELC. The standard error of 4.5 indicates that this coefficient is statistically significant at the 0.05 level. Results from African Americans are computed in an analogous fashion.

As shown in Table C-1, the presence of an EMA is associated with a significant reduction in RWCA Title II funding, but is associated with a significant increase in overall (Title I plus Title II) funding. Few other variables yielded significant coefficients. Controlling for other factors, southern states received about $318 less per case of HIV/AIDS.

The impact of the presence of an EMA is explored in greater detail in Table C-2. For each state that included an EMA, the Committee computed

TABLE C-1 Weighted Regression Analysis of RWCA Resources in FY2001

Dependent Variable	$(Title II) /ELC (Std. err)	$(Title I+Title II) /ELC (Std. err)	$(Title II) /HIV+AIDS (Std. err)	$(Title I+Title II) /HIV+AIDS (Std. err)
State has EMA	–751.4***	1096.6***	–130.6+	560.4***
	(123)	(187)	(74)	(123)
Southern state	280.9*	–111.8	–39.0	–317.7*
	(134)	(204)	(81)	(134)
Percent African American	–6.8	1.5	3.3	13.0+
	(6.9)	(10.5)	(4.2)	(6.9)
Percent Hispanic	–10.2*	12.7+	5.5*	23.1***
	(4.5)	(6.8)	(2.7)	(4.5)
Logarithm of median income	–252.7	–365.1	48.7	72.6
	(501)	(761)	(302)	(500)
R^2	0.70	0.61	0.10	0.71

(+p<0.10, *p<0.05, **p<0.01, ***p<0.001)

the proportion of ELCs who resided in an EMA. Table C-2 expands the analyses in Table C-1 to include this additional variable.

Including the proportion of ELCs within an EMA increases the proportion of variance explained by our regression models. A state with 1,000 ELCs entirely concentrated within an EMA receives approximately $1,814,000 (1000x[2126-312]) more than an otherwise comparable non-EMA state with the same number of ELCs.

The analysis of Table C-2 also accounts for the observed disparity between southern and nonsouthern states. The coefficient drops by approximately one-third of its base value, indicating that nonsouthern states with a high concentration of ELCs within EMAs contribute to the observed regional disparity.

Per-capita income and race/ethnicity appear to play a small role in explaining RWCA formula awards. Although poorer states receive slightly more resources, this effect was small and statistically insignificant. A one-standard-deviation decline in state log (median income) (0.136 log points) is associated with a $50 ($0.136 \times 365$) increase in per-ELC Title I and Title II resources. States with a high proportion of Hispanics also received greater resources. Although this result was statistically signifi-

TABLE C-2 Weighted Regression Analysis of RWCA Resources in FY2001

Dependent Variable	$(Title II) /ELC (Std. err)	$(Title I+Title II) /ELC (Std. err)	$(Title II) /HIV+AIDS (Std. err)	$(Title I+Title II) /HIV+AIDS (Std. err)
State has EMA	–241 (251)	–312 (324)	–66 (160)	–236 (227)
Proportion of ELCs in EMA	–770* (334)	2,126*** (431)	–97 (213)	1,202*** (303)
Southern state	204 (132)	100 (171)	–49 (84)	–198+ (120)
Percent African American	–5.2 (6.6)	–3.0 (8.6)	3.5 (4.2)	10.5+ (6.0)
Percent Hispanic	–4.8 (4.9)	–2.1 (6.3)	6.2* (3.1)	14.8*** (4.4)
Logarithm of median income	–221 (4.8)	–454 (618)	53 (3.0)	22.55 (434)
R^2	0.73	0.75	0.11 (not significantly different from 0)	0.79

(+p<0.10, *p<0.05, **p<0.01, ***p<0.001)

cant, it was also quite small in all specifications. The Committee also examined residuals in the regression analyses in Table C-2. Most outliers (positive and negative) were small states that included small populations of individuals diagnosed with HIV and AIDS.

Tables C-1 and C-2 should be interpreted in light of four principal limitations.

First, HIV and AIDS cases provide an imperfect measure of local HIV/AIDS burden. These measures do not explicitly address distributional priorities or health service delivery concerns that matter to clinicians, policy makers, and RWCA beneficiaries. Differences in costs of care, the severity and complexity of patient needs, and local resources might merit departures from a funding allocation based solely on the number of reported HIV or AIDS cases.

Second, this analysis does not address the underlying quality of case reporting data. This analysis was conducted using the patchwork of reported and estimated HIV cases made available to the Committee. Results should therefore be interpreted with caution. Moreover, the Committee could not directly investigate whether the inclusion of existing HIV case-reporting data provides a superior measure of true known HIV/AIDS prevalence than the sole use of AIDS data. Despite these limitations, both the descriptive analysis and the multiple regression analysis highlight important features of RWCA funding allocation.

Third, this analysis does not address regional medical practice patterns or regional disparities in the costs of AIDS care. As discussed elsewhere in this report, differences in the costs of important inputs might justify additional expenditures in high-cost cities and states.

Fourth, this analysis does not address differences in program quality and outcomes across jurisdictions. Such differences might also justify additional expenditures in jurisdictions that contain the most effective or cost-effective programs and interventions.

REFERENCES

GAO (General Accounting Office). 2000. Ryan White CARE Act: Opportunities to Enhance Funding Equity. GAO/T-HEHS-00-150 Washington, DC: GAO.

HRSA. 2002a. FY2002 Ryan White CARE Act Title I Emergency Relief Grants. (Email communication from Steven Young, HRSA, July 22, 2002).

HRSA. 2002b. FY2002 Ryan White CARE Act Title II Emergency Relief Grants. (Email communication from Steven Young, HRSA, July 22, 2002).

D

Methodological Details of HCSUS Analyses

This appendix provides details of the social area analysis presented in Chapter 5 as a potential method for identifying predictors of resource needs.

SAMPLE

The HIV Cost and Service Utilization Study (HCSUS) (Bozzette et al., 1998; Shapiro et al., 1999) was an interview study of a national probability sample of noninstitutionalized persons with HIV infection. As part of the HCSUS interviews, patients reported where they received care. Using that information, patients were assigned the zip code of the clinic in which they received most of their care. This information was used to identify the county where each patient received care.

Two sources of information were then used to characterize each county. The first is U.S. census data, which are available for geographic units below the Eligible Metropolitan Area (EMA) level. The second is the Area Resource File (ARF), which is a database containing over 6,000 variables for each county in the United States. ARF contains data on health facilities, health professions, measures of health care utilization and expenditures, health status, economic activity, health training programs, and demographic and environmental characteristics. The ARF data are compiled from more than 50 sources, such as vital statistics data and national surveys.[1] Both of

[1]For more information please refer to the following website: http://www.arfsys.com/overviewAccess.htm.

these data sources represent information that is collected and reported in a standardized manner, is publicly available, provided at the county level, and is routinely updated. The U.S. Census is only conducted every 10 years. The Current Population Survey is conducted monthly and updated estimates are provided annually, although those data are not available at the county level. The ARF data are updated annually.

HCSUS interviewed a total of 2,864 patients. Using the location information gathered in interviews, it was possible to attach a zip code to 2,360 of these patients and link information from their interviews to information from the February 1996 ARF (Landon et al., 2002). This ARF was chosen because it corresponds to the time when the patients were interviewed for the HCSUS. These 2,360 patients resided in 82 counties with a mean count of 29 patients per county (ranging from 1 to 260). A total of 504 patients were not linked because of a missing or unmatched zip code either in the HCSUS sample or in the ARF file.

DEPENDENT VARIABLES

As examples of indicators of need, the Committee created two dependent variables using data from the HCSUS study. The first variable measured the number of needs reported by the patients. In the HCSUS interview, each patient was asked the following questions:

1. Did you need income assistance such as SSI, SSDI, AFDC, or health care benefits from Medicaid or the Veterans Administration in the last 6 months?
2. Did you need to find a place to live in the last 6 months?
3. Did you need home health care in the last 6 months?
4. Did you need mental health or emotional care or counseling in the last 6 months?
5. Did you need drug or alcohol treatment in the last 6 months?

The Committee created a variable called "number of needs," which is simply the number of these questions that the respondent answered affirmatively.

The HCSUS interview also asked whether patients had received highly active antiretrovial therapy (HAART). Although this is not a direct indicator of resource needs, differences in use of appropriate therapies might be an indicator of variations in resources and/or difficulties treating patients appropriately. The working definition of HAART use, which is based on the Department of Health and Human Services/Henry J. Kaiser Foundation definition used in the *Guidelines for the Use of Antiretroviral Agents in HIV Infected Adults and Adolescents*, was: taking certain combinations of nucleoside reverse transcriptase inhibitors (e.g., zidovudine and lamuvidine) plus certain protease inhibitors (PIs, e.g., Nelfinavir), combinations of PIs (e.g., ritonavir and saquinavir), or the combination of a PI plus non-nucleoside reverse transcriptase inhibitors (e.g., Nevirapine). Each patient was classified as taking HAART, if he/she reported taking any one of the HAART combinations. According to guidelines published close to the time of the 1996 baseline interview, 99 percent of the sample was eligible for HAART because they had either CD4 < 500, or HIV RNA > 10,000 copies per ml, or they had symptomatic HIV or AIDS (Carpenter et al., 1996).

PREDICTORS

The ARF and census data provide examples of how to characterize the "social area" of the persons interviewed. The ARF file contains thousands of variables, but the Committee selected several that it considered representative of the kinds of variables that are likely to be related to resource needs for HIV care. Specifically, the following variables were selected for the regression models:

1. Total general practitioners in 1996 divided by the total population in 1990,
2. Total number of medical specialists in 1996 divided by the total population in 1990,
3. Percent of the population that was black in 1990,
4. Percent of the population that is foreign born in 1990,
5. Percent of population that lives in urban areas in 1990,
6. Percent of population who live in poverty in 1990,
7. Percent of population who are college graduates in 1990.

In addition to the variables specified above, dummy variables representing region (Northeast, Midwest, South, West) were included in the models to control for general regional differences.

ANALYSES AND RESULTS

To find potential predictors for reported needs and HAART use, the Committee estimated two regression models. The model that predicted reported needs was a linear regression model, estimated using ordinary least squares. The model that predicted HAART use was estimated using a logistic regression. Given that many of the counties had multiple patients, a hierarchical model (Bryk and Raudenbush, 1992) was used, in which the county was specified as the second-level cluster (Landon et al.,

TABLE D-1 Results of Regression Analysis in HCSUS sample

	Regression Coefficient (Standard Errors)	
Predictor Variables	Reported Needs	HAART Treatment
Number of general practice MDs per 100 persons	–10.58 (4.04)**	–36.51 (10.20)***
Number of medical specialists per 100 persons	2.45 (0.65)***	–2.29 (1.90)
Percent African American	0.00 (0.00)	–0.03 (0.01)**
Percent foreign born	–0.65 (0.53)	–1.41 (0.87)
Percent urban	–0.46 (0.36)	0.58 (0.91)
Percent of families below poverty level	0.01 (0.01)	0.08 (0.03)**
Percent of persons over 25 years of age with 4 or more years of college	–3.27 (1.05)**	3.74 (2.56)
Midwest	0.07 (0.14)	1.29 (0.32)***
South	0.14 (0.09)	0.59 (0.30)
West	0.22 (0.15)	1.10 (0.37)**
R-Square	0.02	0.05

(*$p < 0.05$, **$p < 0.01$, ***$p < 0.001$)

2002). Because measures of association, rather than estimates of central tendency, were of interest, the data were not weighted prior to analysis. Results of the analyses are reported in Table D-1. Standard errors are shown in parentheses.

Results

The models indicate that the education in an area, the number of general practice physicians, and the number of specialists in an area are statistically significant predictors of the number or needs reported by individuals. Specifically, persons reported more needs if they lived in areas with fewer college educated persons, fewer general practitioners, and more medical specialists. The relationships with education and general practitioners seem reasonable. The relationship for medical specialists is counterintuitive, but it might be a reflection of an emphasis on more expensive care at the expense of more basic services. The strongest predictors of not receiving HAART therapy were living in a county with a high percent of African Americans, a high percentage of families below the poverty level, and an area with more general practitioners.

Discussion

The HCSUS study was not designed to collect information about patient needs thought to be most related to resource needs and the sample was not designed to support analyses of the relationships between county characteristics and needs. Thus, these results do not necessarily describe relationships that could be used to guide allocation decisions. Rather, these analyses were conducted to illustrate the kinds of modeling that could be done to assess whether publicly available measures of area characteristics could be used to predict intercounty variability in resource needs. Assessing the usefulness for such an approach for RWCA allocations would require measures of need directly relevant to RWCA allocation decisions and data that could be aggregated to the level used for allocations, such as EMAs.

REFERENCES

Bozzette SA, Berry SH, Duan N, Frankel MR, Leibowitz AA, Lefkowitz D, Emmons CA, Senterfitt JW, Berk ML, Morton SC, Shapiro MF. 1998. The care of HIV-infected adults in the United States. HIV Cost and Services Utilization Study Consortium. *New England Journal of Medicine* 339(26):1897–904.

Bryk AS, Raudenbush SW. 1992. *Hierarchical Linear Models. Applications and Data Analysis Methods.* New York: Sage Publications.

Carpenter CC, Fischl MA, Hammer SM, Hirsch MS, Jacobsen DM, Katzenstein DA, Montaner JS, Richman DD, Saag MS, Schooley RT, Thompson MA, Vella S, Yeni PG, Volberding PA. 1996. Antiretroviral therapy for HIV infection in 1996. Recommendations of an international panel. International AIDS Society-USA. *Journal of the American Medical Association* 276(2):146–54.

Landon BE, Wilson IB, Wenger NS, Cohn SE, Fichtenbaum CJ, Bozzette SA, Shapiro MF, Cleary PD. 2002. Specialty training and specialization among physicians who treat HIV/AIDS in the United States. *Journal of General Internal Medicine* 17(1):12–22.

Shapiro MF, Morton SC, McCaffrey DF, Senterfitt JW, Fleishman JA, Perlman JF, Athey LA, Keesey JW, Goldman DP, Berry SH, Bozzette SA. 1999. Variations in the care of HIV-infected adults in the United States: Results from the HIV Cost and Services Utilization Study. *Journal of the American Medical Association* 281(24):2305–15.

E

Tables of HIV/AIDS Quality Measures from Selected Sources

TABLE E-1 Commonly Used Quality Measures by Measure Type

Measure Type	Measure	Source
STRUCTURAL MEASURES	The committee found no explicit structural measures in use; however, certain process measures such as visits with HIV specialists imply the availability of appropriate health care resources.	
PROCESS MEASURES	*Prevention*	
	Counseling and testing	HIVQUAL
	Counseling on high-risk behaviors	RAND
	Tobacco use assessment	HIVQUAL
	Screening & Monitoring	
	CD4+ cell count	HCSUS
	CD4+ cell count	IHI
	CD4+ cell count	UHC
	CD4+ cell count and HIV viral load	FACCT
	CD4+ cell count and HIV viral load	IDSA
	CD4+ cell count and HIV viral load	QUERI
	CD4+ cell count and HIV viral load	RAND
	CD4+ cell count and HIV viral load	RAND
	CD4+ cell count and HIV viral load	UHC
	Cervical cancer	EQHIV

Eligible Population	Measure Criterion/Definition
Pregnant women	The number of pregnant women with counseling offered and testing performed during the prenatal period
All	Counseled regarding high risk behavior at time of HIV diagnosis and within one month of presentation with an initial infection of STD
All	Number of patients with whom tobacco use was discussed during the past year
All	At least one CD4+ cell count determination per studied 6 month interval, by chart review or interview
All	Percent with CD4+ cell count taken in the past 6 months
All	Semi-annual CD4+ cell count attainment (most recent 6 months)
1) If CD4+ cell count > 300 cells/μL; 2) If CD4+ cell count <300 cells/μL	1) CD4+ cell count and HIV viral load every 6 months; 2) CD4+ cell count and HIV viral load every 3 months
Patients being followed actively (having at least 1 visit in last 6 months)	Percent with CD4+ cell count and HIV viral load; every 3–4 months when CD4+ cell count is <350/μL or every 6–7 months when CD4+ cell count is >350/μL
1) Patients on HAART; 2) All	1) CD4+ cell count or HIV viral load test every 3 months; 2) CD4+ cell count or HIV viral load test every 6 months
CD4+ cell count > 300 cells/μL	Offer of CD4+ test (count or percent) and HIV viral load every 6 months
patients with detectable HIV viral loads	Offer HIV viral load every 4 months
All	1 each (CD4+ cell count and HIV viral load) in 2 consecutive 6-month periods
All females	Documentation of Pap smear or colposcopy

Continued

TABLE E-1 Continued

Measure Type	Measure	Source
	Cervical cancer	EQHIV
	Cervical cancer	FACCT
	Cervical cancer	HCSUS
	Cervical cancer	IDSA
	Cervical cancer	IHI
	Cervical cancer	UHC
	Cervical cancer and other pelvic disease	HIVQUAL
	Complete blood count	FACCT
	Complete blood count, CD4+ cell count, HIV viral load	RAND
	Complete blood count, CD4+ cell count, HIV viral load	RAND
	Cytomegalovirus disease	FACCT
	Cytomegalovirus disease	HCSUS
	Cytomegalovirus disease	RAND
	Hepatitis A	QUERI
	Hepatitis B	FACCT
	Hepatitis B	QUERI
	Hepatitis B	UHC
	Hepatitis B and C	IHI
	Hepatitis C	EQHIV
	Hepatitis C	EQHIV
	Hepatitis C	FACCT

Eligible Population	Measure Criterion/Definition
Females with abnormal Pap smear	Repeat of Pap smear
All females	Annual Pap smear
All females	All Pap smears according to guidelines (currently baseline, 6 months, and every 12 months thereafter if normal)
HIV-infected adult and adolescent women being followed	Percent who had at least one Pap smear done in the past year
All females	Percent with Pap smear in last 6 months
All females	Percent with Pap smear (between 9/2000 and 9/2001)
All females 18 years or older AND sexually active female patients 13 to 18 years of age	Number of patients with a pelvic exam recorded in the last year (pelvic exam includes Pap smear; chlamydia screen; gonorrhea test)
All	Complete blood count at first visit
All	Offer baseline laboratories (complete blood count, HIV viral load, CD4+ cell count) within one month of initial diagnosis
Patients on antiretroviral therapy	Offer CD4+ cell count or percent, HIV viral load and complete blood count within past 4 months
1) All; 2) CD4+ cell count less than 200 cells/μL	1) Cytomegalovirum IgG determination; 2) Annual fundoscopic exam
All, as indicated	Fundoscopic exam by eye care provider
Lowest recorded CD4+ cell count of less than 100 cells/μL	Receipt of yearly fundoscopic exam
All	Receipt of hepatitis A test (ever)
All	Hepatitis B antibody determination
All	Receipt of hepatitis B test (ever)
All	Hepatitis B serology attainment (ever)
All	Percent with hepatitis B & C screening
All	Hepatitis C status was known (whether positive or negative)
All	Appropriate hepatitis C screening
All	Hepatitis C antibody determination

Continued

TABLE E-1 Continued

Measure Type	Measure	Source
	Hepatitis C	HIVQUAL
	Hepatitis C	HIVQUAL
	Hepatitis C	HIVQUAL
	Hepatitis C	QUERI
	Hepatitis C	UHC
	HIV Specialist Visits	HIVQUAL
	Lipid screening (for disease and drug related metabolic abnormalities)	HIVQUAL (optional measure)
	Lipid screening (for disease and drug related metabolic abnormalities)	QUERI
	Oral Health / Dental exam	HIVQUAL (optional measure)
	Outpatient visits	IHI*
	Outpatient visits	EQHIV
	Syphilis	FACCT
	Syphilis	HCSUS
	Syphilis	HIVQUAL
	Syphilis	HIVQUAL
	Syphilis	HIVQUAL

Eligible Population	Measure Criterion/Definition
All	The number of patients for whom hepatitis C was document in the medical record
HCV+ patients	The number for whom alcohol counseling and HCV education was provided
All	The number of patients for whom hepatitis A status was documented.
All	Receipt of hepatitis C test (ever)
All	Hepatitis C serology attainment (ever)
All; with exception of those either incarcerated or hospitalized and with no ambulatory clinic visits during 4-month review period	Number of patients who are seen by an HIV specialist at least once every 4 months
Patients receiving antiretroviral therapy	The number of patients for whom lipid screen was performed during the past year
Patients on protease inhibitors (PI) or non-nucleoside reverse transcriptase inhibitors (NNRTI) for consecutive months	Receipt of lipid panel testing
All	The number of patients with a dental exam documented during the past year
All	Percent with visit(s) in last 3 months
All	Have outpatient visits in 3 or 4 quarter during review period.
All	Serologic test for syphilis measured at least once
All	Any serologic test for syphilis performed
All patients 18 years or older AND sexually active patients 13 to 18 years of age	The number of patients for whom syphilis screening was performed in the last year
Patients with reactive RPR/VDRL	Number with RPR/VDRL titer result verified (FTA-ABS)
Patients with positive serology	Number of patients that have been addressed in the chart

Continued

TABLE E-1 Continued

Measure Type	Measure	Source
	Syphilis	QUERI
	Syphilis	RAND
	Toxoplasmosis	FACCT
	Toxoplasmosis	HCSUS
	Toxoplasmosis	QUERI
	Toxoplasmosis	RAND
	Toxoplasmosis	UHC
	Tuberculosis	EQHIV
	Tuberculosis	EQHIV
	Tuberculosis	FACCT
	Tuberculosis	HCSUS
	Tuberculosis	HIVQUAL
	Tuberculosis	IDSA
	Tuberculosis	IHI
	HIV viral load	HCSUS
	HIV viral load	HIVQUAL
	HIV viral load	IHI
	HIV viral load	RAND
	HIV viral load	UHC

Eligible Population	Measure Criterion/Definition
All	Receipt of VDRL test ever
All	Documented serologic test for syphilis (VDRL or RPR)
All	Toxoplasma IgG antibody measured at least once
All	Toxoplasma IgG antibody determination noted in chart
All	Receipt of toxoplasmosis test (ever)
All	Toxoplasmosis serology should be documented
All	Toxoplasmosis serology attainment ever
All	Documentation of PPD (skin test for TB) during the review period
All	Documentation of PPD (skin test for TB) during the review period and that it was actually read
All	PPD (skin test for TB) if no prior positive test
All	1) PPD (skin test for TB) ever documented in chart or by interview. 2) periodic PPD tests (skin test for TB) documented in chart or by interview
All	The number of patients whose PPD (skin test for TB) was placed and results read during the past year
HIV-infected persons being followed	Percent who had a documented tuberculin skin test at any time
All	Percent with PPD (skin test for TB)
All	At least one HIV viral load determination per measured 6 month interval, by chart review or interview
All; with exception of those either incarcerated or hospitalized and with no ambulatory clinic visits during 4-month review period	The number of patients for whom HIV viral load test was performed every 4 months
All	Percent with HIV viral load tests taken in past 3 months
Patients on antiretroviral therapy	Offer HIV viral load measurement within 2 months of initiation or change in antiretroviral treatment
All	Semi-annual HIV viral load attainment (most recent 6 months)

Continued

TABLE E-1 Continued

Measure Type	Measure	Source
	Treatment (Antiretroviral)	
	Appropriate management of patients on antiretroviral therapy (ART)	HIVQUAL
	Appropriate management of patients on ART	HIVQUAL
	Appropriate management of patients on ART	HIVQUAL
	Provision of adherence counseling and/or monitoring	IHI*
	Provision of adherence counseling and/or monitoring	HIVQUAL
	Provision of adherence counseling and/or monitoring	IHI
	Provision of adherence counseling and/or monitoring	RAND
	Provision of adherence counseling and/or monitoring	UHC
	Provision of indicated ART	IHI*

Eligible Population	Measure Criterion/Definition
Patients who are receiving ART therapy, received ART therapy in the past, or are eligible for ART therapy based on New York State ART therapy guidelines; virologically stable	The number of stable patients for whom HIV viral load is monitored every 4 months
Patients who are receiving ART therapy, received ART therapy in the past, or are eligible for ART therapy based on New York State ART therapy guidelines; virologically unstable	One of the following four management options is documented in the medical record in every 4-month period that the patient is considered unstable: (1) regimen was changed and HIV viral load assay performed within 8 weeks of decision; (2) justification provided not to change therapy and HIV viral load assay performed within 8 weeks of decision; (3) documentation that patient decides not to take medication and HIV viral load assay performed within 4 months; (4) decision made to discontinue therapy and planned clinical follow-up plan noted in record within 4 months
Patients who are receiving ART therapy, received ART therapy in the past, or are eligible for ART therapy based on New York State ART therapy guidelines; end stage or patients with no other therapeutic options	The number of patients for whom a follow-up clinic visit is recorded every 4 months
Patients on HAART	Percent with adherence counseling/intervention at their last visit
Patients prescribed antiretroviral therapy	Adherence is measured and described quantitatively at least once every 4 months
Patients on HAART	Percent who self-report adherence to prescribed regimen according to some standard method (3 months)
Patients started on protease inhibitors	Documented counseling regarding compliance with therapy within 1 month of the start of therapy.
Patients on antiretroviral therapy	Documentation of adherence to ART at most recent visit
All	Percent on HAART

Continued

TABLE E-1 Continued

Measure Type	Measure	Source
	Provision of indicated ART	EQHIV
	Provision of indicated ART	EQHIV
	Provision of indicated ART	FACCT
	Provision of indicated ART	HCSUS
	Provision of indicated ART	IDSA
	Provision of indicated ART	IHI
	Provision of indicated ART	QUERI
	Provision of indicated ART	RAND

Eligible Population	Measure Criterion/Definition
Patients with CD4+ <500 cells/μL or HIV viral load >20,000 copies	On HAART (defined as three or more antiretroviral medications)
Patients with CD4+ <500 cells/μL or HIV viral load >20,000 copies	On ART (defined as two or more antiretroviral medications)
Patients with AIDS diagnosis or symptomatic HIV disease; or patients with no symptoms, but CD4+ cell count <500 cells/μL or HIV viral load >20,000 (using RT-PCR)	Initiation of ART—Preferred treatment (1 highly active protease inhibitor + 2 nucleoside reverse transcriptase inhibitor) or Alternative treatment (1 nonnucleoside reverse transcriptase inhibitor or Saquinavir + 2 nucleoside reverse transcriptase inhibitor)
Proportion of patients with indications for antiretroviral therapy according to prevailing DHHS guidelines (CD4-cell count <350/μL or HIV viral load >30,000 at the time of the study) documented by chart review or interview over a 6-month period	Receipt of any DHHS recommended combination antiretroviral regimen during that time period or in the following 3 months
Patients with CD4+ cell count count <350/μL now or in the past	Percent who have taken part in a discussion about prescription of HAART, as indicated in the medical record.
Patients on HAART	Percent who are on first HAART regimen
Patients with CD4+ cell count < 350/μL and/or HIV viral load >20,000 copies	Percent on HAART for at least 3 out of 6 months (not necessarily consecutive)
Patients with any of the following conditions: CD4+ cell count count ≥ 500 cells/μL and HIV viral load > 30,000 copies; CD4+ cell count count 350–499 and HIV viral load >10,000 copies; CD4+ cell count count <300; any AIDS-defining condition; thrush	Receive adequate antiretroviral treatment (or be enrolled in a clinical trial with documentation of informed consent) within 1 month of conditions being met

Continued

TABLE E-1 Continued

Measure Type	Measure	Source
	Provision of indicated ART	RAND
	Provision of indicated ART	UHC
	Provision of indicated ART	UHC
	Regimen change	IHI
	Treatment (Prophylaxis)	
	Hepatitis B	FACCT
	Hepatitis B	UHC
	Influenza	EQHIV
	Influenza	FACCT
	Influenza	HCSUS
	Influenza	IDSA
	Influenza	UHC
	Mycobacterium avium complex (MAC)	FACCT
	Mycobacterium avium complex (MAC)	HCSUS
	Mycobacterium avium complex (MAC)	IDSA
	Mycobacterium avium complex (MAC)	QUERI

Eligible Population	Measure Criterion/Definition
All	Protease inhibitors should not be prescribed concurrently with astemizole, terfenadine, rifampin, or cisapride.
Patients with CD4+ <200 cells/µL	Taking at least three antiretroviral agents
Patients on antiretroviral therapy	Regimen contains at least three antiretroviral agents
All	Percent who had their medication regimen changed in the last month
Hepatitis B antigen and antibody negative	Received three injection series of hepatitis B vaccine
All patients without prior infection	Hepatitis B vaccination series completed or in progress
All	Documentation of influenza vaccine during review period. Patient refused was included as having documentation
All	Receipt of influenza vaccine annually
All	Receipt of influenza vaccination during the year under study
All	Monitoring of CD4+ cell counts and HIV HIV viral loads
All	Receipt of influenza vaccination
Patients with a CD4+ cell count of less than 50 cells/µL	Taking arithromycin, clarithromycin, or rifabutin in recommended doses for recommended duration
Patients with a CD4+ cell count of less than 50 cells/µL noted in chart or interview period in the previous 9 months	Receipt of any CDC/IDSA recommended form of prophylaxis against Mycobacterium avium complex infection
Patients whose current CD4+ cell count is <50/µL	Percent who have been offered chemoprophylaxis with clarithromycin or azithromycin within 2 months of determination that the CD4+ lymphocyte count is <50/µL
Patients with CD4+ cell count <50/µL	Receipt of at least one MAC drug class in prior 6 months

Continued

TABLE E-1 Continued

Measure Type	Measure	Source
	Mycobacterium avium complex (MAC)	RAND
	Mycobacterium avium complex (MAC)	UHC
	Pneumococcal pneumonia	FACCT
	Pneumococcal pneumonia	HCSUS
	Pneumococcal pneumonia	IHI
	Pneumococcal pneumonia	RAND
	Pneumococcal pneumonia	UHC
	Pneumocystis carinii pneumonia (PCP)	FACCT
	Pneumocystis carinii pneumonia (PCP)	HCSUS
	Pneumocystis carinii pneumonia (PCP)	HIVQUAL (optional measure)
	Pneumocystis carinii pneumonia (PCP)	IDSA
	Pneumocystis carinii pneumonia (PCP)	IHI
	Pneumocystis carinii pneumonia (PCP)	QUERI
	Pneumocystis carinii pneumonia (PCP)	RAND

Eligible Population	Measure Criterion/Definition
CD4+ cell count dropping below 50/μL	Offer of MAC prophylaxis within 1 month of drop in cell count below 50 CD4+ cells/μL
Most recent CD4+ cell count <50/μL	Receipt of MAC prophylaxis
All (optional if CD4+ cell count <200/μL	Receipt of Pneumovax® (pneumococcal vaccination) (once)
All	Receipt of Pneumovax® (pneumococcal vaccination) (ever)
All	Percent with documented Pneumovax® (pneumococcal vaccination) in last 5 years
Patients with lowest recorded CD4+ cell count > 200/μL	Documentation of Pneumovax® (pneumococcal vaccination) receipt
All	Receipt of Pneumovax® (pneumococcal vaccination)
CD4+ cell count 200/μL or CD4% <15%. Or oral thrush or fever for ≥2 weeks	Receipt of trimethoprim-sulfamethoxazole, Dapsone, or Aerosolized pentamidine in recommended doses for recommended duration
Patients with a CD4+ cell count of less than 200 cells/μL noted in chart or interview period in the previous 9 months	Receipt of any CDC/IDSA recommended form of prophylaxis against *Pneumocystis carinii*
Patients with CD4+ cell count <200/μL (patients with CD4+ cell count >200/ μL for less than 6 months are also eligible for review)	The number of patients prescribed PCP prophylactic therapy
Patients with CD4+ cell count currently <200/μL	Percent who were prescribed PCP prophylaxis within 2 months of determination of the CD4+ cell count to be <200/μL
Patients with CD4+ cell count <200 μL at last visit (within 3 months)	Percent with PCP prophylaxis (within last 3 months)
Patients with CD4+ cell count <200/μL	Receipt of at least one PCP drug class for 2 consecutive months in prior 6 months
CD4+ cell count less than 200 cells/μL, completion of active treatment of PCP, or CD4 below 15%.	Offer PCP prophylaxis within 1 month of these conditions

Continued

TABLE E-1 Continued

Measure Type	Measure	Source
	Pneumocystis carinii pneumonia (PCP)	UHC
	Toxoplasmosis	FACCT
	Toxoplasmosis	RAND
	Tuberculosis	FACCT
	Tuberculosis	RAND
	Social and Support Services	
	Benefits advocacy	HCSUS
	Emotional counseling	HCSUS

Eligible Population	Measure Criterion/Definition
Most recent CD4-cell count <200/μL	Receipt of PCP prophylaxis
Positive antibody (IgG) to toxoplasma present and CD4+ <50 cells/μL	Receipt of trimethoprim-sulfamethoxazole, or Dapsone plus pyrimethamine, in recommended doses for recommended duration
Patients who do not have active toxoplasmosis and who meet either of the following conditions: Toxo IgG positive; or completion of therapy for active toxoplasmosis	Offered toxoplasmosis prophylaxis within 1 month of meeting all these conditions
Patients with tuberculin skin test >5ml or prior positive without treatment or contact with active case of tuberculosis	Receipt of isoniazid plus pyridoxine or rifampin in recommended doses for recommended duration
Patients who do not have active TB and who have not ever previously received TB prophylaxis with current PPD (skin test for TB) >5 mm; or provider noting that patient has had PPD (skin test for TB) >5 mm administered at anytime since HIV diagnosis	Offer of tuberculosis prophylaxis within one month of these conditions
Patients with a need for help in obtaining income assistance such as SSI, SSDI, AFDC, or health care benefits from Medicaid or the VA in the last 6 months as reported at interview	No unmet need
Patients with need for help in obtaining mental health or emotional care or counseling in the last 6 months as reported at interview	No unmet need

Continued

TABLE E-1 Continued

Measure Type	Measure	Source
	Home Health Services	HCSUS
	Housing	HCSUS
	Mental Health Assessment	HIVQUAL
	Self-management goal setting	IHI
	Substance abuse services	HCSUS
	Substance abuse services	HIVQUAL
	Substance abuse services	HIVQUAL
	Substance abuse services	HIVQUAL
	Support Service	IHI
OUTCOME MEASURES	Health Outcomes	
	CD4+ cell count	IHI
	CD4+ cell count	IHI*
	CD4+ cell count	IHI

Eligible Population	Measure Criterion/Definition
Patients with need for help in obtaining home health care in the last 6 months as reported at interview	No unmet need
Patients with a need for help in finding a place to live in the last 6 months as reported at interview	No unmet need
All	The number of patients for whom a mental health assessment was performed during the past year. Assessment components include: cognitive function; screening for depression and anxiety; psychiatric history; psychiatric medication review; psychosocial assessment; sleeping and appetite assessment
All	Percent with self-management goal setting
Patients with need for help in obtaining drug or alcohol treatment in the last 6 months as reported at interview	No unmet need
All	The number of patients with whom substance use was discussed in the past year
Patients with current use (0–6 months from date of review) and not in treatment	Number for whom referrals are made for substance use treatment
Patients with past use (6–24 months from date of review)	Number with whom relapse prevention or ongoing treatment has been discussed and substance use within the last 12 months assessed.
All	Percent with Support Service Assessment
All patients with CD4+ cell count in last 3 months	Average of the last CD4+ cell count
Patients on HAART	Percent with CD4+ cell count >200/μL
All with at least two CD4+ cell count in last 6 months	Percent with CD4+ cell count rise of >50/μL in the past 6 months

Continued

TABLE E-1 Continued

Measure Type	Measure	Source
	CD4+ cell count	EQHIV
	CD4+ cell count	EQHIV
	Emergency room visits	UHC
	Hospitalization	UHC
	Hospitalization	IHI
	HIV viral load	IHI*
	HIV viral load	EQHIV
	HIV viral load	EQHIV
	HIV viral load	EQHIV

NOTES:
[1]Treatment regimens were recommended at the time that the studies were done and may be outdated according to current standards. Readers are referred to Department of Health and Human Services and International AIDS Society-USA guidelines for the most current treatment guidelines and recommendations.
[2]Only indicators for adults and adolescents > 13 were included in this table.
[3]IHI* denotes a key measure; IHI denotes additional measure.

SOURCES:
EQHIV = Evaluation of Quality Improvement for HIV Care (Cleary, 2003).
FACCT = Foundation for Accountability (Wu and Gifford, 1998; Wu et al., 2000).
HCSUS = HIV Cost and Services Utilization Study (Asch, 2003).
HIVQUAL = HIV Quality of Care Program (NYSDHAI and HRSA/HAB, 2003).
IDSA= Infectious Disease Society of America (Gross et al., 2000).
IHI = Institute for Health Care Improvement HIV/AIDS Collaborative (IHI, 2003).
QUERI= Quality Enhancement Research Initiative (Anaya, 2003).
RAND = The RAND Corporation (Asch et al., 2000).
UHC = University Health Consortium (UHC, 2002).

Eligible Population	Measure Criterion/Definition
Patients with CD4+ cell count <200/μL	CD4+ cell count increased to >200/μL at the last visit
All	Last CD4+ cell count recorded were <200/μL
All	Non-injury-related emergency room visits per patient per year UHC categorized this measure under Resource Utilization
All	Non-injury-related hospitalizations per patient per year UHC categorized this measure under Resource Utilization
All	Percent with hospitalizations within the last month
Patients on HAART	Percent with undetectable HIV viral load
Patients on HAART (defined as three or more antiretroviral medications)	HIV viral load between 0 and 399 copies
Patients on HAART (defined as three or more antiretroviral medications)	HIV viral load between 400 and 19,999 copies
Patients on HAART (defined as three or more antiretroviral medications)	HIV viral load > 20,000 copies

TABLE E-2 Frequency of Process and Outcome Measures by Source

	EQHIV	FACCT
PREVENTION		
Counseling and testing (pregnant women)		
Counseling on high-risk behaviors		
Tobacco use assessment		
SCREENING & MONITORING		
CD4+ cell count		√
Cervical cancer and other pelvic disease	√	√
Complete blood count		√
Cytomegalovirus disease		√
Hepatitis A		
Hepatitis B and/or C	√	√
HIV specialists visit		
Lipid screening		
Oral health/dental exam		
Outpatient visits	√	
Syphilis		√
Toxoplasmosis		√
Tuberculosis	√	√
HIV viral load		√
ANTIRETROVIRAL TREATMENT (ART)		
Appropriate management of patients on ART		
Provision of adherence counseling and/or monitoring		
Provision of indicated ART	√	√
Regimen change		
PROPHYLACTIC TREATMENT		
Hepatitis B		√
Influenza	√	√
Mycobacterium avium complex		√
Pneumococcal pneumonia		√
Pneumocystis carinii pneumonia		√
Toxoplasmosis		√
Tuberculosis		√
SOCIAL AND SUPPORT SERVICES		
Benefits advocacy		
Emotional counseling		
Home health services		
Housing		
Mental health assessment		
Self-management goal setting		
Substance abuse services		
Support services		

HCSUS	HIVQUAL	IDSA	IHI	QUERI	RAND	UHC
	√					
					√	
	√					
√		√	√	√	√	√
√	√	√	√			√
					√	
√					√	
				√		
	√		√	√		√
	√					
	√			√		
	√					
			√			
√	√			√	√	
√				√	√	√
√	√	√	√			
√	√	√	√	√	√	√
	√					
	√		√		√	√
√		√	√	√	√	√
			√			
						√
√		√				√
√		√		√	√	√
√			√		√	√
√	√	√	√	√	√	√
					√	
					√	
√						
√						
√						
√						
	√					
			√			
√	√					
			√			

Continued

TABLE E-2 Continued

	EQHIV	FACCT
HEALTH OUTCOMES		
CD4+ cell count	√	
Emergency room visits		
Hospitalization		
HIV viral load	√	

NOTE: No structural quality of care measures were identified in this review.
SOURCES:
EQHIV = Evaluation of Quality Improvement for HIV Care (Cleary, 2003).
FACCT = Foundation for Accountability (Wu and Gifford, 1998; Wu et al., 2000).
HCSUS = HIV Cost and Services Utilization Study (Asch, 2003).
HIVQUAL = HIV Quality of Care Program (NYSDHAI and HRSA/HAB, 2003).
IDSA = Infectious Disease Society of America (Gross et al., 2000).
IHI = Institute for Health Care Improvement HIV/AIDS Collaborative (IHI, 2003).
QUERI = Quality Enhancement Research Initiative (Anaya, 2003).
RAND = The RAND Corporation (Asch et al., 2000).
UHC = University Health Consortium (UHC, 2002).

HCSUS	HIVQUAL	IDSA	IHI	QUERI	RAND	UHC
			√			
						√
			√			√
			√			

REFERENCES

Anaya H. 2003. QUERI Indicators. (Email communication, Henry Anaya, Department of Veterans Affairs, May 12, 2003).

Asch S. 2003. Table 2: Adherence to Quality Indicators in HIV. (Email communication, Steven Asch, The RAND Corporation).

Asch SM, Kerr EA, Hamilton EG, Reifel JL, McGlynn EA, Editors. 2000. *Quality of Care for Oncologic Conditions and HIV: A Review of the Literature and Quality Indicators*. Santa Monica, CA: Rand Health.

Cleary P. 2003. EQHIV Chart Review Dependent Variables. (Email communication, Paul Cleary, Harvard Medical School, December 9, 2003).

Gross PA, Asch S, Kitahata M, Freedberg KA, Barr D, Melnick DA, Bozzette S. 2000. Performance measures for guidelines on preventing opportunistic infections in patients infected with human immunodeficiency virus. *Clinical Infectious Diseases* 30(Suppl 1):S85–S93.

IHI (Institute for Healthcare Improvement). 2003. Improving Care for People Infected with HIV. [Online]. Available: http://www.ihi.org/collaboratives/breakthroughseries/HIV/charter.asp [accessed July 31, 2003].

New York State Department of Health AIDS Institute and Health Resources and Services Administration, HIV/AIDS Bureau (NYSDHAI and HRSA/HAB). 2003. [Online]. Available: http://www.hivguidelines.org/public_html/center/quality-of-care/qoc-ny-indicators.htm.

UHC (University Health System Consortium). 2002. *HIV Ambulatory Care Clinical Benchmarking Executive Summary*. 12.

Wu A, Gifford A. 1998. Quality of Care Indicators for HIV/AIDS: A Discussion Paper for the Foundation for Accountability. [Online]. Available: http://www.facct.org/facct/doclibFiles/documentFile_302.pdf [accessed July 31, 2003].

Wu AW, Gifford A, Asch S, Cohn SE, Bozzette SA, Yurk R. 2000. Quality-of-care indicators for HIV/AIDS. *Disease Management and Health Outcomes* 7(6):315–30.

F

Biographies

Paul D. Cleary, Ph.D. (Chair), is Professor of Health Care Policy in the Department of Health Care Policy at the Harvard Medical School. His research interests include developing better methods for using patient reports about their care and health status to evaluate the quality of medical care and studying the relationships between clinician and organizational characteristics and the quality of medical care. He has published over 200 research articles on these topics. Dr. Cleary's current research includes a study of how organizational characteristics affect the costs and quality of care for persons with AIDS and a national evaluation of a continuous quality-improvement initiative in clinics providing care to HIV-infected individuals. He also is Principal Investigator of one of the Consumer Assessment of Health Plans Studies (CAHPS) funded by the Agency for Health Research and Quality to develop survey protocols for collecting information from consumers regarding their health plans and services. Dr. Cleary is a member of the Institute of Medicine and previously served as a member of the Committee on Prevention and Control of Sexually Transmitted Diseases. Dr. Cleary received his M.S. and Ph.D. degrees in sociology from the University of Wisconsin.

Ronald Bayer, Ph.D., is Professor in the Division of Sociomedical Sciences at the Joseph L. Mailman School of Public Health at Columbia University. Since 1982, he has been involved in the study of the ethical and policy dimensions of the AIDS epidemic. He served on the National Research Council's Committee on the Social Impact of AIDS and more recently, the Committee on the Elimination of Tuberculosis in the United States and on the Committee on Immunization Safety Review. He is author of numerous articles on ethical issues posed by AIDS and tuberculosis, including *Private Acts, Social Consequences: AIDS and the Politics of Public Health,* and *Blood Feuds: AIDS, Blood, and the Politics of Medical Disaster.* His most recent co-authored book is *AIDS Doctors: Voices from the Epidemic.* Dr. Bayer received his Ph.D. in political sciences from the University of Chicago.

Eric Bing, M.D., Ph.D., M.P.H., is the Director of the Center for AIDS Research, Education and Services at Drew University of Medicine and Sciences (Drew CARES), the Director of the Drew Collaborative Alcohol Research Center, and the co-director of the UCLA Center for HIV Identification, Prevention and Treatment Services (CHIPTS). Dr. Bing is a psychiatrist and epidemiologist with extensive expertise in HIV disease. Dr. Bing received his M.D. from Harvard Medical School and his Ph.D. in Epidemiology from UCLA. Following his training in psychiatry, he completed 6 years of training in health services research, initially as a Robert Woods Johnson Clinical Scholar and then as a Scholar in the UCLA Faculty Scholars Program. Dr. Bing's research primarily focuses on developing and evaluating interventions to improve health care and health outcomes for disadvantaged populations, particularly those affected by HIV, mental illness, and/or alcohol and drug problems. In addition to Dr. Bing's research programs, he also directs an HIV social services center, which has programs in mental health, case management, treatment education, and peer support.

Samuel A. Bozzette, M.D., Ph.D., an internist and infectious diseases physician, is Professor of Medicine at the University of California San Diego, Chief of the Health Services Research Section at the VA San Diego, and a Senior Natural Scientist at RAND Health. Dr. Bozzette, an author of over 125 scientific publications and reports, has worked extensively in clinical trials of new drug treatments and in bringing comprehensive outcome assessment into trials. He now works on several facets of clinical epidemiology, medical care, outcomes, quality measurement and improvement, and cost. He is a Principal Investigator for the HIV Cost and Services Utilization Study at RAND, and directs both the Center for Research in Patient-Oriented Care at the VA San Diego and the VA's national Quality Enhancement Research Initiative (QUERI) for HIV/AIDS. He holds degrees from Georgetown University (B.S.), the University of Rochester (M.D.), and the RAND Graduate School of Policy Studies (M.Phil., Ph.D.; Policy Analysis).

David D. Celentano, Sc.D., M.H.S., is Professor and Director of the Infectious Diseases Program in the Department of Epidemiology at the Johns Hopkins Bloomberg School of Public Health. He previously served as Professor and Head of the Division of Behavioral Sciences and Health Education at Johns Hopkins School of Hygiene and Public Health. His research interests include psychosocial and behavioral factors in HIV/AIDS and other sexually transmitted infections; reproductive health and epidemiology; cancer control and community epidemiology; and alcohol and drug epidemiology. Dr. Celentano served on the Institute of Medicine's Committee on Prevention and Control of Sexually Transmitted Diseases. He received both M.H.S. and Sc.D. from Johns Hopkins University.

Victor De Gruttola, S.M., Sc.D., is a Professor of Biostatistics at Harvard School of Public Health. His research activities focus on developments of statistical methods required for appropriate public health response to the AIDS epidemic. His current research focuses on developing new statistical methods for clinical research on treatments for HIV infection, especially with regard to the causes and consequences of resistance to antiretroviral drugs. Since 1996, he has served as the Director of the Statistical and Data Analysis Center (SDAC) of the Adult AIDS Clinical Trials Group; he also serves on the Antiviral Drugs Advisory Committee of the FDA. Prior to serving as Director of SDAC, Dr. De Gruttola worked on projections of AIDS incidence using data from the New York City Health Department. A special focus of this work was estimation of the risk of AIDS that children of HIV-infected mothers experienced in the first 10 years of life, prior to the development of potent antiretroviral drugs. Dr. De Gruttola received his Sc.D. from Harvard University.

Carlos del Rio, M.D., is Professor of Medicine at Emory University School of Medicine and Chief of the Medical Service, Grady Memorial Hospital. Dr. del Rio is a native of Mexico where he attended medical school at Universidad La Salle. He did his Internal Medicine and Infectious Diseases residencies at Emory University. In 1989, he returned to Mexico where he was Executive Director of the National AIDS Council of Mexico (CONASIDA, the federal agency of the Mexican government responsible for AIDS policy throughout Mexico). His research interests include opportunistic infections in HIV and other immune deficiencies; epidemiology and transmission of HIV and other STDs; early diagnosis of HIV and access to care and compliance with antiretrovirals; impact of HIV in developing countries; and the optimal use of antiretrovirals in limited resource settings.

Aida Giachello, Ph.D., is currently an Associate Professor at Jane Addams College of Social Work at the University of Illinois at Chicago. She is also Director of the Midwest Latino Health Research, Training, and Policy Center, where she has been conducting outcomes research on health disparities and has been training new minority investigators on health research, following a participatory research and community empowerment model. While working at the University of Chicago's Center for Health Administration Studies in 1983, she began her work on Latino health research focusing on issues of financial, institutional, and cultural barriers in accessing health and medical care. Her research agenda focuses on issues of efficiency and quality of care related to chronic conditions including HIV, asthma, diabetes, cancer, hypertension, and maternal child health. She has a Master's degree in Social Services Administration from the University of Chicago and a Ph.D. in Medical Sociology from the University of Chicago with a specialty in health and ethnicity.

William L. Holzemer, R.N., Ph.D., F.A.A.N., is Professor and Associate Dean of International Programs in the Department of Community Health Systems at UCSF School of Nursing; prior to this, he served as Department Chair, CHS (1995–2001), and Associate Dean for Research (1990–1995). Dr. Holzemer is also the Director of the International Center for HIV/AIDS Research and Clinical Training in Nursing. His program of research has examined quality of nursing education, quality of nursing care, outcomes research, variation in practice, self-care symptom management, and quality of life, with special emphasis on people living with HIV infection. He has had continuous extramural funding as Principal Investigator or Co-Principal Investigator over the past 20 years. He recently completed 6 years as a chartered member and Chair of a National Institutes of Health study section. Dr. Holzemer has published more than 100 refereed databased research articles, edited 6 books, and authored 13 book chapters. His current work is focusing upon adherence, symptom management, HIV/AIDS stigma, and quality of life. Dr. Holzemer is a member of the Institute of Medicine, Fellow of the American Academy of Nursing, and a member of the Japan Academy of Nursing. He is a former Fulbright Scholar (Egypt), a Project HOPE Fellow (USA-Mexico Boarder), and is a Visiting Professor at St. Luke's College of Nursing, Tokyo, Japan. He has served as an external adviser in nursing science at the University of Botswana, School of Education, University of Tokyo, School of Medicine, and many universities throughout the United States.

Sandral Hullett, M.D., M.P.H., is acting CEO of Jefferson Health System in Birmingham, Alabama. She was formerly the Executive Director of Family HealthCare of Alabama, a not-for-profit community health center serving 20 rural counties throughout Alabama. Her interests include rural health care and health care planning and delivery to the underserved, underinsured, and poor. She was awarded the University of Alabama School of Public Health's first Public Health Hero Award for her work providing compassionate care to people living in Alabama's rural, impoverished Black Belt communities. Dr. Hullett is a member of the Institute of Medicine and has served on several IOM committees including the Committee on the Changing Market, Managed Care, and the Future Viability of Safety Net Providers. Dr. Hullett received her M.D. from the Medical College of Pennsylvania and her M.P.H from the University of Alabama.

Wendy K. Mariner, J.D., LL.M., M.P.H., is a Professor of Health Law at Boston University Schools of Public Health, Law, and Medicine. She has been a member of the AIDS Program Advisory Committee for the National Institutes of Health, the Executive Board of the American Public Health Association, and the Massachusetts Health Facilities Appeals Board. Ms. Mariner served previously on the IOM's Committee on the Children's Vaccine Initiative: Planning Alternative Strategies Toward Full United States Participation. Her research interests include patients' rights, health system reform, and managed care. Ms. Mariner received her J.D. from Columbia University, her LL.M. from New York University, and her M.P.H. from Harvard University.

Beth Meyerson, M.Div., Ph.D., is President of the Policy Resource Group, LLC, a health policy research consultancy specializing in STD and HIV policy with domestic and international emphases. Dr. Meyerson is adjunct faculty at Saint Louis University where she teaches health policy in the School of Public Health. She was formerly the AIDS and STD director for the State of Missouri. Her current research includes the impact of federal interventions on the STD program infrastructure; state agency coordination of HIV, mental health, and substance abuse programs; and public health involvement in the policy process. Dr. Meyerson's most recent research appears in *Sexually Transmitted Diseases* and *Public Health Reports*. She received her Ph.D. in Public Policy Analysis and Administration from Saint Louis University.

A. David Paltiel, Ph.D., is Associate Professor and Chair of the Division of Health Policy and Administration in the Department of Epidemiology and Public Health at the Yale Medical School. Dr. Paltiel also holds a faculty appointment at the Yale School of Management and is affiliated with the Yale Center for Interdisciplinary Research on AIDS. He has served as a Trustee of the Society for Medical Decision Making and as a member of the Editorial Boards of both Medical Decision Making and Value in Health. Dr. Paltiel's research deals broadly with issues of resource allocation and decision making in health policy. His AIDS-related research includes a host of model-based cost-effectiveness evaluations in HIV prevention and patient care. Dr. Paltiel received his Ph.D. in Operations Research from Yale.

Harold Pollack, Ph.D., was Associate Professor of Health Management and Policy at the University of Michigan School of Public Health during the preparation of this report. He is now Associate Professor of Social Service Administration at the University of Chicago. His main research interests concern substance abuse, HIV prevention, and Medicaid policy for pregnant women, infants, and special needs children. Dr. Pollack served as a member of the Institute of Medicine Committee on Nutrition Services for Medicare Beneficiaries. He is currently researching substance abuse among welfare recipients, and the cost-effectiveness of harm reduction in the prevention of HIV and hepatitis C. Dr. Pollack's recent policy research appears in *Medical Decision Making, Journal of the American Medical Association, American Journal of Public Health,* and other publications. He received his doctorate in Public Policy from Harvard University.

George W. Rutherford, M.D., is Salvatore Lucia Professor and Head of the Division of Preventive Medicine and Public Health in the Department of Epidemiology and Biostatistics at the University of California, San Francisco (UCSF) School of Medicine. He also serves as the Interim Director of the Institute for Global Health at UCSF and the School of Public Health at the University of California, Berkeley (UCB). Dr. Rutherford is a leading expert on the epidemiology of AIDS and HIV infection and the public health aspects of the AIDS epidemic. He served as State Health Officer and State Epidemiologist for the California Department of Health Services from 1990 to 1995. He also formerly served as the Director of the AIDS Office in the San Francisco Department of Public Health in the 1980s and as Director of the Division of Immunizations for the New York City Department of Public Health. His principal research interests are the natural history of HIV infection and the epidemiology of AIDS and HIV infection in California and Latin America. He also has interests and projects in the epidemiology and prevention of coccidioidomycosis, the epidemiology and control of tuberculosis, the elimination of syphilis, and the interface between public health and managed care. He is the coordinating editor for the Cochrane Collaborative Review Group on AIDS and HIV infection, an international effort to systematically review intervention trials in the treatment and prevention of AIDS and HIV infection, and the Chair of the Department of Veterans Affairs' National Research Advisory Council. Dr. Rutherford received his M.D. from Duke University.

Eileen Salinsky, M.B.A., is Principal Research Associate at the National Health Policy Forum at George Washington University. Her current research is focused on public health preparedness and the health care safety net. Ms. Salinsky formerly served as the Director of the Division of Public Health Policy in the Office of Health Policy at the Office of the Assistant Secretary for Planning and Evaluation (ASPE) in the Department of Health and Human Services. During her tenure at ASPE, she co-chaired the Committee on HHS Data Strategy. Ms. Salinsky was also formerly Vice President at The Lewin Group where she directed studies on states' efforts to integrate health data, information technology, public health infrastructure, and the costs of uncompensated care.

David R. Smith, M.D., is Chancellor of the Texas Tech University System and was previously the Interim Chancellor and president of the Texas Tech University Health Sciences Center. Prior to his tenure at Texas Tech, Dr. Smith was the Commissioner of the Texas Department of Health from 1992 to 1996. He received the American Medical Association's Dr. Nathan Davis Award and the American Public Health Association's Award of Excellence for outstanding contributions to medicine and public health. Dr. Smith has served on several IOM committees including: the Committee on Immunization Finance Policies and Practices, Committee to Study Outreach for Prenatal Care, and the Committee on the Health and Adjustment of Immigrant Children and Families. He is currently chairing the Committee on Immunization Finance Dissemination Workshops. Dr. Smith received his M.D. from the University of Cincinnati and is board certified in pediatrics.

Liaison from the IOM Board on Health Promotion and Disease Prevention

Robert Wallace, M.D., is Professor of Epidemiology and Internal Medicine at the University of Iowa Colleges of Public Health and Medicine, and Interim Director of the University's Center on Aging. He has been a member of the U.S. Preventive Services Task Force (USPSTF) and the National Advisory Council on Aging of the National Institutes of Health. He is currently a member of the Board of the Medical Follow-Up Agency of the Institute of Medicine, National Academy of Sciences, and a senior advisor to the USPSTF. He served on the Executive Committee of the Association of Teachers of Preventive Medicine, and was Chair of the Epidemiology Section of the American Public Health Association. He is the author or co-author of over 240 publications and 22 book chapters, and has been the editor of 4 books, including the current edition of Maxcy-Rosenau-Last's *Public Health and Preventive Medicine*. He is a member of the Institute of Medicine. Dr. Wallace's research interests concern the causes and prevention of disabling conditions of older persons. He leads the Health Working Group of the Health and Retirement Study, a long-term prospective sample of older Americans exploring health, social, family, and economic policy issues. He is the site Principal Investigator for the Women's Health Initiative, a national intervention trial exploring the prevention of breast and colon cancer and coronary disease. He has been a collaborator in several international studies of the prevention of chronic illness in older persons.